How to Cope Better
When You
Have Cancer

WILLIAM PENZER, Ph.D.

Esperance Press Inc.
150 South University Drive
Plantation, FL 33324
954 475 1371
cancerville.com

This book is available at special quantity discounts for bulk purchases, fundraising, educational, or institutional use. Contact media@cancerville. com

ISBN-10: 0983501718

ISBN-13: 9780983501718

Library of Congress Control Number: 2012946098

Printed in the United States of America

10 9 8 7 6 5 4 3 2 1

Better to light a candle than to curse the darkness.

–Confucius

If I can stop one heart from breaking,
I shall not live in vain:
If I can ease one life the aching,
Or cool one pain,
Or help one fainting robin
unto his nest again,
I shall not live in vain.

–Emily Dickinson

Of all the forces that make for a better world, none is
so indispensable, none so powerful as hope.
Without hope man is only half alive.

–Charles Sawyer

Dedication

My book is first and foremost dedicated to my wonderful daughter, Jodi, a breast cancer survivor who showed me how to take on cancer full tilt when I was initially drowning in a sea of depression, despair, and disillusionment. Her quiet determination and graceful "dance" with the enemy is a model for all who face this difficult disease.

It is also dedicated to Jake Santoriella, who, with the help of his fraternal twin brother and best friend Chase's perfect bone marrow match, defeated the most aggressive form of childhood leukemia against all odds. For boys only eight-and-a-half years old, they showed the highest levels of bravery, courage, and compassion I have ever witnessed.

It is also dedicated to Susan Berkofsky who did not win her Cancerville battle, despite her strong "Brooklyn" fight. She read the draft of my book for the family and friends, *How to Cope Better When Someone You Love Has Cancer,* [1] and said, "You must write one for the patient too." This helped me to see things so much more clearly and I am not even the target audience."

Each of them, in their own unique way, motivated me to write this book. They will pop in and out on the following pages and you will get to know them well.

It is also dedicated to all the other warm, welcoming, and wonderful people you will meet on the following pages, whose experiences dealing with cancer guided my understanding and writing journey.

William Penzer, Ph.D.
April 2012

Acknowledgements

I have been blessed to have had a solid team of support throughout my career, as far back as my first job as a psychologist for the IBM Corporation, my time as Assistant Director at The Institute for Human Development at Nova University in Ft. Lauderdale, throughout my almost twenty years as Director of the Center for Counseling Services, up to the present time. I thank you all for contributing to my life and my work in meaningful ways.

As for this book, the following deserve special recognition and thanks:

My wife and loving partner for more than fifty years, Ronnie, who not only coped well with my "obsession" for both of these books, but also sat side-by-side with me and dutifully added her gentle touch in editing in her detailed and methodical manner. We have made a good team in life, love, family, and editing. She spent over five hundred hours reading every word and comma aloud to me, helping me revise, revitalize, and finalize both books.

My special daughter, Jodi Mi, and my son-in-law, Zev, who together made a powerful and positive tag team in their journey through Cancerville, which continues in their life together all these years later.

My son David and daughter-in-law, Lisa, for their continued help in the media and marketing of my books.

My son Michael, who facilitated our very special Modern Day Fairy Tale trip.

My grandsons, Jarrett and Dillon, for making me happy and making me laugh whenever I see them. I am pleased to say they seem to have inherited my sense of humor.

Bernie Siegel, M.D., who generously took me under his wing; guided my journey into miracles, angels, blessings, and the like; and warmly wrote the Foreword.

Kerri, who helped us edit both books, adding her English teacher's touch by untangling some of my twisted sentences into coherent, grammatically correct, and well-punctuated prose.

My friend Rob, who contributed his edits to smooth and add to my words.

My childhood friend Howard, from Rockwood Hall in the Bronx, who had his own bumpy journey through Cancerville, and who also read and edited a draft of this book.

My longtime friend and colleague Harvey, a psychologist, author, businessman, and publisher, whose wise and seasoned advice and encouragement guided me through this complex process once again.

Brad, who worked tirelessly into the night to keep my writings organized, graphically aligned, and together in ways my computer illiteracy would not allow me to do.

Jose, who skillfully redesigned the cancerville.com website.

Babs, who artistically designed the cover of this book.

Aishling and Justin who, assisted me by doing research on many different cancer-related topics.

All of the people who gave of their time, energy, and emotions to provide their stories for the "Real People Facing Cancer" sections.

All the unnamed people in South Florida who entrusted me with their minds all these years. Together we learned how minds work, why they sometimes don't work well, and most importantly we learned how to help repair them. The courage and confidence they displayed in the face of adversity helped me to strengthen my resolve in my life and in Cancerville.

My heartfelt thanks and sincere gratitude goes out to all of you.

With love and much appreciation,

Bill

Table of Contents

Foreword by Bernie Siegel, M.D   xi
Preface   xvii
Introduction   xix
An Opening Letter of Hope   xxvii

Part I: Getting the Lay of the Land

1. Welcome to Cancerville   3
2. Turning Down the Spotlight on Catastrophe   17
3. Converting Rapidly from Powerless to Powerful   29
4. Striving to Adapt to a Place from which You Really Want to Run   45

Part II: Understanding the Land

5. Making Eye Contact with Cancerville   59
6. Meetings with the Dedicated Doctors   75
7. Hair Grows Back: Coping with the Physical Effects of Cancer   91
8. Minds Come Back: Coping with the Emotional Effects of Cancer   105
9. Lives Come Back: Coping with the Impact of Cancer on Your Everyday Life   119

Part III: Making the Land Your Own

10. How Minds Work   133
11. Embracing a Really Simple Philosophy: Realistic Optimism   151
12. The Power of Positive Self-Talk   163
13. Dealing with Depression, Debilitation, and Distress   187

14. Calming Your Fears and Anxieties 197
15. Reining in Your Rage 211

Part IV: Tools That Help You Tend the Land

16. Relaxing Tools for Natural Healing 225
17. Cognitive Tools for Taking Charge of Your Mind 241
18. Traditional and Alternative Treatments and Complementary Support Options 259
19. Having a Counselor and/or Support Group in Your Corner 281
20. Big Boys and Girls Do Cry 299
21. Laughter in Cancerville 311
22. Communication in Cancerville 321

Part V: Putting Distance Between Yourself and the Land

23. No One Really Knows Where the Road Goes 347
24. Helpful Life Lessons You Can Learn from Your Cancerville Experience 359
25. A Modern Day Fairy Tale 373
26. On Becoming Even More Empowered 381

A Closing Letter of Caring 397

References 401

Foreword

I found this book to be an easy read because Bill Penzer and I agree with one another. We may have a few differences of opinion, which I will also discuss, but basically we have learned the Cancerville lessons, which help people to not just cope with cancer, but to survive it as well.

My reorientation as a doctor came from one of my patients with breast cancer telling me she needed to know how to live between office visits because she couldn't take me home with her. As I helped more cancer patients learn how to live, I realized that the side effects of learning how to live, cope and survive provided them with a longer healthier life.

Woody Allen shares the key point in a dialogue between two friends, one of whom is very depressed about the bleak, absurd cosmos. When his buddy asks him, "What are you doing Saturday night?" he answers, "Committing suicide." His friend responds, "How about Friday night?"

It reminds me of the letters I have that describe how people changed their lives when their mortality became very evident, by being at risk, and so they started to live a new life they could love, and loved their body as well. Their letters end with, "I didn't die and now I'm so busy I'm killing myself. Help, where do I go from here?" I prescribe what they need, a nap, because they are burning up and not out. We all need to accept our mortality and not wait for a disaster to get us to truly live our authentic life and not the one imposed upon us. Rather than becoming strong at the broken places, we need to learn from those who preceded us and from the lessons shared in the following pages.

It is basically about our potential and feeling enough self-esteem to not be afraid to participate in our lives and health. When we fear failure and are dealing with the guilt, blame, and shame imposed upon us, we are fearful of trying to achieve what we are potentially capable of by participating and taking responsibility.

Many years ago one of our children, at age seven, was diagnosed with a bone tumor. I was sure from the X-ray he had a sarcoma and about a year to live after his leg was amputated. I went home and shared this with my wife and his four siblings and basically informed them about the depressing future. The next morning he came to me and asked if he could talk to me for a minute. I said "sure" and he said, "Dad, you're handling this poorly." From then on he became my therapist by teaching me about living in the moment and enjoying the day rather than worrying about or being depressed about an unknown future. The good news is that he had a very rare benign tumor and he taught me a great deal in the week before his surgery.

He also taught me about the difference between the native and the tourist. If you have not experienced cancer you are the tourist and should be listening to the native and not giving them directions because you haven't been to Cancerville. He taught me that lesson after the surgery I performed upon him. After showing him everyone and everything in the hospital he would see and meet, he woke up and said, "You didn't tell me it was going to hurt." Yes, I was a tourist in his land as the patient. So when you lose your health, find the people with experience to help you find it just as you do when you lose your car keys and need a ride home. Bill is definitely a native guide, so you can trust his lead. Follow his umbrella as he takes you through this complex but manageable maze.

In our family we have experienced MS, cancer, Lyme disease, and many more problems. I have seen how much better I am at living the experience than I was decades ago. This is where Bill and I share some common ground as we both learned how to cope better. The doctor in me and the psychologist in him are the problem. I was trained to cure and prescribe for the disease rather than care for the person and help them to cope and heal their lives. When I learned to love my fate and the lessons going through Hell were teaching me, things changed for my family and me.

I learned by observing my "exceptional" patients, especially those that were not supposed to survive, but did. When Bill learned to follow his instincts, his knowledge, and what he would have encouraged his clients to do things changed for him. We both needed to get out of our professional roles and into our loving, caring, and healthy hearts and out of our heads that only served to confuse us.

What follows in this book can help you to learn in a much healthier way. Bill consistently offers you a horse named Hope upon which to saddle up. You may fall off from time to time, but he will help you get back up and enjoy her stride.

I have seen what hope, love, peace, and faith can do. Things I was not taught about in medical school but now have an open mind to and have experienced and, therefore, can believe in. When I talk about learning from one's feelings and problems let me share what helped me. A friend asked me, during a difficult time, what I did if I was hungry. I told her I get something to eat. She then said, "Then ask yourself what nourishment you and your life need to help you to respond to these feelings and heal your life and body." That advice has helped me many times.

The mind and body are a unit and must be treated as such. When people believed they were being treated with chemo or radiation but weren't, due to medical errors, they still had side effects and their tumors shrank none-the-less. One doctor noticed that the chemotherapy program entitled EPOH, based upon the first letter of the four chemotherapy drugs, could be reversed and he could give his patients the HOPE protocol. With that title more of his patients responded to the chemotherapy than those being treated with the EPOH protocol, though they were identical except for the name.

So remember to make your therapeutic decisions based upon your intuitive wisdom as well as your intellectual decision so there is no internal conflict creating more side effects. You decide how you are treated, not your family or your doctor prescribing for the good patient, or submissive sufferer. I want you to be a respant, my word for a "responsible participant." I recall a doctor at a major cancer center apologizing to me in his book. He told me that his wife had cancer and he was apologizing for what he had thought of me and my work and that now that he was living with the problem I was an enormous help.

One more little bit of advice. If you want a good doctor, find one who, when you ask, "Are you criticized by patients, nurses, and family?" says, "Yes." Why? Because they are learning from their mistakes and lack of experience. As a doctor my patients taught me how to be a better doctor. They were my coaches and guides just as I was theirs. So keep your power related to therapeutic decisions, finding the right doctor, and training him or her. When you love your life and body, your internal chemistry lets your body know you are choosing life and it does all it can to keep you alive.

Basically it is to choose life and not try to avoid dying since that is impossible and there are many vegetarian, meditating joggers who are very bitter people in Heaven. So choose life-enhancing choices, which benefit everyone and allow miracles to happen. If they do happen your doctor will probably not be interested in what you did, while the nurse and social worker are. So become a character your doctors are aware of so that you are not just a diagnosis, and then they will learn from you about the benefits of integrative medicine, meditation, laughter, and the potential, which resides within all of us.

The healing mechanisms are built into us by our creator, but they have to be turned on for our genes to get the message. I call it survival behavior because I have learned the qualities from people who exceeded expectations, and this is related to all kinds of afflictions we have to deal with. Survival behavior is what all the great sages of the past have taught us.

As a woman wrote, her life was now BC and AC, or Before Cancer and After Cancer. You have to abandon the wounds of the past related to parenting distortions. Genes don't make decisions, but our internal environment and chemistry gives them the message. So find healthy growth in your life and don't let your growth go wrong. Our childhood is stored within our bodies and needs to be dealt with by our not evading the truth and having the body present its bill. Bill's model of the mind sums it all up simply— vent cess and be "DAM STRONG!"

If you did not grow up with mottos, which help you to let your heart make up your mind, and see difficulties as God's redirections, you have to reprogram yourself. When you do, your energy changes and amazing things can then occur. In his book *Cancer Ward,* Solzhenitsyn describes self-induced healing as a rainbow-colored butterfly. He understands it is not a spontaneous remission or miracle but self-induced. The rainbow represents a life in order created by transformation, the butterfly symbol. I recited this passage from the book to Bill when we met in my backyard, and he captures these images clearly in Chapter 26. I am pleased to have been a spiritual guide to him as he reached to expand his views on love, medicine, and particularly miracles.

This is not about winning or losing, but participating. This is an area Bill and I may not agree about. I find that when people see cancer as a battle or war, they focus too much on killing the enemy and not enough on healing their lives and bodies. I like to eliminate the disease and heal lives. A Quaker friend, a conscientious objector, walked out of his oncologist's office because the doctor said, "This treatment will kill your cancer." His words became swords and Dave said, "I don't kill anything" and walked out of the office to live twelve more years doing his thing and in his imagery he carried his cancer cells away. Mother Teresa said it very well when said she would not attend an anti-war rally, but if they ever had a peace rally to call her. We may not always follow the exact path, but Bill does build many bridges across which he and I are able to walk together.

In many ways the side effects of cancer are not all bad or problems. For some, cancer becomes a gift, wakeup call, or new beginning. So ask yourself what words you would use to describe your experience and see what those words tell you. If they are negative words, then eliminate from your life all the things that cause words like pressure, confusion, draining, failure, and more. Then find words that help nurture and heal your life—body, mind, and spirit.

In closing let me say hope and your future are not controlled by statistics. It is about your potential and desire to participate. Be sure to pay attention to your dreams and drawings so your intuitive wisdom and intellect can communicate and you can learn from your imagery and visualize what you desire, so your body expects good results from treatment and more. Do not be afraid to discuss death. Let it teach you about life and be comfortable with the word so you can speak freely to friends, family, and physicians. Death is not a failure and the only thing of permanence is love. So if you want to be immortal love someone.

To sum up, what you have to do is to create the person you want to become by rehearsing and practicing just as an actor would do. See the changes you need to make and your treatments as your labor pains. When you see them in that way you will have fewer pains and find they are worthwhile because the result will be your giving birth to a new and healthy self. Get your friends and family to help coach and direct you so when you are not performing well they will be there to correct and guide you. Actors in a comedy enhance their immune function and lower stress hormone levels, while those acting in a tragedy have the opposite happen.

So become the person you want to be and if you have a problem finding a role model ask yourself WWLD? or What Would Lassie Do? Animals and children live in the moment and are great teachers. I know of and have seen miracles and energy healing of cancer in our pets when they were loved and touched and not euthanized as the vet suggested. So love and treat yourself as well as you do your beloved pet, and if you don't have one get one because they improve relationships and increase survival rates.

You are always a work in progress, and as long as you are alive the canvas is never finished, as there is always more color on the palette.

Bernie Siegel, M.D.
Author of Love, Medicine & Miracles, A Book of Miracles and Faith, Hope, & Healing
July 5, 2012

Preface

As I began to write *How to Cope Better When Someone You Love Has Cancer,* I created a personal image of excellence. I wanted it to push me to write an exceptional book about a less than exceptional topic. I decided to use the same image for this book as well because it needed to be just as good, if not better. The image I chose was symbolic of my goal. I was determined to write a clear and powerful book that would truly help people. I wanted to "knock it out of the park."

As a kid who grew up in the Bronx, New York, in the 1940s and 1950s, I was an avid baseball fan who spent a fair amount of time at Yankee Stadium. I therefore picked the following image to motivate me to write the very best book that I could.

It is the seventh game of the World Series, and the Yankees are playing their hearts out in their old stadium on Jerome Avenue. It is the bottom of the ninth inning, and we are down by three runs. There are two outs, and the count is three balls and two strikes. The bases are loaded, and I am at bat. I need to hit a home run—nothing less. That walk-off hit will give us the game and the series.

I want to hear the Yankee announcer of old, Mel Allen, screaming at the top of his lungs, saying, "There is a high fly ball to deep, deep center field. That ball is going, going, and it's gone. The Yankees win the championship. What a hit, what a game, what a series, what a win!"

That was the image I kept in mind while writing this book. I swung as hard as I could and aimed it right at you. I sincerely hope you will catch the ball and that my words will help you to stand tall during a difficult time. That is much more important than the outcome of a baseball game.

I want you to win. That is really all I care about.

Introduction

One of the greatest victories we can achieve is defeating a life-threatening illness such as cancer. Please try your hardest to assume that is exactly what you are going to do. Right from the beginning, see yourself as becoming a member of that elite "green beret" group of survivors. Embrace that thought and image every single day—allow it to both enable and empower you.

I have no doubt that cancer will test your strength by pushing you to the limit every step of the way. But you will be both surprised and pleased with the strength and resilience that you will mount to fight back; and I will help you do just that. I will walk by your side every step of the way. You and I will walk this beat together like two tough street cops in a crime-ridden neighborhood.

I am sincerely sorry that you need to read this book. I wish you could be reading Danielle Steele, John Grisham, or any other book of your choice. I so wish that your life were lighter, brighter, and free of suffering and worry. I hope you get back to that space soon. In the meantime, you have made a good choice. My words will help you through. They have helped many before you and they will help you too. I will walk you through this most difficult situation, while helping you hang tough and remain strong.

Most authors, I would imagine, want everyone to read their books. Oddly enough, I want no one to need to read this one. My sincere hope is that this book will become obsolete very soon. I want cancer to be a thing of the past and cancer centers to become empty ghost towns. That may not happen in my lifetime, but I am hoping it will happen. We are closer than ever before—we will get there! For now, I hope you will choose to read this book as a way to gain added support at a very difficult time in your life.

Nothing—and I mean nothing—prepares a person to deal with a cancer diagnosis. The person diagnosed as well as family and friends are all caught off guard. On July 8, 2005, I knew that someday, if I lived long enough, I would write a book to help family and friends of cancer patients. That book, *How to Cope Better When Someone You Love Has Cancer,* spawned this one.

On that torturous July day, forever etched onto my brain like a permanent tattoo, I sat in the waiting room of Memorial Sloan-Kettering Cancer Center in New York City. I realized many things that day as we sat with our thirty-one-year-old daughter, Jodi, awaiting her surgery for breast cancer. I already knew from my work as a psychologist and psychotherapist that life wasn't always fair, but my experience helping others did not immediately prepare me for helping my family and myself. I was as lost as a tourist in a strange and foreign land, unable to get my bearings or even speak the language. At that very moment, I realized that cancer was not only a horrible and hated medical diagnosis, but it was a place as well. I knew then that my daughter, my wife, and I had entered what I came to call Cancerville.

As we sat there quietly waiting for our daughter's procedure to begin, my mind was numb, as if frozen by an icy cold frost on a winter's morning in Montana. When the nurse called Jodi's name, signaling her turn, she, dressed in a gray hospital gown, stood up quickly and bravely. A single angry thought shot through my head in outraged indignation: "This cannot be my daughter's turn!"

As Jodi took the first steps toward the operating room, elephant-sized tears began to fall down her checks as if she were a prisoner on her way to execution. Yet in reality she was an innocent victim of cancer. My frozen mind thawed and instantly overheated, as if I had been thrust headfirst into an oven. I was helpless, as was she, to prevent the ensuing barbarism. Though the surgeon was just trying to save our daughter's life, it felt much more like a dirty trick than a treatment. It was a macabre Halloween scene, without costumes or candy. There are so many different, difficult, and dark images that can immediately come to mind when you enter Cancerville. Slowly but surely, you and I will work together to eliminate or minimize them, one by one.

Consider this book a guide to a place you really never wanted to visit. Like Jodi, you were never given a choice—just a by-invitation-only command in the form of an X-ray, MRI, blood test, biopsy, or any combination of the above. To get through this very difficult territory, you need a strong voice to lead the way. I am honored you are allowing me to be that voice for you. I take that responsibility very seriously. I will teach you how to provide that added strength for yourself.

As you probably know, the majority of cancer-related books are written by medical doctors or by cancer survivors. I am neither, as I am a psychologist by profession and, most fortunately, I never had cancer. People have understandably asked me, "How can you help people cope better with cancer when you are neither a medical doctor nor a cancer survivor?" That is a fair question, and here is my response:

- I understand the emotions of Cancerville from my entrance, by proxy, in 2005 when my daughter was diagnosed. Despite my training and experience, I did not cope well. In Chapter 10, "How Minds Work," I will explain how my past life experiences led me to enter Cancerville kicking and screaming on my emotional knees. It took me a while to get to a better and stronger place. I want to help you get there much more quickly than I did.

- A mental health professional does not need to have personally experienced something to be able to help others deal better with that something. As an example, I have never been divorced. However, I have helped hundreds, if not thousands, of people through that troubling and painful maze.

• Similarly, I have helped many people facing cancer throughout my forty-year career as their counselor and life coach. I understand the emotional dynamics of Cancerville almost as well as if I had gone through it myself.

• In addition to the people I have helped all these years, as research for these books, I have spoken to many, many people who have been to Cancerville. This has helped fill in many gaps in my understanding of the experience. I came to learn about the range of reactions and coping strategies, as well as those experiences common to all people in Cancerville. On the pages that follow, you will learn how the people I have spoken to all dealt with their Cancerville experiences, as well as how they are doing now.

• Having cancer or being a physician doesn't automatically qualify someone as an expert on emotional coping, nor does it enable someone to translate experiences, thoughts, and feelings into understandable words. Therefore, some Cancerville books fall short of their good intentions while others are excellent. I will reference many of the latter as we go along.

Thus, I believe you will find the words that follow helpful and appropriate. My expertise pertains to matters of the mind in many different and difficult life zones, and Cancerville qualifies as majorly difficult in just about every way. I am also able to explain complex emotional issues in simple terms. I am very confident that the words that follow will resonate with you and will be helpful to you.

I assure you that you will find ways to take Cancerville on. You will rise to every challenge and fight back with all your might and moxie, and I will help you to do that. Together we will, slowly but surely, climb to the top of the slippery Cancerville mountains with an agility and balance you never knew you had. Once you get to the top of the highest peak, you will silently shout, "I have beaten cancer. I am a survivor—I now own the land that tried to own me!" Picture yourself in your mind's eye standing on top of the mountain and planting a flag with your name on it into the salty soil, moistened by your tears of joy.

Holding on to powerful, positive images is one way to keep your mind strong. I will teach you many more tools to do that as we go along. Once you have made it through the obstacle course I have come to call Cancerville, it will be a triumph of grand proportion—a very powerful "Yes!" moment. Toward the end of our journey together, I will tell you about the fairy tale "Yes!" experience my family and I enjoyed a few years after our difficult trek through Cancerville. In many ways, it was the highest mountain peak we ever climbed.

Know in advance that on our way up to the top of the mountain, we may fall off its slippery slope from time to time. That won't mean you are failing "Penzer's Positivism 101 course"; it is simply par for the Cancerville course. We will just pick ourselves up, dust ourselves off, and return to continue our climb. Cancerville teaches patience and perseverance like no other place I have ever been.

What we quickly learn there is that we are much more able to cope, adapt, and rise to the challenges of life than we think. Just as necessity is the mother of invention, survival is the mother of any and all action. We do whatever we have to do and whatever it takes. You may not always be happy doing that, but you will be driven to do just that. You will keep taking it on the chin until your cancer takes it on the lamb.

Know that not all professionals agree about promoting positivism in Cancerville. They are concerned about people being unrealistic. They may also be concerned that people will feel that they are "failing" when they can't sustain a hopeful, positive attitude. As you will learn, my beliefs are based on a philosophy I call realistic optimism. As I've said, be aware from the onset that few people can be consistently positive and optimistic in Cancerville or in other complicated situations. That is why we fall off the mountain from time to time. It does not matter how many times we fall off. What matters is that each and every time, we get back on and resume our journey in a proactive and positive way. This complex issue will be revisited in Chapter 12, "The Power of Positive Self-Talk."

Know that even though I have changed the cover of this book from the first edition, my original choice of the yin and yang symbol was not an accident or merely a design choice. The yin and yang symbol stands for polar opposites that are connected in some way—like life and death. As I sat on the beach in Jupiter, Florida, writing these words, I observed the brown, textured grains of sand and the white, fluffy, frothy waves; they are about as opposite as two elements of nature can be. Yet they kiss and embrace at the shoreline like lovers, becoming integrated partners in their magnificent and timeless marriage. They soothe us while they get to smooch regularly and rhythmically. For me, watching this over and over is as mesmerizing as a metronome—even more so.

So it is with the two very different parts known as our bodies and our minds. Though that yin and yang is not always as gracefully aligned as the tide and the beach, the body-mind marriage is undeniable. To the extent that I can help you maintain a strong and healthy mind while your body is dealing with all of the effects of cancer and the side effects of treatment, you will be much better positioned to take on the physical challenges, heal, and get well. My goal is to help lighten your journey while increasing the likelihood that you will join the millions of people who are cancer survivors.

Yet another yin and yang of Cancerville is health and illness. Most people tend to assume their health and deny their disease potentials. Most do not focus on the possibility of getting sick until they receive feedback that they are. All of a sudden, the yang of a serious illness crashes into the yin of wanting to be okay. This is similar to giant waves pumped up by a major storm crashing into and crushing the shoreline;

the once gentle embrace quickly becomes a disruptive and destructive chokehold. The same is true of cancer and other serious diseases.

Understandably, we do not process and experience a serious and life-threatening diagnosis the way we do a cold, stomach flu, broken bone, or the like. We easily absorb these minor illnesses with our health-based self-image and see ourselves as getting back to health soon. We see the yang as temporary and anticipate the rapid return of our health-based yin.

I want you to strive to do the same in Cancerville. Though the process is longer, more demanding, and much more risky, see yourself returning to health in a reasonable time frame. Try to see yourself as having an illness that is far more complicated than a head cold or broken ankle, but treatable and curable. Eventually the storm moves on and the waves return to quietly kissing the shore once again. Hopefully, the same will occur for your Cancerville storm; try to just assume that will be the case.

There is another yin and yang pairing with which I would like you to be familiar. It is the strength of people and the strength of cancer. Both are formidable in their force; it is a struggling tug-of-war all the way. At some point these opposing forces meet head-on. Know that you will do your very best to prevent cancer's yang from winning and to help your yin of powerfulness ultimately prevail. Your doctors will be pulling on your side of the rope as well, with everything they have and then some, which will add much power to your side. You and your team of support are a force with which cancer must reckon. Your goal is to stay pumped and powerful.

Understandably, people's moods in Cancerville have a yin and yang aspect as well. Emotions there are often in flux and tend to go up and down as events unfold. Sometimes in a flash, the yin of good feelings can switch and sink to the yang of mental misery. My goal is to teach you many tools that will help you return to positive or at least neutral feelings whenever you can.

Clearly, it is my goal to help you draw upon your many yins to counter Cancerville's many yangs. I do not expect you to be a robot, but I hope I can contribute to your being as robust as you can be. My goal right now is to reach out to you so I can help you find that positive place more quickly and more often. A hopeful and positive mindset is key to making this very unpleasant experience a little easier to bear. As many research studies have demonstrated, an optimistic belief can also influence the results in a positive way.

Now, please reach out and grasp my hand. Though it seems silly, I mean it seriously; indulge me for a brief moment. Instead of feeling foolish, try to feel empowered. Every little bit of support helps in Cancerville. Close your eyes and imagine my tight grip leading the way so we can get going. We have a long and demanding journey ahead.

I am firmly convinced that in or out of Cancerville, hope is essential; without hope we are lost and doomed to despair, depression, and defeat. As Barbra Streisand so beautifully sang, "Walk on, walk on, with hope in your heart, and you'll never walk alone." As Maya Angelou so beautifully wrote, "Hope slips through the tangle of our fears and evicts despair."

With hope, you have a fighting chance—in today's world, a very good chance at that!

William Penzer, Ph.D.
July 8, 2011

An Opening Letter
of Hope

Dear Cancerville Patient,

Arriving in Cancerville is a little like getting drafted by the military years ago when you could receive a letter in your mailbox indicating where and when to report to duty. Similarly, without much warning, you are now a green soldier in the boot camp of Cancerville. That is why you need to increase your troop size and strength to help you fight this battle. This book is a manual on how to get through this war zone in one piece. Let me tell you a little more about this war and my book before you proceed.

In many respects, Cancerville is a theater of war. It is, like the battlefields of World War II, the stage upon which a war on cancer is waged. It is where all the action takes place. I wrote these war-related words only to later discover in the comprehensive, 2011 Pulitzer Prize winning, historical book about cancer, *The Emperor of All Maladies*, [2] by Siddhartha Mukherjee, M.D., Ph.D., that they are not original. Post-WWII pioneers promoting cancer research and seeking funding used the metaphor of a war zone to make their case. Other writers in Cancerville have used this image as well. I neither borrowed the idea nor, as I came to learn, invented it. Sadly, that only underscores the tough nature of this disease. It has been a war zone forever. At least now our medical soldiers are winning more battles.

One theater of this war is behind the scenes, where active research is taking place all over the world. A 2010 *Time Magazine* article estimated that in America, $5.6 billion is invested in cancer research every year—more than all other common diseases combined.

In this zone, highly trained and knowledgeable medical teams join you at cancer centers, hospitals, and private practices around the world. They are the frontline troops in the theater of operations, literally and figuratively. The only difference is that in this war, your medical troops are not at risk, while you, innocent as you may be, are in the line of fire. You did not volunteer for this war—fate and other forces drafted you into it.

Doctors deploy harsh but powerful ammunition to fight the Cancerville insurgency that has attacked you. As insurgents do, they fight back hard and dirty under the cover of night. This is what can keep you staring at the ceiling at 3 a.m. Please allow me to help you get to sleep at a more reasonable hour. Try to assume that you, with the help of your family, friends, and medical support team, will win this battle. Although not everyone does win, I encourage you to assume that you will.

Not everyone is comfortable with warring words. As was spelled out by Bernie Siegel, M.D., in the Foreword, he himself is strongly opposed to war-related images in reference to cancer. He believes that just empowers the enemy. Though he feels anger and its release in a variety of forms are appropriate and healthy, he emphasizes loving yourself and focusing on healing your body as more helpful than battling and fighting.

In *Faith, Hope, & Healing,* [3] Bernie says, "I get tired of all the battles and wars people wage against cancer. It's like giving power to the fire...." He encourages "not wasting your life force fighting an enemy." He cites Mother Teresa refusing to go to an anti-war meeting, but pleased to attend a peace rally. Out of respect for Bernie's ideas, my intended subhead, "Real People Facing and Fighting Cancer" sections at the end of each chapter were changed to "Real People Facing Cancer."

I think the approach you take depends upon your nature and I believe Bernie would agree. Take Terry for example. A father who was an NYPD homicide detective raised him to be tough when he needed to be. He became a star athlete, ring-winning lacrosse player, and now successful high school lacrosse coach.

Terry said to me, "Bill, the only way for me to fight cancer was like a vicious pit bull!" And he has, every step of his bladder cancer way. Terry and Mother Teresa share only one thing in common—they are both Catholic. He would go to an anti-war rally in a heartbeat and be the strongest speaker there.

My point is that we are all different and our approach to cancer needs to be tailored to our individuality. Fight it hard, pray for yourself, heal from it, and love yourself throughout. In some cases, all of the above and more may very well apply. As I will say more than once, there is no right way to take on Cancerville, so take it on any way that works for you.

The purpose of this letter is to tell you a little bit about this book and how it might be helpful to you. As for my book/guide/war zone manual, it is often easier to say what something is not about than to describe what something is about. I want to do both so you will know my goals and can decide whether it will be helpful and appropriate for you to continue reading.

I am sensitive to the fact that in Cancerville your time is a very precious resource and needs to be managed well. I know how time-limited you are right now. You most likely are managing all you previously had to deal with along with the demands of Cancerville. It is definitely not easy to handle all of that going on simultaneously, but know you will do just that. This was one of my main goals in writing this book—to make your journey and time in Cancerville a little easier and more manageable.

This book was written for you if you have reason to believe that there is hope despite your cancer diagnosis. It was also written for you, if you are open to miracles, even in the most challenging of circumstances. This book will support and strengthen your optimism. It will help you find hope at moments when you are feeling none. My words will walk and talk you through this strange and scary place.

This is not a book to help you focus on the many details and decisions that you face in Cancerville. It may help you with some decisions, but there are many other books that deal with the details of your specific situation. It's also important for you to know that this book is not medically based, nor is it filled with data or statistical probabilities. Many books are available that cover that level of medical and scientific detail.

My book is much more the words of a wounded but surviving parent-warrior on the Cancerville battlefield. I have been there, done that, and thrown away the ill-fitting tee shirt, as did Jodi. I will also share the words of many survivors whose Cancerville journeys are most inspiring. I will help you over the giant emotional speed bumps that will come at you because if ever there was a time for support, this is it. The devil himself could not have designed and built a more diabolical obstacle course.

That said there is some good news. We humans are amazingly resilient despite all of our doubts, insecurities, and fears. I am hopeful and confident that you will be able to rise to the challenge. Even without this book, you can do that, but in Cancerville you need all the help you can get and I am here to support you. Rest assured that you will be, and perhaps already are, impressed with your own strength and capacity to adapt. You will be equally impressed with those same characteristics demonstrated by your family and friends.

My words come right from my heart and head to yours. As we walk the rough and tumble streets of Cancerville together, we may experience a special form of chemistry. We may never meet face-to- face, but I am hopeful that we will develop an empowering relationship that will do Cancerville and yourself proud. I can almost guarantee you that.

This book is not situation specific. No book can take into account the wide range of differences in its population of readers. This is especially true given that cancer cells do not discriminate— they are equal opportunity exploiters. Race, religion, and nationality do not matter to cancer cells; whether one is rich, poor, or somewhere in the middle is also irrelevant. You may be young, middle-aged, or older. Politically speaking, Cancerville is truly a multi-partisan place. We are all potential targets!

This book speaks to the commonalities that bind us together in our journey through Cancerville. We all have direct lines wirelessly connected from our heads to our hearts, and that is the territory with which I am very familiar and the one I address in this book.

As a psychologist, I strive to simplify rather than to confuse. I will offer you some easy to understand philosophies and ideas that can help you more clearly know the workings of the human mind. These will help you keep yours strong and healthy, despite the pressures of Cancerville. The ammunition you need to fight in the war zone of Cancerville must be lightweight, portable, easy to use, and relieving of your burdens. It needs to be powerful without being heavy.

This is not a book you need to read from cover to cover, so feel free to pick and choose as you like and need, as your time allows. I know that your time and attention are limited in Cancerville. However, the Gestalt school of psychological thought teaches us "the whole is greater than the sum of its parts." Therefore, if you do have the time, I encourage a full read for more complete and helpful support. In addition, some parts may be more relevant for you, so you may want to revisit them from time to time.

Keep in mind that the reason you don't have to read everything is that there is no test at the end of Cancerville. The test has already begun and I want you to do as well as you can. To do well, you will need to manage, stretch, cope, adapt, be hopeful and positive, and take care of yourself. This book will help you do all of that and more.

Unlike many self-help books and just about all Cancerville support books, I did not include quotes from famous people at the beginning of each chapter. It would be easy to find relevant ones from Hippocrates to current day writers. But I didn't want to imply, by association, that the words of famous people validate mine. Believe me when I say that Hippocrates has not read this book and never will.

I did opt to begin every chapter with an affirmation to help you validate yourself, which is far more important. View this book as one long letter with me talking to you directly. In fact, that is precisely what it is. Each chapter builds upon the previous ones and adds another dimension of support. By the conclusion, you will have a comprehensive roadmap guiding you through Cancerville.

In the pages that follow, you will meet many different people who have all been to Cancerville. I have read about some of them and had the pleasure of meeting many others. Each chapter concludes with a section called "Real People Facing Cancer." A few people, like Susan and Jake, will pop in and out as we go along.

Please know that they are all real people whose experiences, stories, and comments are true without embellishment on my part. Nor have I cherry-picked; I have wandered the Cancerville streets and randomly discovered their stories for the "Real People Facing Cancer" sections. Every person who accepted my invite made it into the book. Intriguingly, I have become friends with some of them. Just tonight, we had dinner with Harvey and Carol, whom you will meet in Chapter 2. In many ways, all of their stories have helped me to better help you. Telling tales has been a timeless teaching tool.

One of the many things you will learn in the pages that follow is that though you have cancer right now, you are not cancer. Susan taught me this better than anyone as she said over and over to herself and to me, "I have cancer, unfortunately, but I am not cancer!" All that defines you and your life is what defines you right now. I hope I can help you see cancer as a strong but curable footnote on one page of your book of life—and not as your entire biography.

Unfortunately, cancer is not always so easy to keep in perspective. It is different from many other medical disorders. Cancer has a very scary association. We will cover this in more detail in Chapter 2, "Turning Down the Spotlight on Catastrophe." However, it does feel like an intruder and invader has snuck past your defenses and is camping out on your property. It is, in fact, doing just that. Your medical team is strategically working to make sure those invading cells vacate your property—permanently. Believe that like a Sheriff's Deputy armed with an eviction notice, your team will succeed.

Because Cancerville has so many understandably strong emotional associations, it can easily dominate your mind with negative thoughts and feelings. They reverberate and ruminate like a slow moving rickety, clickety railroad train of old. As it clatters along, it carries a payload of unpleasant and unhelpful messages and images. My goal is to push that train right off its tracks before it pushes you off yours. I want to help you face Cancerville with even more strength, courage, determination, and dignity than you already have. If you are an optimist, I will help you become even more optimistic. If you are a pessimist, I will do my best to convert you to my simple philosophy of realistic optimism; I won't only encourage positivism—I will teach you tools to help you accomplish that.

In surveying the Cancerville literature, I found that it can become complicated and contradictory. Some writers advocate for exactly what others protest. I will do my best to present a realistic, reasonable, and rational perspective. I am not an adamant advocate of extremes, as I believe balance tends to win out in the long run. That said I absolutely respect your undeniable right to approach, enter, and journey through Cancerville any way that feels right for you. You are free to reject any of my suggestions and go with your own. People need to live their lives their way as long as it doesn't hurt others.

Please know that if you compare *How to Cope Better When Someone You Love Has Cancer* to this book, you will find some similarities. This is because the person wrestling with cancer and his or her family and friends face many similar emotional issues. Yet there are some very significant differences as well.

You, the patient, are clearly on the front lines of this battleground. Cancer has hit you and you are experiencing the physical and emotional demands directly. Those who love you take some hits, too, but they are different. You, like Jake, Susan, Eileen, Dani, my daughter, Jodi, and so many others whose stories I tell, have had to take those difficult and emotionally demanding treatment steps on your own. Terry said that for him the definition of being alone was just before he was wheeled into the OR for bladder surgery. Jodi's elephant-sized tears as she walked into surgery screamed out that very same message.

Therefore, your experience and those of your family and friends are different in many ways. That is precisely why I wrote this book for you. It may follow the footprint of the book for family and friends, but it isn't the same. You are the foot soldier in the Cancerville war zone, while your family and friends are your important back-up and support troops. Many call them caregivers, but that term is too cold and sterile for me. It needs to be reserved for professionals—nurses, doctors, technicians, and the like. When Ronnie and I were in that position, we were "heart and soul givers." I am hopeful your family and friends are there for you like that too.

So, my reader friend, as we embark on our long and winding journey, you will find that we will laugh and cry together. We will walk, at times jog, and occasionally run together. But have no doubt that we will get through this together.

Think of me as an excellent tour guide, umbrella and chin held high, leading you as best as I know how through a place that is not at all excellent. I am hopeful that by following my umbrella, we will be able to make your journey through Cancerville a little easier.

Right now, please close your eyes, take a deep breath, and feel my gentle grip leading the way. Trust me that I know the territory well, as I've been here by proxy before, sad to say.

Your new Cancerville friend,
Bill

PART I

Getting the
Lay of the Land

I will learn how to cope better in Cancerville.

Welcome to Cancerville

I t may seem strange to be welcomed to a place where you do not want to be; not wanting to be here is more than understandable. No one volunteers for this assignment, but unfortunately, you are now here. You are going to need to make the most of it in order to take Cancerville on full tilt. I wrote this book to help you do just that.

My goal is to be sensitive and supportive in an empowering way. I will help you find ways to smooth Cancerville's rough edges and level the playing field just a bit. Eventually, my hope is for you to own Cancerville in a take-charge manner so that you can feel as comfortable and powerful as possible.

Nothing in your life prepares you to receive a cancer diagnosis. It comes at you unexpectedly, like a bullet shot from a 357 magnum aimed directly at your body and mind. The word itself can send a chill up and down your emotional spine—even when you are not the one dealing with a cancer diagnosis. But when that word becomes associated and attached to your name, social security number, and medical ID, it jolts you with the force of a lightning bolt; it is a sizzling, agonizing, gut-wrenching moment. My goal is for this book to serve as your better late than never lightning rod. It will bring the jolt of that emotionally charged current down to a bearable level. It will help you take charge of yourself and your situation, and it will give you a much greater sense of being in control and slowly taking charge of Cancerville.

No One Wants to Be in Cancerville

When I first arrived in Cancerville by proxy as the father of my adult daughter, it was very hard to accept that I was actually there. It took me quite a while to face Cancerville head-on. The reason that people look and are tense, terrified, and teary-eyed in Cancerville is that its streets are dark and mean. Hooligans hang out on every corner and try to make trouble whenever and wherever they can. They have no conscience and show no mercy.

Let's assume the medical team will prevail and beat them one of these days. In the meantime, you need to get ready to rumble and start pumping emotional iron. It is a rough and tumble place. You need to be strong to take it on. I assume you will be and do just that.

If you have recently entered this territory, you are probably overwhelmed, exhausted, frightened, and wrestling with a Heinz variety of strong negative emotions. This is to be expected given the lay of the land. Cancerville is a scary place even on a good day. Your challenge is to turn the tables on Cancerville and own it. It will take a little while for you to get there, but rest assured you can and will do just that.

You may have had the disappointing experience of booking a hotel that turned out to be a dump. If so, you most likely tried to move to a better place as soon as possible. As self-protective people, we do our best not to remain in undesirable places for very long, but sometimes there is no other option available and we have to make the best of a not so pleasant place. That is precisely the case when we are in Cancerville.

No matter how upscale the surroundings in which you receive treatment, it is still in Cancerville. The menu can be three-star, the duvet can be soft and comfortable, and the TV can be a forty-inch HD, but those perks don't make up for the fact that you are still in Cancerville. The likelihood is that the place where you are receiving treatment does not remotely resemble the Ritz; it is probably more like the pits. But that is not important.

What is very important is that the medical team in Cancerville is as dedicated as they come. They will work tirelessly to fight back against the delinquent cells that are the driving force of your cancer. They want to save your life and, thankfully, now more than ever before, they succeed.

The Unpredictability of Cancerville

For most of us, daily life tends to be orderly in many basic ways. Public transportation runs on a published schedule. The garbage in my neighborhood is picked up every Tuesday and Friday. Traffic lights run predictably. This is how the world and we operate. Most people, but for a dare-devilish few, thrive on predictability. Many, if not most of us, require structure, clarity, and reliability to feel "safe" and "in control."

What would it be like if trains, planes, and buses followed no clear schedule or routes? What would life be like if we didn't know what time to arrive for school or work or what time we were supposed to leave? How about not knowing what to expect each day and what was expected of you? I think by now you get my drift. In all of these instances, random and unpredictable forces would create chaos, confusion, and controversy.

Welcome to Cancerville—a very unpredictable place! In Cancerville nothing is certain and just about everything is subject to change without notice. Medical tests you never expected to have? Maybe. More chemo than anticipated? Possibly. A revised treatment plan based upon updated test results, infection, or who knows what? Absolutely possible.

Unfortunately, once you are in Cancerville, you are riding on a bumpy train that has already left the station. The route and destination are less than clear. All you can do is assume it will finally get to where you want to go so you can get off. It is a little like getting driving directions on a GPS. They are not always totally accurate, and can lead us astray, but eventually we get to where we are going.

All of this uncertainty will demand your patience, flexibility, and tolerance for ambiguity. Although these traits may not come naturally, you can acquire them with practice and support. For the moment, grab the strap above your head and hold on tight. Cancerville is a day-at-a-time place, so try to stay focused on the moment without looking too far ahead.

Our Healthy Denial

Cancerville, like an approaching car not seen in our side or rearview mirrors, catches us on our blind side. We never think that we will be diagnosed with cancer. We have heard others' sad stories, but we exclude that possibility for ourselves.

It's not so different from a horrible head-on crash. We know that life-threatening highway accidents happen all the time, but we never think they will happen to us. This is actually a good thing. If we didn't have this helpful denial mechanism, we would spend much too much time and energy thinking about all of the potential tragedies that might occur. We would probably never leave the house or ride in a car.

It is easier, safer, and healthier for us to use that anticipatory anxiety to take care of our day-to-day responsibilities. So we tend to focus on bills, work issues, kids' school projects, Little League practice, and the silly squabbles among family and friends that occasionally crop up. Most people restrict their worries to relatively benign areas of life.

When tragedy, or its potential, leaps out at us like a nightmare, it is a whole different story. We are caught off-guard, become shocked and enraged, and engage in endless "not fair" inner discussions. As we all know, life is not always fair. It will take you a while to get past the shock. There is a part of me that still finds it very hard to believe that cancer struck my family, and it has been quite a while now. It is okay to remain shocked, just not shell-shocked. There is no time for that, as you need to be alert and active on your own behalf in every possible way.

You may also think, like I did, that it is a case of mistaken identity: "This cannot be my daughter's turn!" Eileen, upon receiving her cancer diagnosis said, "Are they sure it isn't Sally's or Jane's test results, not that I wish anything bad for them?" She was also concerned about the integrity of the process. After all, the test results had gone from doctor to nurse to lab to technician and back again. In the ER, Susan was given the results of her CT Scan that diagnosed her cancer. She reviewed it like the devoted nurse she was, thinking and feeling it was about someone else. Terry knew something was not right in his body, but never imagined he could have cancer. My friend Howie said, "I Googled kidney tumor and it kept coming up kidney cancer and each time I did that I said: 'WRONG!' I did that over and over until my voice got lower and lower, until it was completely silenced by the reality of my search."

The immediate need to detach from Cancerville and deny the diagnosis is a very typical event. Who can really blame people from wanting to believe it is a case of mistaken identity? You may have initially done the same.

My hope is that my words, like a racecar driver's fireproof suit, will insulate you from the inferno of Cancerville. But equally important, I want you to focus on all that you can do to make a difference for yourself and on how you can cope with your experience in a more comfortable way. I want you to drive that racecar like a pro on this very curvy Cancerville course.

I called my friend and colleague Eileen a few days after she learned of her cancer to see how she was feeling. You will meet her shortly in the "Real People Facing Cancer" section. "I went rollerblading this morning at Hollywood Beach, Florida. I just needed to do that," she said. She could just as easily have slept in with a mood on. Instead she chose to be active, to breathe in the fresh air, enjoy the morning sun, and get in touch with her vitality. She put herself out there in a positive and forceful way for a fifty-something woman. I hope you do, too, in whatever way works for you.

Your Mind as a Slingshot

There is no denying that at times battling cancer will feel like a David and Goliath mismatch. At those times, try to remind yourself who won that inequitable battle. Think about that for a moment or two. Envision yourself holding a powerful weapon that will help you win.

In this case your "slingshot" is your mind. It is the most powerful weapon you possess and it can help you defeat cancer. It has already helped you in other challenging situations. I encourage you to think about times throughout your life when your mind helped you to overcome obstacles, achieve your goals, and succeed. Those memories will help to "power up" your mind to be as strong as it can possibly be at this time. Strong minds can leap tall emotional buildings in a single bound—superman or woman style.

To be sure, Cancerville is filled with different forms of kryptonite that can weaken your resolve. That kryptonite can come from the following sources:

- overwhelming awareness that you have cancer

- constant focus on your health and mortality

- body and mind draining treatments

- always scary and sometimes grim doctor meetings

- interference with your routine, schedule, and life

All of the above and then some combine to wear your mind down, leaving you vulnerable to bouts of anxiety, depression, demoralization, pessimism, and negativity. These, in turn, work to neutralize, if not negate, your strength and power. This is why I plan to help you understand how minds work in Chapter 10.

I will also teach you many tools throughout these pages to keep your mind as strong as you possibly can as you run Cancerville's challenging maze. You will also need to draw on all of the life skills you have built all these years with discipline and determination. All of this combined will help you use your "slingshot" to blast those rocks or boulders of kryptonite into another stratosphere so they do not get in your way.

Cancerville demands an unequivocal commitment to yourself to suck it up, take it on, and rise to its demands. It also requires that you take care of yourself, and try to sneak some fun in along the way. Chapter 21 speaks to the importance and healing power of laughter.

For now, let's just assume that your innate and intuitive compass of strength will help you find your way through the corridors of Cancerville. Let us also remember that even Jake, at eight-and-a-half years of age, was able to take Cancerville on. His father, Rob, called him "The Warrior" in his blogs for good reason. People of all ages have an amazing adaptive potential that shows itself in many ways, but especially when faced with adversity, and most especially when faced with a serious illness such as cancer.

Everything is Truly Relative

The following is a chart I give to people I help with anxiety, depression, or the like. I call it Penzer's Theory of Relativity. This is not to be confused with the more incomprehensible one by some guy named Einstein, who also started a bagel company:

SEEING THINGS MORE CLEARLY

we need to assess what happens to us along a realistic impact scale

	1	2	3	4	5	6	7	8	9	10
	Irritation		*Frustration*			*Aggravation*		*Trauma/Tragedy*		
Health:	Cold		Flu			Pneumonia		Lung Cancer		
Finance:	$50 Late Fee		$100 Late Fee		$1000 + Loss			Bankruptcy		
Accident:	Fender Bender		Car Totaled No Injuries			Head-on Collision With Injuries		Head-on Collision With Death		
Work:	Disagreement With Peer		Disagreement With Boss		Poor Evaluation			Fired		

The interesting thing about human nature is that we tend to see experiences in the 1 to 4 range as if they were 8 to 10+. This is not only true of the people who visit my colleagues and me, but of most people. There are a few cock-eyed optimists out there, but they are not in the majority. In addition, they all seem to be married to pessimists.

Being in Cancerville slowly changes how we look at and measure life events. We develop a newfound appreciation for these distortions and begin to adjust accordingly. What once seemed oh so important and worrisome now seems oh so silly. You will keep running into these interpretive shifts repeatedly, and at some point you will begin to wish for the lower-level stresses you once dreaded. Nonetheless, here you are, much as you didn't expect to and don't want to be.

I am a great believer in the strength, courage, and perseverance that people bring to the battlefields of their lives. I have had the privilege of repeatedly observing that in my office all these years. I am also a great believer in the power of words that feed and fuel those very characteristics. My sincere belief is that the following words will be powerful enough to help you cope a little better in the place I have come to call Cancerville.

Take a very deep breath, let it out very, very slowly, and then do it again. Our journey is about to begin. You may have already started, but I've only just joined your team. Welcome to Cancerville—one hell of a place!

Real People Facing Cancer

Eileen

"Surreal" is the way my friend and colleague Eileen, the "roller-blader," described her experiences in Cancerville. I had emailed her about my working hard to finish the book for family and friends of someone with cancer. I wrote, "I feel as if I'm in a footrace with destiny and I need to finish this book." Less than a month after that email, Eileen's destiny brought her into Cancerville. I came to realize that in a very real sense we are all in a footrace with destiny, whether we are in or out of Cancerville. Our goal is to stay one step ahead for as long as we can.

After her initial thought, "I don't believe this is really happening to me—it all feels like I am having a not-so-pleasant dream," Eileen was unusually calm and unemotional. "I wasn't angry and neither was my mother," she told me. "I wasn't overwhelmed with any emotion. I didn't feel particularly anxious, nor did I think I was going to die. It was a process and I just decided to follow it along; I accepted it all and tried to go with the flow."

"In fact, my friends were the ones flooding out with emotion, hysterics, and drama. Their worry and anxiety was caring and loving, but seemed very exaggerated to me." Important for you to know is that, in my observation, Eileen is not unemotional or cold—in fact I would say the very opposite. Clearly, what I call her inner voice of reassurance was strong and robust.

Obviously, Eileen's reactions were atypical and she and others like her would not likely need to read this book. They seem to have a learned ability to stare adversity down and deal with it calmly—like patiently dusting some furniture until it is clean. Certainly, for most of us, finding inner peace while simultaneously entering Cancerville is not the norm. That Eileen's Mom did the same suggested to me that it was a familial character trait.

Roberta

I was surprised and intrigued when, at a recent meeting, Eileen mentioned that her sister had an aggressive form of breast cancer a few years back. The researcher in me immediately said, "I'd like to interview her." I was curious to know how Eileen's sister, Roberta, dealt with Cancerville. As it turned out, her reaction was just as atypical, if not more so. She said that as soon as she felt the small lump on her right breast, she said to herself, "I have breast cancer." Once her doctor confirmed that, she took the position, "Okay, let's move on and do what we have to do."

She goes on to say:

> I couldn't be serious about it. Never once did I think I was going to die. I laughed and joked all the way through. The techs at radiation fought over who would take me because I was so much fun.
>
> My husband was very serious about it because his sister had died from breast cancer. At one point I told him, 'If you are going to

act like this, I don't want you here.' He quickly lightened up and was a great support to me. If anything, my having cancer strengthened our relationship.

The only time Roberta remembers crying was when she had her hair cut short prior to chemo. But she quickly liked it and enjoyed having wigs where she could have short hair one day and long the next. She kibbitzingly wondered what would happen if she rode in a convertible. Once again, Roberta would not need to read this book and probably could have written Chapter 21, "Laughter in Cancerville," even better than I.

Of interest is that her sister Eileen's experience was pretty straightforward—diagnosis, surgery, done. Eileen is quick to admit that her reactions may have been different if she needed chemo and/or radiation, though I tend to think she would have "skated" on by just the same. Roberta also makes her Cancerville journey sound very straightforward, but nothing could be further from the truth.

Roberta initially had a lumpectomy, followed by strong chemo, followed by seven weeks of daily radiation to which she drove herself. She said, "Through it all nothing shook my spirit." As if all that wasn't enough, at the end of her radiation treatments, their mother, Doris, was diagnosed with breast cancer. This led to a BRCA gene test for which Roberta was positive. As many women in that position do, she chose a double mastectomy and hysterectomy.

As you may have guessed, she faced these with the same strong and smiling spirit. Six plus years later, she reports feeling and doing very well. Clearly, just like Eileen, Roberta drew upon a very strong inner voice of reassurance that served her well throughout her time in Cancerville.

Doris

Intrigued by both Eileen's and Roberta's unusually strong and positive reactions when they entered Cancerville, I asked permission to speak to their eighty-one-year-"young" mother. I just got off the phone with Doris. She laid it out pretty simply for me in as atypical a "Jewish Mother" way as could be. Portnoy would have no "complaints" if he grew up in Doris' home:

> I am that way and my parents were that way so my daughters never saw hysteria. We think good is going to happen, not bad! We are positive people just like my parents were. We get the news, find a reliable doctor, assume the best, and do what we have to do. If it would do good to worry we would, but it won't. It only makes things worse. I'd rather be positive and happy. So far, it has worked for all of us, don't you think?

All I could say to Doris was, "Absolutely!"

Certainly, I don't expect you to initially be like Eileen, Roberta, or their Mom, unless a Doris-esque mother raised you too. Please note that the key word in the last sentence is "initially." My hope is that by continuing to read this book you can get closer to their positive-minded, go-with-the-flow attitude. In addition, in the following pages you will meet many more inspiring role models who faced Cancerville squarely and ultimately won their battles.

In Sum

Cancerville has many rough and bumpy roads on which you have to travel. It reminds me of the difficult and unpredictable terrain I encountered in East Africa where many boulders and rocks blocked the unpaved roads. Though you may have to go into the emotional equivalent of four-wheel drive, you will make it through. The good news is that you can, and likely will, rise to the challenge of being in Cancerville with strength, courage, and dignity. As you keep reading, my goal is to help make your journey a little easier and a lot smoother.

It is very important that right from the beginning you lower the spotlight on catastrophe. Our minds can automatically go for "worst-case scenarios." Let's see if in the next chapter I can help you go to "better-case scenarios." Let us move on to do our best to help you turn down the spotlight on catastrophe so you can sleep more peacefully at night and face each day with more vigor, vitality, and an optimistic vision of your future.

CHAPTER 2

I will be a survivor.

Turning Down the Spotlight on Catastrophe

s soon as you hear a diagnosis of cancer, your first question is, "Am I going to die?" Obviously, there is a very powerful association between being in Cancerville and death. Many cancer patients have told me that nothing awakens one's sense of mortality as much as a cancer diagnosis. Susan said, "It's like getting hit in the face with a mortality pie and it doesn't taste good. It is very bitter and really hard to swallow." The same raised consciousness is true for those close to the patient.

Nonetheless, I want you to try to lose any thoughts of losing your life. The only way to exist comfortably in Cancerville is to be "balls to the walls" positive. That goes for females too. I believe that both males and females have them and women's are invisible, but bigger. Repeat these words every day: "Cancer can be cured!"

There is little room for doubt, even if others' words, books, research, or statistics feed into fearful feelings. Instead, try to leave your fears out of your emotional equation. The unpredictability of Cancerville can work in your favor as well. No one knows for certain what the future will bring in or out of Cancerville. For now, repeat the following as often as you need to: "I will be a survivor!"

Many who were told they had a limited time to live are still alive and well years later. For example, my friend Tom was told his leukemia would take him out of the game within six to twelve months. He was supposed to be the late Tom back in the late 1980s. All these years later, he still smiles about beating that dire prediction. We will encounter many similar stories as we go along.

Renowned psychologist and researcher, Martin Seligman, Ph.D., said it best. In his book *Learned Optimism,* he states, [4] "Life inflicts the same setbacks and tragedies on the optimist as on the pessimist, but the optimist weathers them better.... Even when things go well for the pessimist he is haunted by forebodings of catastrophe." Seligman's research reminds us of the value of being positive-minded, and his writings can help us on the path to becoming more optimistic. You will hear more about his work in Chapter 12, "The Power of Positive Self-Talk."

A Less Than Healthy Denial

But for a select few like Eileen and her family, it takes time to absorb and embrace the fact that you have cancer. It is important, however, to quickly accept reality so you can move forward. I have heard some stories of people who stayed in their denial for too long. They denied their situation and diagnosis, avoided treatment, and ultimately passed away without giving cancer a fight.

Though that was their choice for their own reasons, I would not encourage your following their path. My advice is to accept your situation as quickly as possible and fight like hell to survive. The sign in my office reads: "Never, Never, Never Give Up." That is my philosophy in life and that is my belief— I hope it is yours as well. Cancer is neither a slam-dunk of survival nor a *fait accompli* of loss of your life. It is, at best, a crapshoot and all I ask is that you keep rolling the dice and assume no snake eyes!

In his exceptional book, *Love, Medicine and Miracles*, [5] directed at his "exceptional" patients, Bernie Siegel, M.D., said, "No one lives forever; therefore, death is not the issue. Life is. Death is not a failure. Not choosing to take on the challenge of life is." Throughout this book I encourage you to take on the challenges of Cancerville. At the end of the day, that is really all you can do.

Illusions of Safety and Predictability

Terrible misfortunes happen many times every day somewhere or other. House fires, car accidents, assaults, abductions, and much more happen to random people. Mother Nature periodically shows her wrath in many devastating ways. However, we typically don't walk around worrying about these disasters and catastrophes. Try to use your healthy denial mechanism in Cancerville. Remind yourself that many people survive these days. Clearly, Cancerville does not have a monopoly on taking your life. There are many paths to heaven, only one of which is cancer.

You can't predict outcomes in life or in Cancerville. After all, if you were really good at predicting the future, you would be a billionaire by now and not too many of us can claim that title. In reality, most people, including myself, have amazing hindsight and limited foresight. So what makes you think that you can predict your outcome in a place as complicated as Cancerville? You are much better off believing that somehow or other you will walk the streets of Cancerville and survive. Of course, you do need to be realistic in this regard, which will be discussed in more detail in Chapter 11, "Embracing a Really Simple Philosophy: Realistic Optimism." Then again, there is room for a leap of faith, which will be discussed in Chapter 26, "On Becoming Even More Empowered." Your nature and your beliefs will guide you through this complex and confusing territory.

Obviously, walking around Cancerville fearing your premature demise is an exercise in self-torture. This fear serves no useful purpose. Rather, it inflicts pain, torment, and high levels of anxiety upon you. These will not serve you well. They will drain you of energy and weaken your "slingshot." To keep your mind strong, please do your best to reduce the candlepower of that scary spotlight.

I have sold hope with the tenacity of a drug dealer my entire career. Not only has it helped people free themselves from their inner torments, but it has also paid multiple dividends. Being positive, hopeful, and optimistic generates more of those same feelings. Those feelings can, in turn, increase your energy to tackle whatever challenges you face in the future. In the same way, fostering hope in Cancerville will help you make better decisions for yourself.

On Loss

People don't like to lose—ever! I can recall playing indoor racquetball for many years until my angioplasty in 2001 prematurely ended my competitive fun. Before I had to hang up my racquetball outfits and give away my racquet, I played as if I were going to win a gold medal, rather than just trying to beat a friend or neighbor.

Even today, I do not like to lose a silly board game, even when playing with my grandchildren. My Bronx Yankees played for the pennant in 2010 and for a shot at it in 2011. Even though my serious fan days are long gone, I didn't want them to lose. They did lose, however, despite their well-paid roster, and I was disappointed. We humans are seemingly programmed to root, root, root for the home team, even in situations without great significance or meaning.

If seemingly irrelevant losses can be upsetting, you rapidly realize how the possible loss of your life can be so devastating. I am not denying the seriousness of the situation. I am not insensitive to your innermost fears. I am simply trying to teach you a lesson that took me a while to learn. Your more than understandable fears need to be bypassed via emotional open-heart surgery so that you can endure your experience in Cancerville. There is just no time or energy for such torment. You need to table the notion of anything other than your survival. This book is intended to help you do just that.

Assuming Survival

In the final analysis, you just never know how your story will conclude until you get there. So don't sell yourself or your army of protectors in Cancerville short. Assume and embrace the enduring belief that you will become a survivor, just like the millions of people who are part of that strong group. Believe that you will spit in the face of the ugly cancer cells, survive the ordeal, and get back to your life all the stronger for squarely facing the challenge of Cancerville and for overcoming it.

During Jodi's treatment time in Cancerville, I would often say to myself: "The world could end tomorrow or the next day and we would all be gone, so I won't worry about my daughter anymore than I worry about that." I worked very hard to keep turning down the spotlight on my fear of losing my daughter. One of the ways I did this was by reminding myself of many other potential dangers that we know of but choose to ignore. I again became reacquainted with how fragile human life is, both in and out of Cancerville. I also came to appreciate and feel a full measure of gratitude for every day. I hope you can do the same.

As if to highlight and underscore my thoughts, my friend Ben called me after Jodi began chemo. He said, "Billy, I envy you." I said, "How can that be Benjy? I told you what's going on and I am miserable about Jodi." He said, "I am much more miserable. My daughter Jessica, who just turned eighteen, was taken from us last night in a horrific car accident. She was an innocent passenger sitting in the backseat. At least Jodi has a chance, a good chance." I rest my case about life and death, Cancerville, and all the other vile "villes" that can hurt or kill us.

That you are alive at this very moment is what matters. All of the rest is unknown. Yours could be a sorrowful ending or a positive one. Why not assume that like ours, yours will be a happy one too, and root, root, root for your "home team"— YOU!

I encourage you to think beyond Cancerville to a time in the future when your life will return. Picture a calmer, quieter, less stressful time. See routine returning. Believe that your nightmare will conclude and that you will be a cancer survivor.

Most minds, not just yours or mine, tend to gravitate toward negative anticipations. I would like you to try to block yours from going there and to try to make positive and hopeful assumptions. If this is too large a jump for your mind to make, then at least strive for neutral. Say to yourself: "Self, I don't know what the future will bring. I will wait and see and try to assume I will be okay." That's all you can really do.

In Cancerville, if things get really mean and scary, it can be hard to imagine a positive outcome. Yet over and over, we see people surviving. Every victory in Cancerville is huge and beyond description. The good news is that it happens more and more every day. Please allow me to correct myself. That news is not just good, it is great! Hold onto that headline and strive to make it your own. Believe that your tee shirt will read, "I Survived My Cancerville Journey." I sincerely hope that is exactly what will happen.

Real People Facing Cancer

Harvey

Soon after sitting down for lunch, Harvey, a person I had just met, said, "Cancer is the least of my problems!" He is a sensitive and emotional person who seems to have taken on Cancerville without any angst. "It's the constant pain that gets to me, not the fact that I have cancer," he said.

Cancer has stalked Harvey and his family like a serial killer on steroids. There are too many Cancerville-related deaths within his family for me to list them all. Sadly, he and his wife, Carol, lost their forty-five-year-old son to cancer.

What impressed me even before meeting Harvey was learning from our mutual friend who introduced us that he carried the following message in his wallet:

> *The present moment is the only thing that exists.*
> *The past is gone, the future uncertain.*
> *Right now is the only time and place we can be happy.*
> *If you are not suffering right now, enjoy the feeling*
> *while it lasts.*
> *Regrets will not change the past, nor will worrying*
> *affect the future.*

That is an excellent message for life in general, and particularly for Cancerville.

My previous reference to falling off the mountain, dusting yourself off, and continuing your journey is metaphorical, but for Harvey is very real. He and Carol, like Ronnie and I, are travel lovers; they have been all over the world. Wherever they go, unlike Ronnie and I, they look for mountains to climb or trails to hike. A hike in Nepal caused him severe pain. Hiking on a trail in Vermont that he had done twice a year for forty years was not possible. What were once happy trails became signs that something was not right within his body.

The first doctor missed it completely, but the second, a few months later, nailed Harvey's lymphoma of the thigh. Complicated surgery, chemo, and radiation followed, which were subsequently followed by lymphedema—a repetitive painful swelling. Then a screw in his leg broke while hiking in Peru, which necessitated a hip replacement. Harvey "fell off the mountain" once again in body but never, ever in spirit.

There was no rest for the weary as he developed an infection in his hip joint. Somewhere, in the midst of all that, he was diagnosed with prostate cancer and, a couple of years later, lymphoma on his L3 vertebrae. Shortly after our lunch, he went through radiation for a growth in his breast that was not cancerous, but still painful. Just to give you a sense for Harvey as a Cancerville warrior, when I asked if he had serious side effects from all the radiation he has experienced, he dryly and with a straight face said, "I glow in the dark." I can almost believe that. Undeniably, he has also found a way to reduce the candlepower of catastrophe.

The glow that Harvey gives off is not one of irradiation, but one of a quiet and unassuming yet deep-rooted strength. He is a man who has looked cancer in the eyes and said, "Take me if you can, but I won't go easily or quietly." Those were not his words but rather my sense of who he is and how he has faced his ten-plus years in Cancerville.

Harvey says he has climbed or hiked every significant mountain in the world and been just about everywhere he has wanted to go. Believe me when I say he has climbed the mountains of Cancerville with grace, strength, and dignity. In explaining how he was able to take on cancer so strongly and calmly at age sixty-two, Harvey said, "I did just about all of my bucket list. I had a great life. I wasn't ready to go, but if I had to I would with no regrets but for leaving my family." I realize that not all of you reading this book can say those words—but you still can follow his formula.

According to Harvey, his son, Bruce, was the same way. Harvey quotes Bruce as saying, "I can be sick and miserable or sick and happy. If I am happy, people want to be around me, so it is better for me that way." Clearly, Harvey and his family have had to deal with the genetics of cancer—on their side has also been the genetics of strength, hope, and the will to fight back. Try to be like them—if you fall off the literal and figurative mountains, always get back up and continue your climb. You just never know what vistas you might see once you get to the top of the mountain! If you don't believe me, just ask Harvey.

Harvey encouraged me to go to Machu Picchu because he considers it the most spiritual place in the world. I will add that to my bucket list and follow his advice about that trip as well as his way of coping with difficult circumstances. Harvey is a *mensch* (good man), a *starka* (strong person), and a fascinating lunch companion. Our meeting was *bashert* (meant to be).

Stuart

I met Stuart over the phone. The three Yiddish words I used in the last paragraph regarding Harvey apply to him as well. In fact, our mutual friend, Neil, who networked us together, said, "Of all the couples we have met in our life, Stuart and his wife are the best." I wasn't sure if I should be insulted or not, but chose not to take it personally.

Like Harvey, Stuart has been dealing with Cancerville for a long time. Back in 1999 he was diagnosed with prostate cancer. Initially shocked, he faced reality quickly, reviewed his options, and chose a course of action. "I did what I had to do," he said. All these years later his PSA remains fine.

Unfortunately and fortunately, this is not quite the end of Stuart's story. At the time of his prostate cancer diagnosis, they also found that his blood platelet count was very high. A second painful bone marrow biopsy later, he was diagnosed with myleofibrosis, a type of chronic leukemia that causes the bone marrow to dry up. The oncologist he was seeing gave him two-plus years to live—maximum.

Stuart understandably became agitated, but being a reasonably calm, scientifically oriented person, he decided to get a second opinion. Intriguingly, the same doctor at Mt. Sinai Hospital in New York was recommended to him both by people in New York and by our mutual friend who lives in Florida. Clearly, this doctor at Sinai was the specialist Stuart needed.

The new oncologist was emphatic. He said, "You will not die in two years—worst case it will take ten percent from your natural lifespan. Stuart did the math and breathed a long sigh of relief. His parents lived into their 90's, so he had a shot at eighty-one, not fifty-nine. That is a statistically, and more importantly, emotionally significant difference.

From that point on meds that kept his platelet count down stabilized his system—or perhaps it was a combination of those meds and his positive attitude. Or perhaps it was both of those plus his wife of now forty-eight years having been a volunteer cancer counselor for the American Cancer Society for over thirty years. How fortunate for Stuart that he had a built-in, live-in, sleep-with cheerleader to encourage him forward. All went well for Stuart until last year when his blood counts were way off again after all these years. Such is the up, down, and sideways nature of some Cancerville journeys.

With his characteristic determination and will to survive, Stuart made his way into an experimental trial at Mt. Sinai. This required him getting a letter from a cardiologist that his minor heart arrhythmia was inconsequential. So far, so good, and Stuart believes the new medication is working with minimal side effects. This allows Stuart to continue working full-time—some days thirteen hours a day—which he feels is a form of distraction and "therapy." He says, "It distracts me from thinking about my aches, pains, and problems, and gives me a sense of purpose. I will retire or semi-retire one of these years, but not yet."

Stuart admits that when learning of the not-so-good results last year, his hands were shaking so badly he could hardly write his co-pay check. But a few hours later he had calmed down and was able to go to work the next day. Stuart says:

> The mind is an amazing and resilient thing. It is able to block out so much that is disturbing and agitating. My advice is to keep positive, assume cancer won't kill you, stay occupied, and find the very best treatment for you. Perhaps believing you won't die from it helps keep you from dying from it? Being a pharmacist helped me know the lingo better, but talking to seriously ill people my entire career helped me learn how to deal with it better.

I think Stuart is talking about healthy denial here. It helps us all to move forward despite the scary times. To me, both Harvey's and Stuart's experiences provide strong evidence that turning down the spotlight on catastrophe in many, many situations is a helpful thing. Perhaps, in a variety of different situations, including dealing with cancer, we shouldn't count ourselves out until we are out, in which case we are no longer counting!

In Sum

Try to leave the unknown alone for now; none of us can know the future. Right now, this very moment is certain and the rest is unknown—in and out of Cancerville. Assume you will be okay. Believe that the knowledgeable and talented doctors and their medical staff are working and planning on winning, just as you are. Know that hope makes it easier and sometimes even makes it better.

You really don't have the time or energy to waste on the unknown. Right now, you need to begin to understand Cancerville and its land so you can take it on. Let's take a brief look at just how powerful you are—even if you don't exactly feel that way.

CHAPTER 3

I am much stronger than I feel.

Converting Rapidly from Powerless to Powerful

I don't care how important you are, how much clout you have, or how much money you have accumulated. I don't care if your name is Gates, Trump, Kennedy, or Winfrey. You might have the financial resources to buy an organ, a private room, or a Medevac plane to fly to a different cancer center. Once there, however, you will feel as powerless as everyone else.

Cancer is an overwhelming disease and Cancerville is an intimidating place. No one would ever suggest otherwise. However, I want to help you overcome those feelings quickly so you can take cancer on. In many different situations, strength and power are all about attitude. It can be helpful to develop a certain kind of swagger that will carry you through. This is no time to be cocky, but it is a time to be clear-headed and courageous.

As we shall see, the feelings of powerlessness are more illusion than reality. Though you cannot treat your disease without the help of your doctors, you can address your disease in a variety of ways. Any kryptonite that makes you feel powerless only applies to the medical side of the equation.

The Power of Your Thoughts

As we will come to understand more clearly in Chapter 12, "The Power of Positive Self-Talk," how we process our life experiences and what we say to ourselves about these experiences are both very important. Our thoughts and self-talk not only influence our feelings, but also affect our attitude, spirit, motivation, and oftentimes even the outcome of an event. In a very real sense, our inner script and the monologue that follows from it guide our way.

Think about my friend Eileen waking up and telling herself to go rollerblading that morning after she was diagnosed with cancer. There was much power in those words. After all, they pushed her to dress, go to her car, drive to the beach, put on her blades, and blast off into the morning sun. Contrast that with how she would have felt if she had woken up saying the following to herself:

> I feel like crap. I can't believe this is happening to me. I have to have a serious operation and who knows what else. This sucks big time. I don't even want to get out of bed. I think I will

just lay here and cry. Why do things always go wrong for me?

Giving in to this most understandable series of thoughts would have taken Eileen right down the proverbial tubes—a most disillusioning and disturbing way to start the day. Did she and do you have every right to that anguished self-speech? Absolutely! I encourage you, if you must, to have that pity party in whatever form you need and then streak past it like a racehorse on steroids. Here is a possible inner discussion that can follow your personal "Why me?" lament:

> Okay. My life has taken a most unexpected and unnecessary turn. I am not happy about any of this. Who would be? But you know what? I am a pretty strong person and I have always risen to the challenges of my life and given them a run for their money. So I am going to do the same thing now. I am going to suck it up, meet it head-on, and do my best to survive this ordeal and win. I think I'll go rollerblading this morning!

Or how about this inner discussion?

> Okay. Okay. I am really scared right now—crapping in my pants scared! This news caught me way off guard. Whoever thinks they are going to get cancer, especially at my age? That happens to other unfortunate folks. Even though I never saw myself as strong or brave, I have no choice now but to take this on full force and full tilt. I am all in for myself and will muster all the strength, courage, and determination that I can find. And while I am going through this ordeal, I will do my best to live my life, enjoy my family and friends and their support, and make the

most of a sucky situation. I'm going rollerblading this morning!

Or you might want to parallel Susan's inner self-talk:

> Son-of-a-bitch! How the hell did I get cancer
> of all things? How did this happen to me?
> It's just not possible! Well, wait a minute
> here—I am a person no different from any-
> one else. Cancer happens to people. Why
> shouldn't I have gotten sick just like oth-
> ers do? Even though I hate the thought, it
> makes perfectly good sense. What I need to
> do is learn as much as I can about this dis-
> ease and mobilize my resources for a fight
> to the finish. I'm not giving up or giving in.
> I will take it on in any and every way I can.
> I need to get myself together, get dressed,
> and go rollerblading this morning!

Obviously, I'm using rollerblading as an example of taking an empowering action. I'm not encouraging you to actually strap on some blades and start skating—especially if
you have never done that before. I am, however, encouraging you to speak to yourself in a strong and determined way
to enhance your feelings of personal power. You will need to
keep writing your self-talk in a strong voice as Cancerville's
bite and, at times, impersonal nature, can drain you of hope.
My simple maxim is that the more empowering your inner
voice can be, the more powerful your body and mind will be
as well.

The Power of Your Knowledge

In my book *Getting Back Up From an Emotional Down*[6] I
share poems that I wrote during my own emotional down in

the 1970s. We will talk more about that in Chapter 10, "How Minds Work." One of them states:

> Knowledge is power of that there's no doubt,
> Self-knowledge awaits you if you dare seek it
> out.

I am well aware that I have no shot whatsoever at becoming Poet Laureate. Nonetheless, I believe strongly in the power of information, learning, and knowing more about something—especially something as significant and serious as cancer. An informed "consumer" in any life zone is always in a better position to plan, choose from options, make decisions, manage, and cope. The more you know about what you are dealing with in Cancerville, the more prepared and powerful you can feel.

I fully understand that these words won't work for everyone—some will choose to glance at information related to their condition and not dig too deeply. Others will want to learn a little more and some may Google till the sun comes up. The choice is clearly yours. I believe, however, that learning more about your disease and its treatment will not only help you become a more informed consumer, but will also enable you to participate actively in partnering with your medical team.

No one expects you to become an oncologist, surgeon, radiologist, or specialist of whatever type of cancer with which you are dealing. An informed patient is not only better able to anticipate what is involved and contribute to the plan, but is also able to feel just a little more powerful. It also helps you to come up with Plan B if Plan A isn't working for you. Since there are many unknowns in Cancerville, filling in some of the blanks that can be known helps to make it a little less daunting.

Some people like Susan, who was a nurse, or Dani, who was a dentist, have a bit of an edge over those not so scientifically inclined, but it is likely that you can learn more about your situation. I strongly believe that there are times in our life when knowledge can be empowering. In a place like Cancerville you need all the power you can muster.

Susan would chide you to become a fully informed and active manager and advocate of the medical side of your situation. In the Fall 2011 issue of *Cure* magazine, Dr. Len Lichtenfeld, M.D., says:

> Until we arrive at that magical day when our treatment information follows us to where we get our health care, you must be your own advocate. Know your disease, know your treatment, and know what your healthcare team wants you to do and when you should do it. Keep copies of important records and even CDs of scans. If you don't understand something, speak up and ask questions.

I want to wave a yellow flag of caution. Partnering with your doctor is okay— being your doctor is not. My old college hygiene text quoted Hippocrates who said, "He who hath himself for a doctor hath a fool for a patient." Sorry ladies, but it was 1959 and you hadn't burned your bras yet!

There are many stories of people making decisions based on information they researched that came back to bite them. Steve Jobs, for example, delayed his physician recommended surgery for nine crucial months, believing alternatives were better for him. He later regretted that decision.

Roger Ebert, a well-known movie critic, went against his doctor's recommended treatment, which ultimately caused him to suffer severely. The details of this unfortunate result will be discussed in Chapter 18, "Traditional and Alternative Treatments and Complementary Options."

Cancerville treatments are obviously not pleasant, but in most cases they are necessary. I encourage you to learn as much as you can, but always remember that your doctors are the most learned and experienced. Seriously consider their recommendations and heed their advice. When in doubt, feel free to seek second or even third opinions. For example, Rob consulted with two other major pediatric oncology centers to confirm that they completely agreed with the protocol Memorial Sloan-Kettering was using.

The Power of Your Medical Team

I will be speaking much more about your medical team in Chapter 6, "Meetings with the Dedicated Doctors." For now, just know that the doctors with whom you are working are on your side all the way. They want to help you, and they want you to become a survivor. They are totally committed to your well-being and will do everything in their power to add to your power as you fight against cancer.

It is not just the doctors that are all in for you. Every person on your medical team from the receptionists to the nurses to the directors of cancer centers hate this illness and work very hard in every way possible to defeat it. I can't promise that their moods will always be upbeat, nor can I assure you they will always be warm, or even appropriate, and on point. What I can assure you of is that they will always do everything they can to help you defeat cancer. Cancer is their enemy, too, and you are automatically their friend. They are your guides and will hopefully lead you through the Cancerville maze to the cure.

The Power of Your Support Team

Just about all of the medical magic you need rests solely with your medical team. Yet magical or otherwise, hugs, kisses, and emotional support can make your journey much easier. Warmth and love have been found to help strengthen immune systems and overcome a variety of medical problems in and out of Cancerville.

Bernie Siegel, M.D., repeatedly stresses the importance of emotional support in the healing and medical recovery process. He is a strong believer in the power of the patient and his or her family as healing facilitators. He is a lobbyist for love and states, "I am convinced that unconditional love is the most powerful known stimulant of the immune system... The truth is love: heals."

For example, when Jodi was going through treatment, my wife and I did a variety of things to be helpful, supportive, and loving. We flew back and forth from Ft. Lauderdale, Florida, to New York City many, many times. We wanted to meet with the doctors, be there for Jodi's surgery and chemotherapy treatments, and bring support and occasional fun to the scene. I think we saw almost every show on Broadway. We were also there to celebrate and bring warmth to special days. Though we could not be there every day, we were fortunate to be able to be there every time we wanted or needed to be. There were daily phone calls as well. In today's wired world, some of these calls could have been made via Skype, so we could have been "face-to-face."

The day of Jodi's surgery, after she was back in her room, I needed to get out and escape briefly from Cancerville's New York headquarters. I needed some fresh air to clear my mind, and I probably needed another drink, but that's beside the point. Oh, by the way, I forgot to tell you about the BYOB bar that I discovered in the men's room at Sloan-Kettering on the day of Jodi's surgery. It was where I drank at least five airplane bottles of vodka. I was trying to raise my spirits by drinking them. It didn't work. The one advantage of finding a bar in the restroom is that you are not very far from a toilet. That advantage notwithstanding, I do not encourage you to follow my lead. I am not particularly proud of sometimes using alcohol to offset my pain, but in some situations, you've just got to do what you've got to do. On occasion, we humans, smart as we might be, can be pretty dumb. Guilty as charged!

So, needing to escape for a while, instead of having another drink, I went for a walk and wandered into the megastore Bed Bath and Beyond. There was no booze there despite all the B's. I needed to get Beyond, but all I got was Bed and Bath. A few minutes into the store, I saw a small pink pillow with arm- and leg-like appendages that vaguely resembled a person. I instinctively bought it and brought it back to give to Jodi. I later learned that she slept with the pillow at night and sometimes took it in the car with her to cushion the literal bumps in the road on the Manhattan streets. I was completely unaware that it helped her with the figurative bumps as well.

Years later, I received an email from Jodi telling me that she had to retire "Pinky" because he had pretty much come undone: "Better him than my daughter!" I thought. She shared how attached she had become to him and how much he had helped her get through those troubled times.

I was struck and touched that a simple $9.99 purchase could have had such a significant impact on her. Being a psychologist, I wondered to myself whether it wasn't so much "Pinky" as it was that I gave it to her on what was the very worst day of her life. Maybe what "Pinky" represented beyond his cushiness was my comforting, loving, and cushioning support and presence beside my daughter at those times when I wasn't able to be there in person. I'd really like to believe that.

You just never know the impact that words, actions, or small gifts will have on you. In some instances they may be from others. But don't forget you can also give gifts to yourself. Buy a pretty and fun something or other for yourself and see if it helps you to feel just a tiny bit better. It is important for you to remember that sometimes it doesn't take much to make a significant difference. Just a loving hug, a kind word spoken by others or you to yourself, or the equivalent of a "Pinky" at the right moment, can be most significant.

The Power of Taking Action

I have been using "rollerblading" as a metaphor for taking any action that helps give you stronger and more powerful feelings. These help counterbalance the strong feelings of being scared, angry, overwhelmed, etc. that Cancerville can rapidly cause you to feel. Obviously, you don't actually need to roll-erblade. There are so many different actions that can further your cause and contribute to your sense of feeling and being powerful. Taking action can not only distract you from your focus on Cancerville, but also enable you to live your life. Here are some examples of actions that can make a difference:

- seeking out counseling and/or support group assistance

  > Susan felt empowered and more positive from our one-on-one visits, but not from the support groups she tried. She did look to Internet sites for support and experimental trial opportunities. We will talk much more about this in Chapter 19, "Having a Coun-selor and/or Support Group in Your Corner."

- enjoying creative activities such as painting, sculpting, and writing

  > Check out the beautiful picture of a glass sculpture that Antje, a twenty plus year sur-vivor, made that depicts her vision of Can-cerville at www.cancerville.com.

- participating in physical activities such as working out, walking or jogging, practicing yoga, dancing, etc.—if and when you are up to it

- planning ahead for a nice trip post-treatment

- catching up on the classics or other subjects either in book or movie form

- going to shows, concerts, etc, when you are able

- watching TV

- planting a garden or having a few plants around to nurture

- spending time with family and friends rather than withdrawing

- reaching out to help others, which is often very rewarding and uplifting

> Jake was confined to the hospital for many months. When he felt up to it, he would make pretty "get well" cards for the other children staying there. This no doubt distracted him from his own pain and suffering while making him feel good about helping others. Perhaps it also gave him a sense of taking control of something at a time when so much of his young life was totally out of control.

These are merely examples of what you might consider doing as you move through Cancerville. As you well know, there are so many other activities in which you can become involved. My belief is that the more active you are, the more powerful you will feel. I believe this is true generally, but even more so when dealing with cancer.

This is precisely why Geralyn Lucas wore bright red lipstick to her mastectomy. She was taking a small but bold and symbolic action as she faced a traumatizing surgery. We will talk more about her experience in Chapter 5, "Making Eye Contact with Cancerville." It is also why Kris Carr became an orthodox yoga participant, healthy diet convert, herbalist, and pursued any other healthy action she could. We will get to meet her in Chapter 18, "Traditional and Alternative Treatments and Complementary Options."

It is also why Harvey, whom you met in the previous chapter, still travels despite his constant pain and the inconvenience of needing two canes, a motorized wheel chair, and special vans in which to sightsee. He may have completed his bucket list, but as long as Harvey is alive, he is going to live his life and indulge Carol and his love of travel. As always, Bernie Siegel, M.D., said it best when he wrote, "We must realize that people are not living or dying but alive or dead… If you are alive, you can still participate by loving, laughing, and living." I encourage you to try your best to fill that Rx.

If you struggle with that, as many do, read Randy Pausch's book, *The Last Lecture.*[7] We shall meet up with him again in Chapter, 22, "Communication in Cancerville." Upon hearing of his likely passing within three to six months from his caring and compassionate doctor, he reminds his wife, Jai, what he said the day before at a water park after a really fun speed slide:

> Even if the scan results are bad tomorrow I just want you to know that it feels great to be alive, and to be here today, alive with you. Whatever news we get about the scans, I'm not going to die when we hear it. I won't die the next day, or the day after that, or the day after that. So today, right now, well this is a wonderful day. And I want you to know how much I'm enjoying it.

He was simply living in the moment of his life and not looking too far ahead.

Nothing I am suggesting is meant to imply that it will take big, bold actions on your part or by your support team members to make a difference. Almost all of the time little things mean a lot. Roller-blading is not exactly an Olympic event, nor are any of the other activities I suggested as examples.

Real People Facing Cancer

Stuart

Stuart Scott took serious action in his Cancerville fight. He is a popular and well-spoken sports anchor who had the mike when the Miami Heat recently won the championship.

Three years ago he fought off stomach cancer, but it returned. How is he facing it this time around? In his most powerful "tough guy" voice, Stuart says to his cancer cells, "Nah, dawg, I'm better, I'm stronger. You're not going to beat me." This is impressive because many people have told me that it is much harder to muster hope and fight the second time around.

Beyond these strong, in your face words, Stuart practices martial arts a few days after his chemo treatments to further kick cancer's butt. He says:

> It's just who I am so it's not a matter of being impressive, it's a matter of I'm going to win this and this is how I win. It motivates me to win. You can try, but I'm just gonna come harder than you. I'm gonna come harder than you all day long.

Now that's what I call taking action and finding your inner voice of power! Commenting upon all of this, the writer who interviewed him wrote:

> Scott is to journalists what Lance Armstrong is to athletes. He's fighting and excelling during his battle with this ugly disease…. He is showing the world…that cancer isn't an excuse to stop living. It is even more of a reason to start.

I'd really like you to feel that way and start doing that too—in your own way. Whether you "dance with the enemy" or beat it into submission as Stuart is doing is your choice. Whether you "dance" or "karate chop," please engage with it in as powerful a way as possible, if for no other reason than to feel empowered every step of the way.

Nancy

An impressive example of taking action as a cancer survivor is Nancy Brinker. Diagnosed with breast cancer at thirty-seven, she was up on her horse playing polo as soon as the doctor allowed her to resume that strenuous activity. But that was only the beginning. If you are not familiar with her name, I understand, as I was not either until doing research for my last book. Her identity will come more clearly into focus if I tell you that her sister's name was Susan G. Komen, who died at age thirty-six from breast cancer. Nancy promised Susan she would make a difference in raising people's awareness of breast cancer. And my goodness, has she ever lived up to that promise!

The organization Nancy founded, "Susan G. Komen for the Cure," is known world- and corporate-wide and has raised over one-and-a-half billon dollars. As importantly, it has also raised awareness of breast cancer all around the world, thereby promoting prevention and early detection. It has also contributed generously to breast cancer research in the group's never-ending commitment and search for the cure. In every way possible and then some, Nancy Brinker has modeled taking action in Cancerville.

Please do not measure your accomplishments against Nancy's. She is a very unique woman with skills, resources, and a support team that most of us don't have—not even close! Measure yourself, if you must, by your accomplishments and actions and feel proud of them every single day.

Debbie

Debbie, whom my sons grew up with in Plantation, Florida, has accomplished impressive things as well. She was a successful attorney and the mother of three young children when she was diagnosed with incurable, Stage IV stomach cancer. Debbie didn't let that get in her way. While researching her options, she learned that stomach cancer was difficult to detect and treat and not well known; it didn't have the visibility of breast or prostate cancer.

She decided to do something about that and founded Debbie's Dream Foundation (DebbiesDream.org) in 2009. It is dedicated to funding innovative treatment for stomach cancer, stimulating pharmaceutical companies to focus on stomach

cancer and sharing information, as well as providing education and support to people around the world who are dealing
with stomach cancer. Debbie took her cause live when she
appeared on the Dr. Oz show.

Debbie has had more than seventy chemo treatments
since her diagnosis in 2008, but they don't seem to have
slowed her down one bit. Debbie, like Nancy, seems to know
how to take trauma and troubles and turn them into powerful
support for others in Cancerville.

Matthew

In 1995, at age twenty-one, Matthew was diagnosed with
a pediatric brain cancer and told he would not likely make
it six more months—so much for medical predictions! At the
time Matthew was a college senior, a music composer, and
concert pianist. Side effects of his treatments limited his use
of one hand.

Though he still composes and plays music, he turned his
creative juices into founding Stupid Cancer (stupidcancer.
org). This amazing and energetic organization is growing it
by leaps and bounds. Still expanding its reach and outreach
of loving assistance of all kinds, today it is the largest support
organization in the United States for young adults. Clearly,
Matthew and his mighty, albeit small band of organizers, have
turned their respective lemons into a wonderful blend of lem-
onAID!

In Sum

After reading this chapter, I hope you have come away
realizing that you are not as weak or powerless in Cancerville as you might think or feel. You see, the kryptonite really
only applies to the medical side. You are not expected to be
a superman or superwoman in that zone. Leave that to the
super doctors.

There is so much you are doing right now and that you will continue to do to make a difference for yourself. Of that I am very confident. My confidence comes from the fact that, among other things, you are taking an important action by reading this book. Bravo! Please remember that it doesn't have to be a big action to make a big difference. Cancerville is not a competitive event or a reality TV show. It is a realistic challenge to which, I am confident, you will rise in your own way.

Let's move on to talk about adapting to this most demanding place. It is a challenge, but one I am hopeful you will take on with confidence, strength, and much moxie.

CHAPTER 4

*I am an adaptive person and have
a track record to prove that.*

Striving to Adapt to a Place from which You Really Want to Run

If taking action helps you to overcome your sense of powerlessness in Cancerville, then a variety of specific actions and attitudinal adjustments will help you to better adapt to its demands. To demonstrate your power, you will need to adapt to Cancerville by finding ways to cope with all that is expected of you. All animals are programmed to adapt to their environs, as well as significant shifts in the terrain. In my humble opinion, none is better suited to that process and goal-directed purpose than human beings. You will adapt to Cancerville; I have no doubt about that!

People Rise to the Challenge

Catastrophes and crises create chaos, which in turn demands immediate adjustments. Entering Cancerville is obviously a crisis of grand proportion, but one that you will ultimately manage. As people, we adapt naturally and automatically to life's demands. Think of times in the past when you had to cope with and adjust to difficult situations. Reminding yourself how you were able to do it then will help you gain confidence that you can do it again now.

In speaking about crises, I vividly remember November 22, 1963. It was one month to the day before Ronnie and I were to be married, and I was nervous enough! I was teaching a class at New York University as a graduate assistant when a pained voice came over the loudspeaker announcing that President John F. Kennedy had been shot in Dallas, Texas. Everyone stood up and left the room; I didn't even have to say, "Class dismissed." I opened my mouth but no words came out. Like everyone else that day, I made my way home in a daze. We were not used to trauma and tragedy of that magnitude in those simple days.

As word spread of Kennedy's assassination, the world as we knew it changed. People spent the next several days watching events unfold, glued to their tiny black and white TVs. The same, of course, occurred on 9/11. Hardly anyone went to work that day or for days after, and once again, time stood still. I can't recall how many times I watched the color footage of the planes crashing into the World Trade Center before I just couldn't bear to watch anymore.

Those painful news images are really no different from the announcement that cancer cells have invaded your body; it is hard not to replay that news over and over again in your head.

However, I will teach you ways to stop doing that in Part IV of this book.

Such Cancerville news is a clarion call to arms; the chaos that ensues, emotionally and otherwise, is unprecedented. The announcement that you have cancer is nothing short of your own private assassination and 9/11 combined! Your world, as you have come to know it, is dramatically and traumatically changed. It will require major shifts in your routines, priorities, thoughts, and attitudes. Unlike national catastrophes, Cancerville is not for spectators. It won't be on TV and most people will have no idea what you are going through. Some who do know will inadvertently say the "wrong thing," as Lori Hope, author of *Help Me Live: 20 Things People with Cancer Want You to Know repeatedly points out.*[8]

Many in Cancerville report feeling very alone, even if they have a support team around them. But try to remind yourself that you are actually part of a very large network—in America, one-and-a-half-million people are diagnosed with cancer every year. Even if you are the only member of your team, you are not alone.

When Cancerville hits, all of a sudden and out of the blue, you are faced with confusions, questions, major decisions, and logistical adjustments that resemble a space shuttle launch. Yet the likelihood is that you don't have the support team or personnel of NASA. You will start creating a support structure and team out of whatever material and "personnel" are on hand. Creatively taking action, moving slowly forward, talking yourself through each step, researching, and learning will all help you to move ahead into calmer terrain. My recent visit to the World Trade Center site helped me to see that America is resiliently rebounding from 9/11. Let's just assume you will do the same.

The Process of Adapting

Adaptation is an interesting and understudied human experience. The majority of people do it naturally and automatically.

I have repeatedly observed people rise to the challenges of life and of Cancerville. There are only a very few who fall by the wayside. Make up your mind now that you will figure it out as you go along. You need to be there as strong and present as you possibly can for yourself.

This all makes me think of my mother and myself when my father died of a heart attack in 1960, at age forty-nine. After my father's passing, my mom and I adapted. We tightened our belts and she went from part-time to full-time work. I also found a part-time job while attending college full-time.

My father's death left emotional scars on my mom and me, but we coped as best we could and learned over time to accept the painful reality of his loss. Counseling or support groups back then were not readily available. We just sucked it up and moved forward.

Even a successful outcome in Cancerville will leave emotional scars. But remember, nobody dies from those scars. Sometimes you can even learn from them. I know that my mother and I just kept marching on. I haven't stopped yet, and she only did a couple of years ago after having lived to one hundred. In Chapter 24, we will look at some of the positive life lessons one can learn in Cancerville.

In all zones of our lives, much as most of us do not enjoy change, we adapt to it. We suck it up, stare challenges in the face, and do what we have to do. We certainly don't like Cancerville. No—wait a minute here—we absolutely hate it! Be aware, my wife edited out the word I originally had before "hate." I still feel that I should put it back in. Please do that on your own. I am optimistic that you will try your best to do whatever Cancerville asks and expects of you; hopefully you can do it with a smile, simply because your soul needs that warmth. The demands of Cancerville act as a lubricant for change and adaptation. What makes people so special is our ability to do just that.

I believe adaptation is a slow but steady process of determining what is needed and reacting accordingly. It is a fluid and often changing experience that goes with the flow of what is happening in the moment. Therefore, I do not see what follows as steps (as in one, two, etc.), but rather as components to foster your adaptation to Cancerville.

Acceptance

A most important component of adaptation involves your acceptance of the situation. This includes getting past the initial shock and realizing that "it is my turn," hard as that may be to believe. Clearly, all of our beliefs regarding immunity from harm's way are false and illusory.

I know you would like to run out of Cancerville to a much safer and calmer place. Let's assume you will, but not just yet. Acceptance allows you to mobilize your energies and target them directly to address your needs. It also helps you to realize that you are in the safest place you can be under these circumstances. Much support and many medical treatments are available for you in Cancerville. Though you may hate that you need them, it is important for you to accept that you do. Theoretically, you have a choice, but practically speaking, acceptance moves you forward toward treatment and survival.

Attitude Adjustment

Adjusting and readjusting your attitude is a most important component of your adaptation. My hope is that, as we walk through Cancerville together, you will be able to embrace a stronger, healthier, and more positive mindset as quickly as possible. Though I personally experienced a full range of negative feelings as I entered Cancerville as a "heart and soul" giver, I came to realize that such feelings were hurtful and toxic to my family and myself. I wasted too much time and energy on feeling sorry for my daughter and my family's plight. That time and energy could have been better directed toward a more accepting and hopeful approach.

As I have said, adaptation is a process with a slow learning curve. I hope to help you avoid the thinking traps into which I fell—headfirst. Clearly, your positive attitudes about your strength and survival will influence your mindset in ways that will enable you to meet Cancerville's demands squarely and confidently.

Just today I came across a brief story about a twelve-year-old boy in my community who was diagnosed with lymphoma when he was nine. C.J. gave an emotional pep talk to the Florida Panthers hockey team before they left for a game in New York. He said, "I told them to keep their eye on the goal and even if they get frustrated—you have to push through. Their goal is to reach the playoffs; mine was survival." C.J. appears to have achieved his goal as he is in full remission. I can't help but believe that his attitude played a significant role in his recovery. Perhaps his pep talk also helped the team make the playoffs!

Action

In an interactive way, the above components flow into your accomplishing the goals you set for yourself. As stressed in the previous chapter, successfully trekking through Cancerville requires you to personify the Nike, "Just Do It!" theme. It requires the same type of commitment that you have made in other goal-directed areas of your life. It will definitely require a rebalancing of your pre-Cancerville commitments and priorities. The proverbial time pie will have to be re-sliced temporarily to allow for a new world order of disorder. In fact, everyone in your life will have to adjust and adapt to the changes that ensue. Cancerville is a front-burner experience all the way in every way.

Without realizing it, we constantly adapt and plan in order to effectively manage our lives. Think of all the planning and work that goes into the simple goal of having a family picnic. Cancerville, a place where we do not have much experience, certainly requires even more strategic planning. Cancerville is no picnic and no fun whatsoever! Nonetheless, a strategic plan needs to be established. This plan will help you to adapt to Cancerville's demands.

Logistical, financial, attitudinal, and emotional issues need to be thought over and discussed. For example, what needs to be done to mobilize the medical insurance? Who will take you to chemo appointments? What do you need to do to set up necessary schedule changes? Lines of communication all around need to be created. A great deal of planning needs to go into how to approach and ultimately take charge in Cancerville.

Though the specific changes and associated actions required will vary from person to person, their disruptive influence is the common denominator. Your goal is to strategically plan for how to adjust to the shifts that Cancerville needs you to make. My goal is for your plan to not only include practical actions to adapt and accommodate, but also to weave together a variety of activities that will offset the emotional burdens that Cancerville imposes.

Here is a practical and specific example:

Any Weekday Plan

Get the kids off to school by 8:30 a.m.

Arrange for them to be picked up at 3 p.m. and go to aftercare

Light breakfast at 9 a.m.

Listen to relaxing music and do a relaxation exercise—say three affirmations about the next few days (e.g., I will be okay; I will cope well; The side effects will be minimal and I will manage them well)

Shower and dress

Mom picks me up at 11 a.m.

Chemo at noon—remember to bring my head-set, iPad, and book

Mom drives us back— return home by 4 p.m.

Nap while Mom picks up the kids and gives them dinner

Mom leaves at 7 p.m. when John gets home and he gets kids ready for bed

Light bite and watch TV with John

Do relaxation exercise before going to sleep—repeat my three affirmations

Have John get the kids ready for school tomorrow and have Mom pick them up

Rest tomorrow and use distractions and relaxation when I can

Though the above does not need to be written out, some people feel more "in control" when they do. The important thing is to have a clear plan, to make sure all bases are covered, and to include some mind-strengthening tools. In Chapter 10, "How Minds Work," we will learn why these are so important generally, but especially for people going through Cancerville or any other serious life challenge.

A Never Ending Commitment

Much research has shown that, in a variety of adverse situations, persistence wins out. Much can be said for plodding patiently but powerfully along with a "can do" attitude and a "will do whatever it takes" set of beliefs. In life, there are those who say "uncle" and those who say "never!" In Cancerville, try to be part of the latter group. Though there are some situations where saying "uncle" may be appropriate, I encourage you when it is realistic, to take a "can and will do" mindset right from the beginning.

Strength is often measured in the long run—literally and figuratively. People who persevere often accomplish their goals and achieve their dreams, simply because they don't give up. The significant things in life are almost never achieved easily. Much needs to be pursued doggedly, at least for a while. Think of athletes, Olympic or otherwise; they have logged thousands upon thousands of hours doing difficult and demanding things to achieve their goals and to fulfill their dreams. They have sweated it out just as you are now doing.

See yourself becoming a Cancerville athlete and going the distance. As you do, you will adapt faster and easier to its demands. You will begin to see it as another important challenge in your life, similar, but more daunting, to others you have faced and overcome.

Real People Facing Cancer

Shelley

My long time colleague and friend Shelley has a unique story. Little did she know that Cancerville had her in its sights since the age of ten. At twenty-eight she learned that she had a rare form of hepatitis. The origin was ultimately traced back to a close family member. That disease can be a risk factor for liver cancer.

She went along for many years with no ill effects, other than periodic MRIs to check her liver. In 2001, however, her MRI showed that her liver had become "chopped," and there was talk of a transplant, which was never needed. The MRI reading was subject to different interpretations.

Fast forward to November 2009. Her MRI was fine but her tumor marker blood test showed fifteen when nine or less is normal. Her doctors ignored that blood result and based their beliefs on the MRI; they were wrong! Three months later, even before another MRI, a doctor told her, "You have cancer in your liver. How come you didn't know that?" "Because no one told me that and I am not a radiologist!" was her immediate and angry reply. At that time she was scheduled for surgery.

When I asked Shelley how she dealt with that disturbing news, she sounded a little like Eileen from Chapter 1—both are mental health counselors who practice what they teach others. She said:

> I try to bypass my gut and go straight to my head. Sure I had a big knot in my stomach, but I go quickly to 'what do we do next?' My father taught me to use humor to diffuse tension so I kibitzed a lot. When I enter a war zone of any kind, I just put on my uniform, get my marching orders, and do what I have to do. I come up with a plan to cover all the bases I need to in order to just go forward. I try to convert the unknown to known and create a 'to do' list—meet with a surgeon, find the best care and hospital available, get copies of results, and generally take charge. Immediately after the surgery, drugged on anaesthetic, I kept waking up, jumping up, and asking, 'What do I need to do now?'

Shelley was a trooper in all respects—a poster person for adapting to the demands of Cancerville. Retired now, she was back at her Mahjong game the week after being released from the hospital. She rapidly resumed her daily routine. "I got home and recovered quickly. My positive, can do attitude helped me a lot," she says. "I never once went on the Internet. I am me, others are not me so I am not going to find out about other people's experiences or read silly statistics that probably don't apply. It is not that I am so courageous, Bill—it's just how I deal," she shared.

There is yet another twist to Shelley's tale. In November 2011, she was told her MRI was bad and that she had cancer of the liver again and this time would need a transplant—she was back to being "chopped liver" again! Based on her previous MRI experiences, she asked for them to redo her MRI, but they would only do that as part of her in-hospital workup for a transplant. Not wanting to rock the boat and risk being denied a new liver, she reluctantly went along with that plan. They probed and poked her as part of the evaluation and finally did the repeat MRI.

The night before she was to get the results, she told her daughter and sister her fantasy that her MRI would show no cancer and that she would not need a transplant. They both shared her wish but doubted the likelihood. Shelley had her meeting with the doctors and, lo and behold, her wish was granted. It wasn't cancer, and she was denied the opportunity of getting her name on the transplant list. It is a nice group to be rejected by because you don't need an organ anymore.

Then she said, "Do you blame me for not trusting any more MRI results? If I come up positive for cancer again I will have to go to consultants all over the world before I believe it is true—especially France—my favorite place to visit." Notice that even when angry and frustrated, Shelley kibitzes.

Shelley concluded that she tries to stay in the moment and not look too far forward into the future. She does believe that if she needed the transplant, she would have come through fine. "I never believed I would die from this," she says, and "though I am still in the woods, no one is shooting at me so I was able to hang my 'uniform' back up."

Unfortunately, Shelley had to start ironing her "uniform." The MRI was showing problems again, and she went back on the transplant list, even without going to France. In her inimitable fashion, she did just fine? My money was on her all the way.

In Sum

It is likely that you will have to make many adjustments in order to adapt to the demands of Cancerville. All of a sudden, schedules and routines are turned upside down. What once seemed important and of high priority to you might become insignificant, as Cancerville will likely become the main event and your primary focus. Your adaptation to and survival in Cancerville is what matters; not much else feels all that significant. You will do what you have to in all areas depending upon the demands of your life, but overcoming cancer will be your main focus

You will learn how to leap those tall buildings, if not in a single bound, in two, three, or more, as needed. You will pick up whatever emotional kryptonite invades your mind and fling it into another stratosphere far from Cancerville. You may have to do that over and over, but you will each time a challenge presents itself. You need your own strong and unwavering support, and I suspect that you are fit for the role. If not, your support team and I will help you get there.

You will be able to make the necessary logistical adaptations no matter what they are. The challenge will be for you to rise to the attitudinal and emotional adjustments. Please keep reading, as you will find much support for those challenges as we continue through Cancerville together.

Right now, you need to begin to understand Cancerville and its land so you can take it on. Toward that end, we move on to accomplish that in Part II.

PART II

Understanding
the Land

CHAPTER 5

I will be able to play a difficult hand well.

Making Eye Contact with Cancerville

When you first arrive in Cancerville, a part of you will not want to acknowledge that you are really there. If you are like me, you will probably close your eyes and make believe that you are somewhere else. You may even try to do that with your eyes open. You will likely do your best, especially if you are male, to talk to no one else in Cancerville, pretending you are a visitor rather than a resident. Hopefully, that will change soon.

For the majority of people, the transition into Cancerville takes time; but entering Cancerville is really not unlike any other new and difficult situation. There is a learning curve. There is a time frame within which you will adjust and adapt. Obviously, you will never like Cancerville, but you will figure out how to dislike it less. You will also learn how to manage it better. There is probably no one who can immediately go from the shock of the diagnosis to taking on Cancerville full tilt. Sometimes it all happens so quickly that there is little time initially to process your experience. That was Josh's case and you will meet him in Chapter 9.

Becoming Empowered in Cancerville

Eventually, you will need to go face-to-face with Cancerville. Doing so is an important part of accepting this most unfortunate reality. Although acceptance may sound completely undesirable right now, acceptance will allow you to move forward and take on Cancerville's challenges. The sooner you make eye contact with Cancerville, the faster you can be present in an empowered way for yourself. All of this progress will pave the way for you to begin to understand this complicated land and figure out how you can be most helpful to yourself.

By going face-to-face and staring down Cancerville, I don't mean to say that you should be glaring at it, flooded with all of your anger and "Why Me?" resentments. I am referring, instead, to feeling strong and powerful and being able to hold your own by keeping your "slingshot" in the ready position.

In the beginning, Cancerville is a very intimidating place. But soon it will become a place where you will feel more capable of taking on its challenges with strength, courage, and determination. The sooner you face Cancerville directly and begin to stare it down, the better you will feel. Your goal is to own this land for the duration. As we continue to walk through Cancerville together, I will help you to do just that.

Cancerville is Just Another One of Life's Challenges

Diane McKay, Psy.D., when she became president of the Florida Psychological Association, gave some good advice in the Winter 2011 *Florida Psychologist* newsletter. Although she was speaking to psychologists about their frustrations and professional challenges, her advice can be applied to Cancerville or any other demanding situation. Dr. McKay said:

1) Recognize, and accept, that change and adversity are inevitable in life.
2) Build your internal resources. Cultivate your own emotional strength and discipline.
3) Build your external resources. Engage fully with your own support system of colleagues, family, and friends. Look to your own faith and/or spiritual/religious beliefs...
4) Be resilient. Resilience is like any muscle; you need to exercise it.
5) Learn from and be inspired by others who have successfully managed their own adversity. There are stories of people who overcame what seemed like insurmountable odds embedded everywhere... They triumphed over their adversities to live happy and successful lives.

These words fit any and all challenges that run the gamut from professional to Cancerville woes. In these five simple prescriptions, she gives us a guide to follow in any demanding situation. This may be your first visit to Cancerville as a patient, but it is not your first challenge. Please try to draw from the strengths you have already developed in your life's journey. In fact, the playbook is already embedded in your DNA and personal life experiences. Just aim that "slingshot" at Cancerville and begin to take charge of it like the seasoned veteran that you already are.

Being Patient with a Clumsy and Cumbersome Medical System

As you already know, you are entering Cancerville at a very peculiar time in the delivery of medical services in the United States and many other places as well. While the technological side of medicine has never been stronger, the rest of it is in disarray. It is sad to see and say that the entire medical system appears to have lost its way.

We experienced some of this chaos during our journey through Cancerville. One day while visiting Jodi in New York, Ronnie developed strong pains that seemed like those of a heart attack. Given her stress levels at the time, it wouldn't have been surprising if that were the case. So we all jumped in the car, which Zev drove ambulance-style, sans siren (though, come to think of it, he always drives that way) to the ER of St. Vincent's Hospital in the West Village. After several uncomfortable hours of waiting, the doctors told us that Ronnie probably had had a gallbladder attack. It was just another crazy day in Cancerville. Her gallbladder was removed a few months later. Ronnie thankfully recovered but St. Vincent's wasn't so fortunate.

In the October 25, 2010 issue of *New York Magazine*, St. Vincent's Hospital was declared dead on arrival. Better them than my wife the day she went there! The sad news was that St. Vincent's, along with sixteen other hospitals in New York City, had closed since 2000. St. Vincent's, around for 160 years, had treated victims of the Titanic, the Triangle Shirt Waist Factory fire, and 9/11. They had such a strong legacy, but such a weak balance sheet. St. Vincent's was one billion dollars in debt and drowning to the tune of ten million dollars a month. This is just one small example of this strange time in the medical field.

Being Patient with the Process

It is likely that there will be multiple frustrations in Cancerville ranging from lost documents to mis-scheduled appointments, to hurry-up-and-wait times, to short supplies of medications, to a variety of insurance confusions. Cancerville is often a slow experience that demands a one-day-at-a-time perspective. The picture in your mind before you entered Cancerville may have been that it works with precision and in fast motion. In reality, it can be a drawn-out process that moves like a slow golf cart that needs a battery charge. With so much racing through your mind, your frustrations can multiply at each turn, delay, and detour.

If you ever needed patience, you need it now. Know that even when it doesn't seem like it, the medical team is doing their very best. They are lifeguards on a stormy beach. They are focused on the choppy waters and helping the people there get back to shore. The more you can be a patient patient, the better you will feel. Maybe that is where the word originated.

The Impersonal Nature of Medical Practice

Yet another issue to be reckoned with is that in the past many years, the practice of medicine has become more and more impersonal. I remember the days when doctors were like special friends who took care of your whole family. They were involved in one way or another from your birth to your death—they really seemed to care, even making house calls.

Today, it is a whole new world. Some doctors sit at computer screens rather than looking at the patient; some dictate their notes as they walk quickly through the hallways from one examining room to another. Or they are so time-limited that they make the visit a harried, hurried, hassle; after waiting an hour or more to see the doctor, often all you get is a quick glimpse. Try to get the doctor on the phone and it is likely you will be speaking to an assistant or secretary—and that is if someone responds to the voicemail you left yesterday.

This has all led to the VIP medical team. There, for a mere fifteen hundred dollars or more out of pocket uptick a year, you will be given the level of care and communication that you used to get for a three dollar visit—maybe!

I can't blame the doctors for this mess. Insurance companies have become abusive to the point of being disgraceful. As the screws of payments get tighter and tighter, the doctor has no choice, if he or she wants to remain in business. More people need to be seen each day. This leaves less time to spend with each person, and as emergencies and phone calls arise, the wait becomes longer and longer. This is especially true when many people are all scheduled for the same appointment time.

The insurance companies have even created difficulties for the doctors when prescribing medications. Frequently, doctors have to use substitutes that are on the approved formularies of the insurance company but are not necessarily as effective. The money madness game of medicine is maddening, and the insurance companies are to blame. Often even new and improved medicines are limited by insurance company boycotts because of their high cost.

In addition, governmental regulations regarding computerization of records have added much time and distraction. Many doctors complain that they must spend hours in the evening catching up on records and posting results and their explanations on a portal for their patients. The latter often complain that they don't understand what the findings mean. So as doctors are working harder than ever, their patients are more frustrated than ever. What was that I said about medicine becoming impersonal?

What also complicates the present-day medical scene is that it is now driven by the HIPAA privacy act and Risk Management policies. This means that "bureaucrazy" rules in the medical community, and unfortunately, Cancerville is no exception. My goal in sharing all of this information is not to overwhelm you or to worry you in advance, but I have promised to be honest with you. This area of Cancerville is probably best explored sooner rather than later. Clearly, you will need to learn how to manage all the paperwork, insurance issues, and bureaucratic obstacles without letting these things get you down.

So what does all of this mean for you in Cancerville? There will literally be a forest full of trees converted into papers for you to sign. In addition, there will be disclosure statements and releases that sound like they were written by Attila the Hun, Jack the Ripper, and the U.S. Supreme Court.

Please don't go face-to-face or try to stare down these forms. Just close your eyes and sign them. Your attorney might advise otherwise, but this is my opinion. Ronnie recently had to sign a zillion forms for a simple cataract surgery, and I advised her to do the same. I clearly remember the ones specifically created in Cancerville that Jodi asked me to review. I didn't understand a word. I simply encouraged her to sign on the dotted line so she and the process could move forward. Even Rob, an attorney, agreed and did the same with all of the papers related to Jake's treatment.

Please do not personalize that which is not yours to own. Try to accept the reality of medical care in the twenty-first century. In many instances the system is broken and beyond repair. This is why most doctors do not encourage their offspring to follow in their footsteps anymore. It is not the way it used to be, nor is it the way it needs to be.

The good news is that you are not beyond repair. Know that the overwhelming majority of doctors in Cancerville do care and will do everything they can to help, protect, and facilitate your survival. Know that they did not create the present system—they inherited it. Also remind yourself that they did not cause your cancer, but they can and will do everything in their power to get rid of it once and for all and forever. In the final analysis, that is what really matters most!

On Not Displacing Your Angst

Although your nerves are hypersensitive and you may be feeling hyper, try not to let the less important frustrations get to you. It might be helpful to refer back to the Relativity Chart in Chapter 1 and use it as a guide. Please do your best, as well, to not take your frustrations out on staff members who are really just following standard operating procedures and doing their jobs. None of the people you will interact with created HIPAA or the disclosure/release forms you will be asked to complete. In fact, the staff probably finds them just as annoying as you do. At least you will only have to sign them, while the staff will have to sort, staple, and store all those forms appropriately.

Going face-to-face with Cancerville demands patience and courtesy outside the medical arena as well. It is easy to displace all of your angst and frustrations onto the innocent others with whom you interact. For example, I remember speaking rudely to an employee at my gym when he shut the steam room a little earlier than usual one night. This is not my typical style, and after thinking about it, I was sorry for what I had done. The next time I saw him I apologized. I simply shared with him that I was going through a difficult time and didn't mean to take it out on him. Since then we have enjoyed a nice rapport, and he seems to go out of his way to be friendly as he greets me or waves good-bye.

To stare down Cancerville, you need to be comfortably balanced and in charge of yourself. If you have a little slip-up like I did at the gym, make peace and move on. We will talk more about your Cancerville angst and reining in your anger in Chapter 15.

Coping with the Environs of Cancerville

I remember riding the elevator at Sloan-Kettering in July, surrounded by many young, hairless folks who appeared pale and weak. Some were in wheelchairs attached to IV lines; few had smiles on their faces. That scene was neither calming nor comfortable. In fact, it made me want to break down and cry.

Sadly, the imagery is even more difficult, daunting, and draining in the children's wings of Cancerville. However, remember that in the hospitals and medical facilities of Cancerville, you mostly see the people going through treatment at that very moment, rather than seeing all of the survivors who are back to their everyday lives. It can really help to visualize that positive outcome for every person you see going through treatment, as there are millions who have gone through Cancerville and have been cured. The survival rate from cancer overall has almost quadrupled since the late 1970s.

The gray and somber mood of Cancerville sometimes extends to the facilities themselves. Of course, facilities vary widely, but many lack a calming or cheerful ambience or even basic creature comforts. Often, they appear to be cold, even on a hot July day. We decided to take a private room for Jodi's comfort after her surgery. Even so, it was much smaller than we expected. Ronnie, who stayed with Jodi the three nights she was there, had to sleep on an uncomfortable reclining chair. The out-of-pocket charge for such "luxury" was over five hundred dollars per night—yet the Plaza or Pierre it was not!

In the same vein, Rob felt that the facilities for children at Sloan-Kettering were disappointing, to say the least. Moms slept on recliners and showered in shabby community bathrooms. The playroom for the children was inadequate. According to his son Jake, "Even the bingo prizes sucked." In that family's signature style, they brought in toys and crafts for the other children to enjoy. Jake, in the midst of his own challenges, donated all the gifts and money he received from family and friends to the bingo loot bag. The apple does not fall far from the tree!

Clearly, making eye contact with and staring down Cancerville sometimes requires tolerating less than comfortable conditions and making the best of them. It may help to remember that you are not visiting Cancerville for the food and facilities. You are there for a cure. That is all you want and all you need. In reality, it is better for the monies to go into research than into fixing up the place.

You are not being unreasonable if the depressing environs bother you in a cancer facility. Ambience and décor can certainly influence your mood in many positive ways and help lift your Cancerville state of mind. In addition to being there almost 24/7 for the many months he was there, Jake's mom recognized the value of a positive environment for her son and the entire family. As such, she brightly decorated his long-term room at Sloan-Kettering and filled it with warm wall hangings and the ambient equivalent of a happy smile. She changed the decorations weekly and went all out for holidays such as July 4th, Halloween, and Thanksgiving. Now that is what I call taking charge!

Strength comes from making a silk purse out of a sow's ear, as the expression goes. If you have the time, energy, and option of being creative like Cristina, you may want to do what you can to improve the physical environment in Cancerville—especially if you are inpatient. This is a small but significant example of facing Cancerville head-on and taking charge of what you can. You will feel just a little more powerful and your mood will be lifted as well. If upgrading the ambience is not an option for you, try to focus on your dedicated medical team and their powerful ammunition. Please remember that it is their medical expertise rather than the environs that truly distinguishes Sloan-Kettering and so many other cancer centers. My hope is that your treatment will not involve long-term care in a hospital and can be done while you enjoy the comfort of your home.

I learned that Sloan-Kettering holds a prom in June for all of the children and teens who have been treated there during the year. There is food, music, dancing, and fun. Jake and his family attended, as did over one hundred patients, family members, and all of the staff, nurses, and doctors. The latter wore tuxes and prom dresses, while providing the same for the children.

Hearing about and picturing this prom brought a few tears to my eyes, as I envisioned the sometimes grim-faced doctors happily dancing with the children whose lives they had saved. Perhaps some of my tears were for Jake having been voted Prom King. Believe me when I say that he earned that title in every imaginable, and at times unimaginable, way.

Rob asked Jake if he was surprised when they named him Prom King. His reply tells us what really makes cancer centers special. Jake said, "No, not at all. I knew I was going to win when I heard that the nurses were the ones voting—all my nurses loved me." That illustrates at least two things: first, that this young boy finally got to take charge of Cancerville and stare it down in the sweetest of ways—for one magical night, Jake was the King of Cancerville. Second, that a little boy believed so strongly in his nurses' love, clearly shows that the human factor is far more important than the facility. I hope all of this helps you believe in the commitment and dedication of cancer center teams all over the world; the expertise and spirit of the medical staff are what really counts. You can cope with the facilities.

Feeling Stronger

Making strong and serious eye contact with Cancerville requires coming at it with resolve. This means confidently knowing that you will be able to tolerate everything that comes at you and then some. Resolve also implies your determination to keep bouncing back whenever, if ever, you have a momentary meltdown. Meltdowns tend to go with the territory, so don't be upset with yourself if you have one. These happen to the strongest of people from time to time because Cancerville is one tough trek. Yet I am confident that you can meet Cancerville directly and hold your own. Use all of the positive stories coming out of there to support your strong approach.

There is one more way in which you can take on Cancerville and try to make it a more level playing field. Take a lesson from the playbook of Stuart Scott, whom I previously mentioned. In private, look in the mirror and make a tough grimacing face like a wrestler or martial artist. Look mean and bare your teeth as if you were about to bite, fight, and rip into your opponent. Make believe that Cancerville lies beyond the mirror and grunt and growl in a show of power. That's facing Cancerville, staring it down, and hanging tough against a formidable opponent.

Use that strength and draw from it, believing that you will be okay. Keep that in the forefront of your mind as you stare down Cancerville every single day. Aim your "slingshot" right at its hateful head and assume that, like David, you will win this battle too.

When I first wrote the above, I had no idea that people at Columbia and Harvard Universities were researching postures and the effects of what they termed "embodiment." Their research had people assume either high- or low-power poses. An example of the former is someone standing and leaning slightly forward. The latter is someone sitting with hands crossed and head bent slightly down. Harvard and Columbia haven't experimented with my pose of growling into the mirror just yet, but I am confident they will try it soon.

Those who took the stronger power poses had significantly higher post-pose cortisol and testosterone levels of these "fight" hormones, than those who took the more passive positions. This suggests that power posturing promotes the activation of mind and body chemicals that energize our strength. Those inner forces are just what you need to take on and stare down Cancerville. So grunt and growl even louder and show more of your teeth. Embody strength in every way that you can, and the likelihood is, by doing that, you will generate more strength. In Stuart's strong voice and spirit, let me hear you growl!

Real People Facing Cancer

Geralyn

Anyone who puts risky and risqué in the same sentence is my kind of writer. I read Geralyn Lucas' *Why I Wore Lipstick to My Mastectomy* just after Jodi's surgery.[9] It was both an inspiring and unnerving book. It was a young woman's scream in the night at having breast cancer at age twenty-seven. After rereading it many years later, I still found it a disconcerting "booby trap" that brought my "This cannot be my daughter's turn!" lament back to a blood-curdling scream of outraged indignation once again. Nonetheless, Geralyn's words, courage, and bright red lipstick have helped many women face this most demanding challenge. I came to realize that her powerful, descriptive writing style makes her book a difficult yet ultimately rewarding read.

Amid her multiple terrors, identity and treatment confusions, and crashing and crushing self-esteem, Geralyn's bright red lipstick symbolized her determination and strength; it was her "red" badge of courage. It was how she faced Cancerville and was a counterpoint to her drab hospital gown and the red bloodstained sheets covering the surgical table. TMI! In my opinion, it was her middle finger of defiance aimed at Cancerville—one huge hawk of a bird!

Her story begins post-diagnosis but pre-surgery in a Manhattan strip club. There she is doing an in-depth, introspective analysis of the importance of boobs in the "naked city." In the middle we get an in your face description of her mastectomy and chemo "cocktails," as well as her use of affirmations, hypnosis, and positive self-talk to neutralize these negative happenings. She is a poster person for my encouragements and the types of tools that I will describe in Part IV. Her story concludes with her being a survivor and later a mom who took the increased estrogen risk pregnancy entailed back then and succeeded.

Then we come upon her tattoo. She hemmed and hawed about nipple replacement surgery despite her mom being a nipple-promoting nuisance. Ultimately, she opted for a tattoo:

> I want a serious heart to remind me how courageous it is to follow my heart. I want wings on the top to represent all of the angels who showed me I would get my life back...I tell Josh (the tattoo artist) that I want it right at the lower end of my scar, much lower than the nipple would be. It is not replacing the nipple and I do not want it to be perfectly centered. I want the heart to look like it's flying up, soaring away. Where my scar ends, my courage and hope begin.

Then, just when one finally breathes a long-awaited sigh of relief, Geralyn shares in vivid emotional and humiliating detail that she agreed to pose topless and nippleless to show her less than balanced breast reconstruction. The photo was for a *Self Magazine* handbook for women dealing with breast cancer. They were trying to show that despite disfigurement, women can get on with their lives.

Her photo shoot scene is like something out of an avant-garde movie. Reviewing the blown up black and white Polaroid result, the photographer responsible for the in-your-face shot remarked: "LOOK AT YOURSELF! You look so—pause—ballsy! My God. It is so powerful." As I read those words, I couldn't help but think of my "balls to the walls" encouragement. She goes on to say that "I set out to inspire other women that they could be beautiful after this surgery and I ended up convincing myself…. I finally accepted myself."

Geralyn tells the reader that she continues to wear her bright red lipstick to a variety of important places and concludes by saying:

> But there is a strange lipstick residue from that day that I have never been able to wipe from my lips…. Each time I wear lipstick I am emboldened by the memory of that day; the IV line in my arm, my surgical gown on with my butt hanging out, and my perfectly applied lipstick. I swear I can still taste that hope.

Hope is what I hope you can feel, see, and taste every day and forever. Although my words are in black and white, I hope you can see a bright red glow coming off this page and that it helps boost your own strength and courage.

In Sum

I am confident that you will be able to figure out how to make eye contact with and stare down Cancerville. Remind yourself that you are strong enough to take on its burdens and meet them head-on. Have faith in your medical team and work quickly to establish a partnership, despite the bureaucratic hassles. Reach out to talk to others you meet in Cancerville. You just never know where your next moment of inspiration will come from. Above all else, think strong. Cancerville gives you no choice other than to rise to its challenges each and every time.

As part of taking on Cancerville, let's turn to the important subject of meeting with your doctors. These meetings can be difficult, but they are part of slowly accepting where you are and learning what lies ahead for you.

CHAPTER 6

My doctors and I are on the same team.

Meetings With the Dedicated Doctors

As people, we vary in terms of our attention to detail. Some want only a brief overview from the medical team while others expect that every issue be clearly explained. Ronnie's nature is the latter, while I am definitely an "executive summary" type. It may be part of my being from "Mars" and my wife being from "Venus." Or maybe, it's because I am of a personality type that goes for the big picture, while she prefers to know all of the details. Jodi, in this regard, was more like I was during her Cancerville treatment; she showed up, did what she was advised to do, and moved forward.

Your personal style will greatly influence how you approach your meetings with the doctors. You will bring your nature to the consultation and treatment rooms of Cancerville. So will family and friends whom you may choose to accompany you. Because that is the case, nothing I say here should be seen as absolute. I greatly respect your right to conduct all aspects of your time in Cancerville as you see fit. What I do hope to offer here is a game plan for these meetings.

Please keep in mind that the dedicated doctors are people— just like you and me. Like us, they vary greatly in style, sense, and sensitivity. Please remember that the Cancerville doctors, no matter what their natures, are committed to the very same goals that you have for yourself. They want cancer to lose and you to win. At the end of the day, that is really all that matters.

Getting Past Difficult Meetings

I remember our family meetings with the doctors in Cancerville all too well. We would wait hours to see the doctor for ten or fifteen minutes. During those moments, Cancerville intimidated me in a way few places have. The physicians were harried, and we, I couldn't help but sense, were annoying. They were in a rush and made that known to us, but we had hours of questions. In fact, we wanted to move into their offices for the duration. For better or worse, many physicians are more interested in treating than greeting or meeting nervous and distraught patients and their family members. Both positions make sense depending upon the seat in which one is sitting.

I hope that your medical team brings a friendly and encouraging demeanor along with their technical expertise. If you can't have both, I think you will agree that knowledgeable doctors trump cheerful ones. As you already know, not all doctors are created equal. Some, whose bedside manners leave much to be desired, are nonetheless highly skilled and trustworthy practitioners.

In fairness, a doctor's job—especially in Cancerville—is not easy. Having spent my career as a psychologist trying to help a garden variety of unhappy people, I can only imagine how difficult it is to treat and support patients and their family and friends in Cancerville. By two o'clock in the afternoon, many are probably wondering why they didn't go into dermatology. Yet every cancer doctor I have met has been totally dedicated to fighting cancer and being part of an army of hope.

The doctors stand between you and the difficult treatments. They also have the challenging job of standing in front of and blocking the exit door. They don't want you to lose your fight any more than you do. They are determined to minimize your pain and suffering while saving your life. They are on a most serious search and rescue mission and will do everything they can and then some on your behalf.

Approaching Medical Meetings with More than a Pad

Depending upon the specifics, you may or may not attend medical meetings with your family and/or friends. If others do attend, you may prefer that they be quiet listeners or more verbal participants. These choices are part of an unwritten bill of rights that you have as an adult dealing with cancer.

If you are like Ronnie, you bring a comprehensive list of questions along with pen and paper to take notes. If you are like me, you will just wing it. However, the danger of my approach is that, just like white-coat blood pressure elevations, there can also be white-coat dementia. Thank goodness both are temporary. It is, however, possible to forget both your questions and the doctors' answers as you sit there in a funky fog.

A tape recorder may help if the doctor is okay with that and you are not the note-taking type. It is also helpful to bring another set of ears to listen, ask questions, and remember what is said. Rob's dad, Phil, attended every medical meeting about his grandson, both to support his family and to be that additional pair of ears.

Practically speaking, it is important to limit your questions to those that are essential and answerable. You don't wait hours to see the doctors because they are playing cards in the rec room. In fact, there is no rec room! They are as overworked as any other doctor in America today. Being respectful of their time may help generate good will and avoid creating a situation in which the doctor does not take you or your questions seriously.

Receiving Reassurances in Cancerville

I encourage you to accept that you may not get the complete reassurance you want from the doctors. You want to know that you will be okay, but unfortunately, in Cancerville, assurances are not always available; there are just so many unknowns. Instead, give yourself the answer you crave—like a special gift. Assume that "yes, I will be a survivor." On the other hand, as Cancerville's successes mount, more doctors are more able to be more optimistic.

Perhaps you will receive the reassurance you are seeking, or perhaps you will not. It will depend upon the type and stage of your cancer, as well as the doctor's nature. Unless you have information to the contrary, I strongly encourage you to assume that you will be okay. In Parts III and IV, I will teach you tools that can help you influence your thoughts and expectations.

The Information You Will Most Likely be Given at a Meeting

What information and feedback are your doctors responsible for providing? Here is a brief overview that you can adapt to your particular situation:

My doctors and I are on the same team.

Initial Meeting Post-Diagnosis:

- a summary of your test results and confidence in their accuracy

- your diagnosis based on these results, including type and stage (if known)

- the plan for treating your disease

- a brief overview of the impact of your treatment and how to minimize side effects

- the probable time frame of your treatment

- what follow-up testing will be done and when

- whether any genetic testing is suggested to help you determine heritable origins (if appropriate)

- when the next meeting will take place

Follow-up Meetings:

- your progress and any new findings

- unexpected problems that have arisen

- how you have tolerated treatment

- any changes in your treatment plan

- what follow-up testing will be done and when

- what is happening next

- when your next meeting will take place

These Meetings are a Pain

One of the most difficult parts of these meetings is having them at all. Part of me sat through each one saying to myself, "What are we doing here?" I am pretty sure Jodi felt the same way. Another difficult part is listening, sometimes over and over again, to the list of possible negative outcomes of the treatments. This information works against your efforts to be positive. Know that such disclosures and disclaimers represent mandatory risk management and malpractice suit prevention. The medical team is required to disclose the dangers of treatment, just as they are required to have you sign all those forms. Tune it out as best you can, and assume that none of the possibilities will happen to you.

Former football great and member of the Dolphin perfect season team of 1972, Jim Mandich interrupted a nurse who was telling him about the hurtful effects of his medication. He said, "The doctors told me all the good it'll do. I don't need to hear the bad." To his credit, Mandich, known for his partying ways, referred to chemo treatment times as "happy hour." How's that for putting a positive spin on a not so pleasant time?

His story reflects your need to be vigilant in blocking out unhelpful negative news. To be clear, there is an obvious and significant difference between being given helpful vs. hurtful information. "If you run a fever of more than 101 degrees post-chemo, you need to call the doctor," is helpful to know. "Unfortunately, you are going to feel awful after this treatment," is upsetting and puts negative expectations in your mind, which can lead to self-fulfilling prophecies—which often come true. If you are told you will be terribly nauseated post-treatment, the odds are that you will be more likely to feel that way. Better to not be told anything in advance and just wait and see what happens. This is why I never read the information that comes with a prescription; Ronnie, of course, reads every word!

I spoke in Chapter 1 about our tendency to use healthy denial to avoid worrying about a variety of life-threatening events. In your meetings with the doctors you can use that denial to your advantage. For example, one of Jodi's chemo drugs could have caused heart problems, so she had to go for periodic cardiac testing. My initial thought when I learned of that potential side effect was: "Great, my daughter will have a heart condition in addition to cancer. Really terrific!"

I responded to my automatic negativity by saying: "Bull on that! She is young, in great shape, works out regularly, and will be fine. There will be no long-term problems." In fact, that Jodi never developed any heart problems confirmed my optimism. It is very important to catch your mind heading south and redirect it to neutral, if not positive, thoughts. We will discuss this most important issue in Chapter 12, "The Power of Positive Self-Talk."

Communicating with the Doctors is Essential

Usually, feedback meetings are scheduled on a regular basis while you go through treatment and even after it is completed. These may occur more frequently with more complex treatments or when trying to accomplish a specific result. In Rob's case, he and his family met with their team of doctors after each round of chemo. They were struggling to get Jake into remission so that his fraternal twin brother, Chase, could provide his bone marrow, as he was a perfect match. This is why Rob nicknamed Chase "The Hero."

Four grim-faced meetings with the doctors indicated poor chemo results, precluding the possibility of a bone marrow transplant. Rob's emotional knees buckled under the pressure, but he rallied back quickly. After the fifth rough round of chemo, the doctors finally achieved their goal, which they announced in a far more upbeat meeting. Their relief, however, was quickly neutralized by the need for another demanding round right before the transplant. The doctors took this boy to the edge of his life in order to save his life—but save his life they did!

I am quite sure that it was not important to Jodi that we be present at all doctor meetings. In fact, my guess is that at least a few times she would have preferred just going to them with Zev. She knew, however, how important it was to us to be there and was kind enough not to exclude us from them. I recall one time when we flew back and forth from Florida in one day just to attend an important meeting and enjoy lunch with our daughter. I am not sure that would be necessary in today's hi-tech world of video conferencing. Then again, my guess is that my wife would still want to be there in person. That's just who she is and how she is wired as a mom.

Between Doctor Meetings

When you are in between doctor meetings in Cancerville, try to assume that no news is good news. Doctors don't pull any punches there. They don't like to report bad news. However, if there are any complications, physicians are ethically and legally bound to share that information with their adult patients.

In my opinion, the best thing you can do is to let the medical team do their job and wait for them to communicate. They will not leave you out of the equation, as communicating and updating their patients are important parts of their job. As the next section suggests, there may be times when you will want to initiate discussion.

I, myself, felt the need to email Jodi's surgeon twice at Sloan-Kettering with a question. Each time it had to do with something I had read in a magazine or newspaper. He was kind enough to respond reassuringly the same day. He was quick to remind me that a magazine is not a scientific journal and that the information didn't apply to Jodi. That kind of response helps one to get back on a positive track quickly. As I have said, when dealing with Cancerville, remaining positive is an on-and-off process. It is easy for even the most optimistic person to be temporarily derailed by someone's comment, a magazine article, or any other information that hits in a sensitive place.

When calling or emailing the doctor, try to use discretion. Sending daily emails or making frequent phone calls will not be appreciated. Instead, pick your queries carefully and remind yourself that the doctor is helping many patients at the same time.

You can fill in some of the blanks by reading relevant books and checking reliable Internet sites for additional information. I read at least six books on breast cancer as well as others, including Lance Armstrong's inspiring account of his experience in Cancerville, *It's Not About the Bike*.[10] Both you and your family may find Bernie Siegel's book *How to Live Between Office Visits* very helpful as well.[11]

On Being an Involved Patient

There are, however, certain situations that demand your vigilant attention. Ultimately, you have the right to question, obtain second opinions, seek out information, or try to change to a different doctor or setting to ensure the care provided is the best available.

I am encouraging you to trust your medical team. I am also, however, acknowledging your right to thoroughly check out and become informed about each phase of treatment. This is especially true if it is not going according to plan.

As previously mentioned, the medical team and you are partners in your search for the cure. They will most likely support your desire to get second opinions or go to a place where relevant trials are being conducted, etc. In many instances, they will guide you in those directions. But, never hesitate to ask a question or obtain other opinions. Cancerville doctors work together, share, and care.

As far back as 1979, Norman Cousins promoted an informed doctor-patient partnership in his widely acclaimed book, *Anatomy of an Illness as Perceived by the Patient.* [12] He said, "I saw the need to build bridges across the gap that for so long had separated the physician and the public." As those words suggest, all involved individuals need to work together in a collaborative effort. These words are as applicable today as they were back then. They apply as much to Cancerville as they do to any other area of medicine.

Bernie Siegel, M.D., believes that those who challenge the medical system live longer. In *Love, Medicine & Miracles* he encourages patients to:

- Question authority—tests, etc. Speak up for yourself, your needs and comforts in all areas, both before and during tests.

- Make your doctor aware of your unique needs and desires.

- Take a tape recorder and earphones along with meditation tapes and some of your favorite music. Record conversations with your physician for later review and for family use. (This was written in the 1980s when tapes were the rage!)

- Tell the surgeon to speak to you during surgery, honestly but hopefully, and also to repeat positive messages but absolutely avoid negative ones.

Clearly, Bernie is pushing you to have an active voice, not only for surgery, but for all of your meetings and treatments.

Obviously, whether you are buying a car, moving to a new city, or walking the Cancerville beat, an informed consumer is in a stronger position to adapt, cope, know what to expect, and manage all of the demands. In Cancerville, "consumers" are like tourists in a foreign land. They may have read Frommer's and/or Fodor's books on travel, but will eventually put their trust in a local guide who truly knows the lay of the land. Your local guides in Cancerville are your medical team. They walk the streets day and night. So find a team that you can trust and respect, and allow them to lead your way as you walk together back into health.

My doctors and I are on the same team.

Watching Out for Sadistic Statistics

Finally, there is a tricky, sticky wicket involved in your quest for information and hopefulness. Cancerville is filled and often flooded with statistics. When they are hopeful and optimistic, we hold onto them with a lover's embrace. When they tilt the other way, we want to burn the book or article or punch the person citing the statistic.

Statistics can be misleading; therefore, you should treat all statistics with a certain level of cautious detachment. They change all the time as new studies and protocols come into being. They are based on large samples and may or may not apply to your situation; your circumstances are specific to you. No one statistic, or even a battery of them, will predict your experience. Be reminded of what Shelley said in Chapter 4 about how she was unique and couldn't relate to the statistics concerning liver cancer.

I hear of and have met people who were given little chance to survive, but did. Unfortunately, I also know of those for whom Cancerville was supposed to be a slam-dunk and it wasn't. Misleading statistics even apply to the diagnosis itself. Jodi was given a ninety-nine percent probability that her lump was benign. That was reassuring until we learned otherwise. It is best not to get caught up in statistical predictions.

Years ago my doctor friend Bob said, "Bill, in any individual's medical situation, surgery, or disease there is either a one hundred percent chance or a zero percent chance that the person will be okay." In that context, all you can do is assume that there is a one hundred percent chance that you will be okay and leave it at that.

In *Promise Me*,[13] Nancy Brinker says, "Certainly, a key component to managing one's own cancer treatment or the treatment of a loved one is managing expectations, which means chiseling some kind of reality-based tunnel between statistics and hope." I totally agree and encourage you to give greater weight, whenever it is appropriate, to the hopeful parts.

Real People Facing Cancer

Anthony

In 2008, prior to becoming a major league baseball player, Anthony Rizzo, who went to high school not far from my home in Florida, was diagnosed with Hodgkin's lymphoma. In a recent interview, he said that he credits his Boston area doctors for being encouraging:

> They assured me everything was going to be OK and I would beat it, no problem. They told me I would be able to play baseball again and just live a normal life. They gave not only me but my family hope. That's an important part of beating cancer. Maintaining hope.

As if to prove his doctors right, Anthony hit his first home run in the second game he played as a major leaguer. What a difference three years can make: "That ball is going, going, and it's gone!" Rizzo is one of many major league baseball players who won their battles with cancer.

Howie

When my friend Howie was diagnosed with kidney cancer, his doctor told him, "I am going to hurt you to save you, but you will be okay." His doctor delivered on both counts. His painful recovery took quite a while, but he is alive, back at work, and well today—seven years later. He had been in similar situations before. Twenty-plus years ago, as a younger man, he underwent cardiac bypass surgery. Additionally, eight years ago, after a heart attack he had a defibrillator implanted in his chest.

Clearly, Howie's health has not been his strongest suit. Fortunately, he has strength and great survival instincts. Thank goodness for that. Howie's belief in a pre-determined fate has also helped him cope. That philosophy has allowed him to "Let go and let God." Like the nerdy fictional character Alfred E. Newman used to say, "What me worry?"

Sandon

Unlike Anthony and Howie, Sandon Mark Herzlich Jr. was not given much hope for the future of his football career when he faced Ewing's sarcoma, a rare form of bone cancer. At the time, he was in his junior year playing football for Boston College. When he learned of this diagnosis, he said he channeled all of his energy into facing his "toughest opponent" yet. Like Jake, he needed a Hail Mary pass. Who better than Sandon to make it happen!

His football future—as well as his life—hung in the balance. He was determined to rid his body of disease so he could put the uniform back on. He said to his family, teammates, and fans, "Together we will fight this and win…. From what the doctors have been saying, they don't think it's too promising coming back…. The doctors may know the cancer but they don't really know me." This is precisely what I mean when I encourage you to give that important reassurance to yourself.

Sandon returned to excellence in 2010. He worked hard to build his upper body to compensate for the fact that part of his femur bone had been removed and replaced with a titanium rod. He played all thirteen games in his senior year and racked up sixty-five tackles and fifty solo stops. Because of the way he handled and faced cancer and encouraged others to fight with all of their might, he won many awards, including the Disney Spirit Award. The Giants signed him in 2011 as a linebacker, and their team just happened to win the Super Bowl in 2012. Unlike Anthony and Howie, who both received strong reassurances from their physicians, Sandon wasn't encouraged by his doctors, but persevered nonetheless. He won his battle in Cancerville and returned to a successful football career.

Frank

As you will see, Frank may have liked some reassurance, but he wasn't specifically looking for any—rather he was looking for support beyond the medical side of the Cancerville equation. Talking with him reminded me that "medicine" comes in a variety of forms, not all of which are prescribed by a physician.

Frank, a fifty-five year old marketer, was diagnosed with pancreatic cancer right around Thanksgiving. Once getting past that shock and awful diagnosis, he moved right along, and twelve demanding, but not impossible, chemotherapy sessions later, his scans were clear and his stomach pain was gone.

While appreciating his doctor's chemical support, he was disappointed that he was not told about or encouraged to participate in the hospital's wellness center. Frank says, "Doctors are just focused on medicine, and have blinders on about the mind stuff, and that can short-change the patient."

Fortunately, Frank and his girlfriend of five years, Valerie, found out about and started going to the center. There they have drawn from individual counseling, couples counseling, support groups, chair massages and nutritional counseling. Additionally, Frank joined a men's group. Now that is some pretty powerful "medicine."

Clearly, the most potent "medicine" of all (other than the chemo) was the shift in the quality and depth of Valerie and Frank's relationship. Prior to the diagnosis, they lived in separate homes and only saw each other Wednesday nights and weekends. They are both independent people, so that worked well for them. However, upon being diagnosed, Frank moved into Valerie's townhouse for a variety of practical reasons. This seemed to strengthen their love. Frank says:

> I am overwhelmed by how our relationship has moved to a whole new level of intimacy and love. There was always love, but not as strong as it is now. I could not have gotten through this without her kindness, support and outpourings of love.

He goes on to point out yet another yin and yang: "On the one hand we are dealing with this terrible disease, and on the other it is contrasted by this wonderfully empowering love." Frank's response to my substitution of "heart and soul" giver for caregiver was very positive. In addition he has received much support from family and friends who email and call in response to his blogs at caringbridge.org.

Another strong "medicine" that Frank chose to take was a leave from work. He ultimately resigned from his super-stressful, competitive, and difficult job as a salesman. Frank made a financially costly but emotionally necessary decision to take care of himself while healing and to not subject himself to any more angst or unneeded pressure.

Researching his situation initially was another important type of "medicine" that Frank prescribed for himself. Like so many others, this helped him to feel more empowered and in charge, so he could know what he was facing and make appropriate decisions. Frank also read fiction for distraction, which is another healthy form of "medicine," but was also learning more about a chemo pill his doctor wanted him to start taking.

Clearly, from every vantage point, Frank has added many "spoonfuls of sugar" to help the chemotherapy medicine go down and encourages you to do the same. He says:

> Follow your doctor's treatment plan and look at it as one step closer to getting better. Have a positive attitude, as that is very important. Draw from your "heart and soul" provider if you are lucky enough, like I am, to have one. Talk to many people for information and research on your own in the beginning. Take advantage of any wellness center opportunities, and take the best care of yourself that you have ever done. See yourself as special, deserving, and as surviving your Cancerville experience.

Great advice! Unfortunately, despite his all of his efforts things did not go well for Frank, and he passed several months after we spoke by phone. Nonetheless, I am confident that his advice to you would be the same as above.

In Sum

The meetings with your doctors are not easy, as no one really wants to be there. However, they are an important way to gain perspective about the latest results and the doctors' plans for the future. Cancerville treatment is an ongoing process, as are your communications with the medical team. Sometimes positive results come slowly, and these meetings summarize what has occurred so far as well as the updated plan. Other times, it all falls into place smoothly as treatment proceeds, but even these reassuring meetings are important and helpful.

Approach these meetings with an open mind. Know the doctors on your team want to win just as much as you do. They will do everything in their power to achieve that result. What I said in Chapter 4 about people not liking to lose applies to the doctors as well. They do not want to lose anyone on their "lifeguard" watch.

The physical effects of cancer will be discussed in these medical team meetings. It is essential that you understand and know what to expect, so you can deal with these issues. As I reminded myself daily for quite a while, hair does, in fact, grow back! Let's look more closely at this topic in the next chapter.

CHAPTER 7

My survival is the goal.

Hair Grows Back: Coping with the Physical Effects of Cancer

I t is difficult for you to maintain a positive perspective in Cancerville while experiencing pain and weakness as well as other side effects of treatment. Let us agree that feeling down, distressed, and disheartened when you are struggling is both appropriate and understandable. I hope the words that follow, as well as those in Parts III and IV, help you cope better during these most upsetting times.

In reality, it is not very complicated. To ultimately help you, the medical soldiers in Cancerville, unfortunately, have to hurt you first. To eliminate cancer cells they often have to use harsh measures. Thus, their arsenal includes administering very strong medications, radiating, operating, and sometimes even amputating. These are all aimed at delivering a knock-out punch to those invading cells.

Cancerville treatments are a mean means to a life-saving end. Unfortunately, to kick cancer's butt, the doctors have to kick your butt too. Because of this, at times, my words won't always help you stay in a positive space. However, because these emotional speed bumps are intermittent, I hope that my words will be helpful and comforting most of the time.

To me, Jodi's hair falling out in clumps, which sadly began the day of her thirty-second birthday, was a visible symbol of all the indignities to which my young and innocent daughter had been subjected since the day she arrived in Cancerville. Just about all patients report painful experiences. John's allergic reaction to one of his chemo meds caused pneumonia that almost killed him. Almost is the operative word in that sentence. He is cancer-free today, I am glad to say. Jake's chemo rounds pushed him to the edge, but happily he, too, is alive and well today. So many people I have met and you are meeting in the "Real People Facing Cancer" sections have taken the hits and the hurts and healed. Let's assume you will too.

My friend and colleague Harvey has a sign in his office that simply says, "No Pain, No Gain." That is the filter through which your pain and suffering needs to be viewed. That is the way I tried to see Jodi's situation although, at times I am quick to admit, it was a struggle. No one likes to be hurt, and no one can easily bear seeing someone they love hurt either. However, push yourself to see your cancer cells taking a big hit from your treatments. Or hopefully, like Salvatore and others whom you will soon meet, the effects of your treatment will be minimal to none.

Taking Insurance When the Dealer Has an Ace Showing

As I see it, in Cancerville, cancer is the dealer and always has an ace showing. You, I'm sorry and sad to say, have been dealt a poor hand. Therefore, the goal is to outplay the dealer and not to allow him to get blackjack. Your medical team will do all they can to help you do just that. Robert Louis Stevenson said it best when he declared, "Life is not so much a matter of holding good cards, but sometimes of playing a poor hand well." That is exactly what we all need to do in Cancerville.

They called Jodi's post-surgical chemo an "insurance policy." I understood what they meant, but hated that she needed it. It implied that, despite her surgery, those sneaky bastard cancer cells could be hiding somewhere within her. It was helpful for me to believe that there were no cancer cells remaining (my healthy denial), but that the insurance was important, nonetheless. I chose to assume that this chemical insurance was not really any different from all of the insurance I have paid for throughout the years, "just in case." You pay the hefty premiums to avoid the risk—Jodi did just that. You may have to do that, as well, to prevent the dealer from winning.

I had a really hard time watching that liquid insurance flowing through an IV into Jodi's body. I wandered around the hospital in my own self-induced "chemo-brain" dazed state. Ronnie and Zev stayed with Jodi in a small but nicely appointed room, donated by the Lauder family. To both their pride bank credit, and my shame and blame account entry (more about these in Chapter 10), they were able to make small talk and lift her spirit. To my credit, I resisted looking for spirits and gave up any claim to the men's room bar at Sloan-Kettering. Progress in all areas is slow but steady.

Let's be clear that I have been describing Jodi's experience with chemo. There are so many variations when it comes to chemo and other procedural recommendations. In some cases, chemo will occur before additional treatments;

in others, it may not be needed at all. For some types of cancer it may be essential, as it was in Jake's case. Fortunately, he also had an ace in his hand. His brother, Chase, was the "Ace" waiting in the wings to save him.

As I've mentioned, throughout his blogs, Rob referred to his brave sons as Jake the Snake ("The Warrior") and Chase the Ace ("The Hero"). Jake's Snake nickname was given long before he became ill; Chase's Ace was new, but very much needed to counter the dealer's ace. Together, Chase and Jake got 21. The dealer busted! The good news is that in Cancerville, as this story shows, even though the dealer has an ace showing, the doctors have many of their own and other good hands, including those of the surgeons, to help you.

Striving to Accept Your Treatments

Clearly, you might be asked and expected to tolerate treatments that you don't want, but unfortunately need. I am sincerely sorry about that, but the doctors are doing everything in their power to save your life.

Jodi's surgery threw me for a loop. I wouldn't want to see anyone have to go through that—especially someone I love. Whatever the noxious and obnoxious treatment might be, the alternative is far likely to be far worse. Cancerville asks, "What price life?" Your automatic answer needs to be, "Whatever price is asked." This assumes that a medical expert rather than a quack is recommending the treatment. I share much more about this subject in Chapter 18.

It took me quite a while to accept the surgery and to try to accept Jodi's chemo. I came to believe that if there were any remaining cells, those powerful chemicals were attacking them and insuring my daughter's safety. Thus, if I were thrust back in time into the thick of Cancerville, I would have stayed in that room with Jodi. I would have felt relief instead of grief as every ounce of helpful medication entered her body to kick the sorry little opportunistic asses of the cancer cells.

I would have cheered both the chemo and Jodi on, just as she cheered for her team as a young cheerleader at football games in Coral Springs, Florida: "Two-four-six-eight, what and who do we appreciate—cancer treatments, cancer doctors, nurses, and medical teams. Yeah!" If I knew then what I now feel, I would have focused on the importance of that temporarily disruptive, but life-protecting, liquid. I hope you can see it that way, too, and cheer yourself and your medical team on.

The short-term side effects of chemo are a consequence of it doing its job. That is what is important to focus on and that is the point I struggled with when we were in the thick of Cancerville. I want to stress one more time that most side effects are temporary; I don't want you to miss that. I want you to embrace the fact that hair grows back. I remember how excited Jodi was to show Ronnie that she could finally make a very tiny, but for her significant, ponytail. The medicine had destroyed the enemy, but not her hair follicles. Her beautiful long hair grew back, not quickly, but eventually. So did Jake's and everyone else's I know who went through chemo—except for those who were bald to begin with!

You do not have the power to lessen the negative aspects of Cancerville's treatments anymore than you had the power to prevent yourself from getting cancer. Your power lies in mobilizing your hopefulness to lessen the emotional pain of these not so nice scenes when they occur.

Sample Words of Support

If a Cancerville patient and I were talking in my office, here is what it would sound like:

Person: This isn't easy. I am facing some heavy-duty treatments. They all suck. I'm sad and I'm scared.

Me: I understand. Cancerville is one rough place. Everyone there feels those feelings and more. Any angry feelings?

Person: Enough to blow up a small village. I just can't stop thinking about this. It haunts me day and night.

Me: It is often like that initially, but we will help you to not be so haunted. Once you accept this difficult reality, you will be able to take charge of it.

Person: How?

Me: By seeing your struggle and your pain in a different way. Your pain and suffering are not for naught. They are part of fighting your disease and destroying your out-of-control cells. It is a search and rescue mission, even though the search doesn't work as quickly as Google does. It aims at the cancer cells and, unfortunately, hits some of the healthy ones as well.

Your pains will be temporary and your cancer will be temporary and your life will continue on. Hold onto that thought. Let it play out in your mind for just a moment.

My survival is the goal.

Pause

Person:	Okay, but what about my scars from the surgery?
Me:	Scars heal and fade. Even if not, they are the price you pay for winning the Cancerville war.
Person:	But what if I lose the war?
Me:	That thought is off the table and needs to be out of your mind or it will drive you out of your mind. I assume you will win. I want you to do that as well. We have no reason to think otherwise. Your cancer was caught early—thank goodness for that.
Person:	It's not easy.
Me:	I know. That's why we meet and you read, listen to relaxing music, and do relaxation exercises and yoga.
Person:	Despite all of that, I keep falling off the damn mountain.
Me:	Everyone does. What is important is that you always get back up. Feel proud of that, and of being "DAM STRONG!"

Person: I am going to hate being bald.

Me: That is not easy for anyone. It hits us on our vain side. Your beautiful blond hair will be long and thick again.

Person: Are you sure?

Me: I guarantee it. Hair grows back. Let's assume cancer won't. Just try to be hopeful and optimistic when you can. It can make a big difference.

Person: Thank you, Bill, for your support. I always feel better when I leave your office.

Me: You are welcome. See you next week. Call me if you need to. You have my cell number.

Let's Just Move Forward!

I decided to pay attention to the local newspaper for a few weeks to see what trauma and tragedies were occurring outside of Cancerville. I was, frankly, surprised at the extent of these occurrences. It helped me realize that, unlike headlines that appear after a tragedy occurs, Cancerville often prints its headlines in advance. As soon as you receive the diagnosis, the doom and gloom press releases start forming in your mind. Please try your best not to "write" these as they don't apply right now and, most likely and hopefully, never will.

I read many articles involving unexpected tragedies: a pregnant woman and University of Miami student, both killed while crossing the street in separate accidents; a man sitting on a bus bench being hit by a car and having his arm severed; an eight-year-old dying of Tay-Sachs disease; and a golf course worker who died instantly when he was hit in the head with a ball. These were all sad and shocking stories, but an even more poignant one appeared and appealed to my never-ending belief in people's strength.

A seventeen-year-old girl was heading to class at her high school in Ft. Lauderdale, Florida. A car driven by an older woman suddenly swerved out of control and ran her over. She lived, but lost a leg just above the kneecap. Upon her release from the hospital, she showed maturity, wisdom, and courage not typical of a teen who had just suffered a major functional and narcissistic injury.

At a news conference, she thanked all who helped her, including the medical staff, her family, friends, and others who offered their support. Then she said some of the most incredible words I could ever imagine:

> If I keep working at it and practice, I think I'll get through it…. The thought never really occurred to me to, like, wallow in self-pity. I just thought, it's happened. There is nothing I can do. Let's just move forward.

Wow! Couldn't all of us in Cancerville take a lesson from this young woman's accepting and optimistic playbook? As has been said, "The child is the father of the man."

"Let's just move forward!" needs to be a battle cry for all in Cancerville.

Real People Facing Cancer

Evelyn

Earlier, I mentioned that Jodi received her chemotherapy at Sloan-Kettering in rooms donated by the Lauder family. Many remember Evelyn Lauder as an American socialite, philanthropist, and as a typical Jewish grandmother. She was originally from Vienna, Austria, but fled with her family from Nazi-occupied Europe, eventually settling in New York City. She was a public school teacher until she met her husband, Leonard, and rose to become Senior Vice President of the Estée Lauder Company. She also created and was chairwoman of the Evelyn H. Lauder Breast Center at Memorial Sloan-Kettering Cancer Center.

Evelyn was diagnosed with breast cancer in the late 1980s when she was in her early fifties. A few years later, she established the Pink Ribbon campaign and one year after that the Breast Cancer Research Foundation, which has raised over 350 million dollars. Initially, the pink ribbons were given out at Estée Lauder and Clinique retail counters, but eventually the campaign expanded into a global effort that distributed 80 million ribbons worldwide.

Evelyn was described as passionate about working in all ways to prevent breast cancer and eventually finding a cure. In a *New York Times* article, she was described as "an immaculately turned-out, awesomely organized woman." She won many different awards throughout her career.

In 2007, Evelyn was diagnosed with non-genetic ovarian cancer. She passed on to take her rightful place in Heaven in 2011. When she learned in 2009 that her cancer was most likely terminal, she wrote the following verse:

> Shock waves asking circles of questions. How far, how long, how good, how bad? How long? How long?
>
> Shock waves of pain, not for me, but for the loves of my life....

At her funeral, her loving and devoted husband, Leonard, said: "Up until the very end she was smiling, always up." A successful photographer and flower lover, Evelyn once said: "The orchid is the strongest flower; it will survive any tempest. Their beauty comes from within. And when they die, they always come back to life." Clearly, Evelyn was a beautiful orchid who believed in the mantra "Let's just move forward," and in that manner left a "pride bank" filled legacy. It was never about her, but rather about all of the women she wanted to help—and did she ever!

Martin

I came to "meet" Martin by phone after having met his wife, Joanne, a psychologist, at a workshop one Saturday morning in February. In a room of about one hundred fifty people, she chose the seat next to mine. No coincidences, remember! When I asked what brought her to the conference, she simply said, "My husband has cancer, and I am here as his caregiver." With that I handed her a copy of the book for family and friends, which I had in my briefcase.

That led to my having a lovely chat with Martin this morning. Unfortunately, we had difficulty understanding each others' accents, as he is from Yorkshire, England; nonetheless, we had a hearty, heart-to-heart conversation as if we were two old friends.

Though religion never played an important role in his life, Martin has practiced Buddhism since the mid-1990s and finds the meditations he does during this trying period of time very helpful—at least on days he can muster enough energy and focus. He was diagnosed with Hodgkin's Lymphoma several months ago and has been on every-other-week chemo ever since. Though he greatly feared a digestive disaster, he is relieved to say that didn't happen.

However, the law of unanticipated consequences seems to apply. He endures chemo brain, which he says has both cognitive and emotional components—the latter causes him to become very sensitive very quickly. Sometimes that leads to tears when his wife does something special and sometimes to anger and impatience, even though he admits he quickly realizes its irrationality, relative to the stimulus.

In addition, Martin admits to having down days because of his isolation. His oncologist has discouraged him from being out and about with others, considering his weakened immune system. So other than leaving his house for treatments, he spends his days alone at home. He does walk in the evening when he feels up to it. Martin says:

> I am an active man and don't enjoy being so limited and restricted. I like to be around friends and people I know, but I can't right now. I like to take long walks, but I can't right now. My energy is low, and I don't have the physical reserves to do much. For ten or eleven days out of every fourteen the treatment kicks my arse big time. If that is the price I have to pay in order to see out my natural lifespan, well it's a price I'm willing to pay. I am not mad, but this limited lifestyle can be maddening. But I keep reminding myself that this is temporary, my scan is clean, and maybe I can just have one more month of treatment and get back to living my life rather than the very constrained one I have at present.

There are many peripheral pieces to the story. Martin and Joanne met online. At the time, Martin was living in England where he cared for his mother, who had dementia. They "toed" and "froed" (Yorkshire speak for "went back and forth") across the pond periodically for seven long years, supplemented by daily calls and Skype.

When his Mom entered residential care, he moved to the U.S. He arrived in the spring, married in the summer, and was diagnosed with cancer in the fall. Bummer! He became overwhelmed with our medical system, which he says is far more bureaucratic and complicated than the English system. He delegated all that stuff to Joanne, while she also chose to research his situation. He had no interest in researching and was content with his doctor's reassurances that he would become a survivor.

Further complicating things is that his adult daughters from his previous marriage live in England, so Martin had to tell them of his troubles via Skype. That their mom died during cancer treatment didn't help very much—though she didn't die from either cancer or the treatment.

Given the rough spots in Martin's road well before entering Cancerville, it is impressive that he has always been a pretty positive guy. Upon learning he had cancer, his main emotion was curiosity about the experience, which he readily admits may sound and seem bizarre. It is certainly not typical, but is perhaps the same force that led him to Buddhism.

For him it is all about seeds of potential, karma, balance, and self-reliance. As a result he says, "From this perspective having cancer can be seen as positive because it clears negativity from my karma." Whether you can relate to this idea or not, it clearly demonstrates the power of positive self-talk. It also shows that we have the ability to frame things in ways that help us be more comfortable with the challenges of our lives.

Martin started writing a blog about his cancer experience. He says it helps him vent and release his feelings. He enjoys writing and also reading others' blogs dealing with cancer and also likes that he and fellow Cancerville bloggers comment back and forth. Martin shares that:

> I am not a support group kind of guy. I like hanging with friends, not strangers. And I am not supposed to be around people right now. So blogging has created a "germfree" community for me with which I am comfortable. And it lets me vent, share, gain support, and be supportive too. It's all good—amazing really what technology allows you to do.

At least I think that's what Martin said. Those Yorkshire blokes may make great pudding, but they just don't speak English in a way I can readily understand. My guess is that they say the same about us. At least on the computer we can both LOL together.

Martin concluded by saying:

> I hope that my time living in the center of Cancerville (he read my first book and liked my gentle, positive voice) will give me new insights, which I can take with me into the rest of my world and make me a more insightful and compassionate person.... I may have to remind myself of my time in Cancerville's 'prison' complex. To that extent Cancerville will remain with me, but not as a dark or even gray cloud, more as a photograph I keep in my wallet or, these days, on my cell phone.

I sincerely believe Evelyn Lauder would have enjoyed sharing space in this section with Martin. In many ways, they reflect similar ideas and ideals as they turned their cancer experiences into opportunities to learn and help others. They both reflect the notion that hair grows back, just as beautiful orchids do too!

In Sum

Hair grows back. Scars heal. Life, hopefully, goes on. Your pain is difficult to endure, but you will deal with it. Time may not heal all wounds, but it does help. Defeating cancer is undeniably the main focus for all of us in Cancerville. Whatever it takes to do that needs to be tolerated and ultimately accepted. Insurance such as Jodi experienced, or as Martin is dealing with, even though "costly," is a small price to pay for life.

I believe physical scars heal more quickly than emotional ones. As we move on to discuss how to better cope with the emotional effects of cancer, I will help you learn to strengthen your ability to do that. Let's just move forward—slowly, but surely. Using that battle cry will keep your mind stronger in Cancerville.

CHAPTER 8

I will keep my mind strong in Cancerville.

Minds Come Back: Coping with the Emotional Effects of Cancer

Just like hair grows back, minds slowly return close to where they were before you entered Cancerville. It does, however, take a while. Both hair and minds grow slowly.

Perhaps it is because they are one above the other. More seriously, it is because Cancerville packs a wallop to both hair follicles and matters of the mind.

Resilient as our minds are, they were never quite built to withstand the ravages of the war on cancer. In fact, minds were not built to withstand war in general. Witness the many soldiers returning from the battlefields of Iraq and Afghanistan who, while not physically injured, have suffered severe emotional upheaval. The number of soldiers affected emotionally grows even higher when we include those who have sustained serious and disabling injuries.

Those actual war zones, as well as that of Cancerville, play out over months and even years of time. This runs contrary to our fast-paced technological lifestyle, which measures experiences in nanoseconds. Most of us don't do very well with slow rides filled with ambiguity and uncertainty, perhaps all the more so because of our modern accelerated sense of time.

Coping with the Unknown

Just about all of us need clarity and closure. No one wants to be haunted by unanswerable questions. Thus, the unknown outcome of Cancerville becomes a torment unto itself. Tell us all will be well and we will walk to Alaska and back barefoot. Tell us to wait and see, however, and our minds drift toward negative and unacceptable spaces to fill in the blank unknown. It is much better for you to fill in the blanks with strong statements of your survival. The more positive you can be in Cancerville, the better you will manage being there.

Minds buckle when the unknown creates high levels of anticipatory anxiety. That is okay as long as you don't allow yours to become completely undone. Try to go into every meeting expecting positive news and accepting that if you don't get it this time, you will the next. In this regard, think about Rob and his family's fifth, finally positive meeting with the doctors. The previous four very difficult meetings faded as they slowly, but surely, just moved forward!

Despite my pushing hopeful, positive, and optimistic perspectives, I am neither indifferent nor insensitive to the emotional upheaval that Cancerville causes. I am simply trying to help you offset and counterbalance the negatives when you can.

Cancerville and PTSD

I am convinced that many, if not all, of the patients who go through Cancerville develop a form of Post-Traumatic Stress Disorder (PTSD). PTSD usually occurs when someone has a near-death experience from a car or plane accident, fights in a war, or experiences any assault or hostage situation. After writing the above words, I found the following in *Psychiatric Annals*, "Studies have shown cancer treatment can lead to posttraumatic stress disorder-like symptoms." Mortal dangers can create immortal fears.

The symptoms of PTSD, in and out of Cancerville, include depression, anxiety and agitation, difficulty sleeping, nightmares, flashbacks, and other haunting feelings. The person with PTSD has difficulty leaving the traumatic encounter behind. It follows him or her in upending waves that return over and over to the emotions associated with the original experience. It is trauma with a capital T.

This is precisely why I said in the introduction to this book that that very difficult day at Sloan-Kettering would be forever tattooed onto my brain. Though I can help you neutralize and resolve much of the Cancerville emotional residue, there will always be some memories and images that remain with you. I have them and it is likely you will too.

It is clear why this is the case. As people, we do not suffer death potentials gladly or easily; we are programmed for survival. Even when we are not the fittest, we strive to survive and stay alive. Think of Aron Rolston, the man who hacked off his arm so he could free himself from the rocks in which he became stuck while mountain climbing. In 2010, they made a movie, *127 Hours*, about his traumatic, but life-saving, experience.

I want you to try to stay positive and calm, but I am not expecting you to be a robot. We are all sensitive to many issues, especially when it comes to our health and life. It is likely that, at times, your "stiff upper lip" will quiver and temporarily sag. That is okay as long as you regroup, refresh, and remind yourself that there is a war going on that demands an ongoing fight. In Part IV, I will talk about a variety of tools you can use to help lessen the traumatic impact of Cancerville. For now, let's just understand that it will take a while for your mind to calm and heal from the battles that you face in Cancerville.

Bernie Siegel, M.D., has had a powerful and profound influence upon my thinking. I know he will wince when he sees the word "battles" in the previous sentence. As I said in the opening letter, I think that for some people there is room for both mindsets—waging a battle against cancer and healing oneself from cancer through meditation, self-love, healthy habits, re-balancing of priorities, and the like. I am pleased to say George P. Kansas agrees with the idea that some people can draw from both warring and peaceful strategies. You will meet George in more depth and detail in the "Real People Facing Cancer" section of this chapter.

I had the pleasure of meeting George and sharing the stage with him at The Weekend of Hope in Stowe, Vermont. It is a beautiful and positive event, which the City of Stowe hosts every May, generously donating 300-plus rooms to cancer patients and their "heart and soul" givers. Among George's many contributions is his effort to take the sting out of sensitive words in Cancerville. Toward that end, he has written a book entitled, *iCanSir!* [14] It is worth a read, especially for you the patient, as he was one too.

In it he states:

> To describe my condition and my plan to people, rather than using expressions including words like "kill," "destroy," and "battle," I said

things like, 'I forgive my cancer. I'm grateful to my cancer for teaching me what it was meant to teach me. Its work is through and it's free to go.' I would meditate to my cancer cells, 'You may die now. I no longer need you. I will not mourn you as I heal myself....'

You'll notice throughout this book I often went back and forth between the different metaphors. Violence in one reference and peace in another. The reality is that they both can work. The bottom line is that they are both effective at different times and sometimes they are effective at the same time. Just like in life.

I would like to believe, like George, that for some people, like Shelley in Chapter 4, wearing the uniform of a "warrior" is empowering, while carrying and using the "weapons" that soothe their souls is healing. I am willing to bet a small sum that many people in the "Real People Facing Cancer" sections like Eileen, Roberta, Harvey, both Stuarts, Howie, Martin, and others you have yet to meet would agree.

The Emotional Effects of Chemo

There is yet another emotional issue with which you will need to deal. Jodi termed it "my chemo brain," and I know that she is not the first or the last to use that term; just about everyone experiences it. Salvatore, who we will meet shortly, is an exception.

Jodi used the expression chemo brain to explain her shifts in mood and attitude that could literally turn, not so much on a dime, but on what seemed like a relatively minor trigger. She could go quickly from fine and calm, to not so fine and not so calm, to very agitated and angry. All of a sudden, and sometimes for no clear reason, she would flood out emotionally. This would cause a commotion of tears, temper, and tirades that were very uncharacteristic of her typically sweet, kind, warm, gentle, and quiet nature. Martin, whom you met in the previous chapter, shared having very similar experiences.

Clearly, the scenes of Cancerville, comingled with the meds, weakened Jodi's, Martin's, and many other people's minds thereby creating roller coaster rides of emotional ups and downs. I will explain why this occurs in Chapter 10. Be alert to this possibility during your Cancerville treatments. Hopefully, Chapter 22, "Communication in Cancerville," will help you get through these difficult scenes as well as possible.

The Spring 2011 issue of *Cure* magazine featured an article titled "Chemo Brain." It spoke about research showing shifts in cognitive functions as a result of chemotherapy. These included memory loss, difficulty retrieving known words, and problems concentrating. People who have undergone chemo have complained about these things for years, and now these studies have begun to validate their frustrating experiences. Perhaps, in the not too distant future, the emotional effects of chemo will also be studied and will confirm what Jodi, Martin, and many others already know—that harsh medicines affect emotions already sensitized by the demands of the Cancerville experience.

The Resilience of Our Minds

My belief in the potential of minds to bounce back is not based on wishful thinking or idle chatter. It is based on observing the human mind up close and personal for more than forty years. It is based on sitting with thousands of people wounded on the battlefields of life. Some were in Cancerville, while others were in Anxietyville, Depressionville, Divorceville, or some other not so great place.

The majority of these people, especially those who made a serious commitment to themselves, healed and moved forward. In most cases, their experience, painful as it might have been, helped them to grow. From their pain came real and long-lasting gain. The same can, and hopefully will, be true for you.

I have always believed that as a therapist I have helped facilitate personal growth, but that the person I was helping did most of the work. Although we all have our breaking points, people eventually can and do bounce back. They may not do this with the force and speed of a bungee cord, but in their own time and way, most people rebound. I am pleased to share that eventually our family did. As part of our healing, we rediscovered some important life lessons, which will be discussed in Chapter 24.

Real People Facing Cancer

George

As we saw, Mr. Kansas (whose name sounds a bit like a title for a state body-building event, although Kansas is George's real last name) goes both ways when it comes to war and peace metaphors. It is no wonder we got along so well in Stowe.

George's story is compelling in many different ways. He was granted sole custody of his two children in 1995 while divorcing their mother. As part of that adjustment process, he had to transition from a successful attorney with three offices to a stay/work at home dad. His mom was instrumental in helping him deal with the challenges of single parenthood. Among other things, she took on many days of taking care of the children.

Five years later, his mom was diagnosed with pancreatic cancer. Hers was a battle royal and, despite her efforts and her family's loving support, she passed on in five months. This had a profound effect upon George's life and death view—it altered how he approached his life and changed his perspective. My sense is that he expanded his life coaching and consulting practice and scaled down his law practice. He also transitioned into being a record producer, concert promoter, fundraiser, and self-help author.

George's challenges seem to come in five-year incre-ments. Normally robust and athletically inclined, by 2005 he became easily winded while playing on the beach with his children or skiing with his family. He tired too easily, had a hard time getting out of bed, and generally felt weak. Though, like most of us men, he went into denial mode, his father and sister who are doctors, pushed him to get checked out. He resisted well, but finally felt so unwell that he obliged.

Like Stuart, whom I spoke about in Chapter 2, George's blood numbers were way off. Two transfusions later he felt much better, but the question lingered as to what was caus-ing the problems. Once again, like Stuart, the doctors needed a painful bone marrow biopsy. While George awaited the results, he contemplated more than his navel—he contem-plated his life and his death potentials and committed to fol-lowing his own advice as a life coach.

He was "all in" for himself and drew from his meditative playbook to calm his mind, which was jammed with issues ranging from his children, to his work, to a fund raising concert that was coming up. He was swallowing and choking from that mortality pie Susan spoke about, but he was determined to draw from every tool he possessed to fight back, as well as make the most of each day regardless of his health status.

In *Help Me to Heal*, [15] Bernie Siegel, M.D., says, "Think about how you are spending your lifetime, because what you experience and what you feel affects your ability to heal—both psychologically and physically." George gave much thought to these issues as he awaited the diagnosis. That came soon enough. It was Leukemic Reticular-endotheliosis or Hairy Cell leukemia, so named because under the scope the white cells look like hairy tennis balls. George states:

> ...Ultimately there are no two ways about this situation. It sucks. It sucks to have cancer. Diagnosis sucks. Nausea, dizziness, diarrhea, it all sucks. Go ahead and say it out loud, it's o.k. Cancer sucks. It's really o.k. I'm giving you permission. Cancer sucks moose poop! Can-

cer_____(fill in your own explicative here).

But George is quick to say:

> You've got to come to grips with this as quickly as possible.... Try not to beat yourself up for wanting to freak out in the first place. That part, at least, is a natural response to the stress of the news. But we can do better than that! ... A diagnosis is merely a professional observation of the condition of your physical body at a given moment in time.

Remember when I said that George likes to take scary words and transform them into hopeful phrases? He worked hard to do that for himself first, and subsequently for others.

It is evident that George worked the very programs he wrote about and taught to the clients he coached. He meditated and breathed deeply regularly. He shouted out words of encouragement to his body and his mind as he healed from his treatments. He became his own life coach and talked himself through Cancerville one step at a time. He skirted the dark and dismal streets of Cancerville, and when he caught himself going down them, he lifted himself right back up, as did his family and friends. He fought the battles and healed himself and is alive and well today. Now he is invested in helping others make their way through Cancerville and beyond, which is why he has gone to The Weekend of Hope for the past five years.

At the end of the day and weekend, George's charisma trumps it all. He accepted his cancer cells, forgave them, and bid them adios and adieu. My interpretation is that he told himself, Yes, I have cancer, but iCanSir! Something good will come of it and no matter what happens to my body, my soul will always be perfect. He sums it all up by saying:

The harder I worked the smarter I became. The smarter I became the more mindful I remained. The more mindful I remained the luckier I got…. The point is that I remained focused on my health and determined to live true to myself throughout the process…. It is also not coincidental that I thought of the worst-case scenario first. As positive a guy as I am, I'm human and I was scared…. Fortunately, I was able to wrestle the fear into submission long enough and frequently enough to be able to remain focused on the positive potential.

It is important to note that George is fit and robust again. He runs marathons and triathlons regularly, and is in training for an iron man competition. He is no longer easily winded or fatigued. His energy flows and glows, not in the dark like Harvey's, but in his positive and enlightened mind. His body and his mind have come back fully, and he is a role model for us all, especially those battling with and healing from cancer.

At the 2013 opening ceremonies for the Weekend of Hope in Stowe, George lifted his mountain bike high over his head, as he described his rigorous training schedule, and introduced his coach. In that proud and powerful moment, George, in my opinion, was not only speaking to the audience, but also to cancer and his no longer hairy cells. My interpretation was that he was saying "Got You Last," and I would swear as he held the bike over his head for a lingering moment, I saw his two middle fingers in the upright position. Much better than being uptight!

Salvatore

I have come to believe that there are no coincidences in the universe—just opportunities. So perhaps I should not have been surprised when I met Roseanna through a party to launch *How to Cope Better When Someone You Love Has Cancer,* a party which coincided with my 70th birthday. I never expected that there would be a story attached—a story far different from most when it comes to minds in Cancerville.

Rosanna's company provided servers for the event even though she lives in New Jersey and we live in Ft. Lauderdale, Florida. How coincidental is that? Our local caterer recommended them and her employees all did a wonderful job.

When Rosanna found out about the book launch party, she emailed me about her father, Salvatore. That peeked my curiosity and the rest, of course, is his story. It shows that not all people have serious or significant reactions to chemo or other cancer treatments. Sometimes minds maintain their strong and stubborn natures and suffer no trauma—post-traumatic or otherwise. This is why it is important to wait and see how it goes rather than expecting serious side effects from Cancerville treatments.

In traditional Italian fashion, Salvatore yelled at his wife one day, "I don't have cancer!" According to all of the doctors and their medical tests, he was wrong... or was he? Sal is old school traditional. He was born in Italy, became orphaned at age eight, and emigrated to the U.S. all by himself at age seventeen. He knew no one here but eventually established himself as a cabinetmaker from the old school of quality. He met his bride-to-be, Rosa, in Little Italy, New York. She was originally from Amantea, Calabria, Italy, Sal's hometown. It is an interesting example of what seemed to be a chance meeting that was, in my opinion, really meant to be!

In August 2011, at age seventy-four, Sal was diagnosed with Stage IV stomach cancer that, according to all the tests, had spread to his bones, liver, pancreas, and brain. The doctors told his family to say "arrivederci" to Sal by the New Year. His family was frantic, but he was as cool as he could be about his fate.

He never believed his doctors and felt they were just in it "for the money." That's just how "old school" Italians and many others think—perhaps they are better off. During doctor meetings, while his children asked a truckload of questions, Sal just sat there with a peaceful expression on his face. He kept this demeanor for all the months he went through the process that included eight rounds of chemo. He did what he was told to do, never believing there was anything wrong with him. Except for some fatigue, the chemo did not seem to bother him in any way.

The doctors hoped the chemo would make him more comfortable and give him a few more months to live; yet during this treatment time, he was unable to eat and lost twenty-five pounds in a month. His hip and leg hurt when he walked, presumably due to the cancer that had spread to his bones. When his family visited him in the fall, however, he was out raking leaves.

Salvatore, the traditional alpha Italian male, showed no emotion. Though his daughter Rosanna cried daily, he never cried or cursed. "I remained strong and kept thinking there was nothing wrong with me. Being Roman Catholic, I took comfort in praying to St. Pio of Petrocelina," he said. Intriguingly, his daughter said he always had a temper and a short fuse, but during this time nothing bothered him. He was at peace, despite being in Cancerville—then again, he didn't believe he was there.

When his chemo was completed, the doctors did more testing. They searched all over his body and found...nothing. Absolutely nothing! Salvatore was completely clear of any cancer in all of the places it had previously showed itself. He continues on a pill version of his chemo—just in case. Yet he feels fine, eats well, and is regaining his weight. His doctors were amazed, and his family was delighted, and all's well that ends well. Now, more than ever, he thinks it was all a crock.

It is important to note that Sal was not without feelings as he greatly enjoyed the daily visits by family and friends. He enjoyed all of the company and attention while being happy and in a good mood. Rosa, however, was exhausted from feeding the visitors—mangia, mangia. The Jews and Italians share many similarities; whenever there is a celebration or a problem, we throw food at it.

Salvatore never believed he had cancer and perhaps that, along with the chemo, is what helped rid it from his body.

We will never really know what made the difference. We only know that, like Tom, Sal was supposed to pass on but didn't. We have to hand it to those "old school" Italians and follow their strong and stubborn lead.

In Sum

The emotional demands of Cancerville lessen over time and resolve themselves. Patients ultimately adapt to the changes that occur. This is no different from the high school girl who lost a limb when hit by a car but who has moved on. She returned to school just thirty-two days after the automobile accident that traumatically changed her life forever. This accident may have taken half her leg, but it did not take away even half an ounce of her spirit. Perhaps it even spurred her on. I expect to hear great things about her in the future. Her strength, courage, and optimism can inspire us all.

The same needs to be the case for you. Life is always about accepting and adapting to change because no one lives a static existence. "Life," as someone once said to me, "is not always perfect. We make the best and do our best." We were built to be flexible. In Cancerville, perhaps to your surprise or wonderment, you will see that you are able to accept, adapt, and cope even better than you might have expected when all this began.

Clearly, Cancerville can be a very disruptive and intrusive experience for most patients and their families. Eventually, however, lives do return more or less to their previous rhythms. Let's take a closer look at these issues.

CHAPTER 9

I will heal and be healthy again.

Lives Come Back: Coping With the Impact of Cancer on Your Everyday Life

The details of your treatment plan and your reaction to it will determine the impact cancer has on your day-to-day life. The likelihood is, however, that many aspects of your life will be affected initially and, in some cases, inter-rupted. What once was part of your comfortable repertoire and routine will likely become challenging—at times daunt-ingly so—at least for a while.

You may find it helpful to have a verbal and visual perspec-tive of the healing process. As you know, it is a slow trajectory that goes back and forth until your health stabilizes. Think of a bad cold. The old joke says that if you take an antibiotic, a cold takes about a week to go away, but if you don't take an antibiotic a cold will go away in about seven days. With or without antibiotics, Cancerville is a much longer and more dif-ficult journey than a cold.

During crunch times, I encourage you to talk to yourself using statements such as the following:

- I feel like crap right now. But I just need to bear it for the time being.

- There is not much I can do about it. However, this too will pass and I will feel better.

- Unfortunately, this is the way I am supposed to feel right now, but fortunately it won't be like this for too much longer.

- I will try to distract myself when I can. I am going to lie down and listen to some music right now.

Giving yourself permission to not feel so well when that is the case, as well as providing yourself reassurances that you will feel better soon, is helpful and empowering to your body and your mind.

It is easy to lose sight of realistic expectations in com-plex situations because we live in a techno-centered world of instant and immediate experience. It might be helpful to draw upon an image that for you reflects the slow but steady process and progress of personal growth, physical and emotional healing, and overcoming major challenges. Here are some examples:

- progressing from your adolescence to adulthood

- achieving a significant academic goal

- planting a garden, painting a picture, writing a book, etc.

- parenting children

- building a career or business

- developing a healthy and positive partnership

All of the above share common elements that resemble the healing/recovery process. All are slow, evolving experiences that ultimately lead to mastery, accomplishment, and prideful feelings. They also involve ups and downs—forward progress followed by regress and then progress again. They all encourage and demand patience and the trite, but true, awareness that "Rome wasn't built in a day." It will take more than just a day to regain one's health and get back on one's feet after a serious illness and extreme treatments, but recovery will happen. Our bodies and our minds are amazingly resilient.

As you already know, Cancerville is no seven-day cold or even a few months broken limb. It is a royal and prolonged pain in much too many ways. Healing will undeniably take time; but the more positively and patiently you can accept the down times, the faster it will go—although it will probably still go much too slowly for you. That is, most unfortunately, the nature of the Cancerville territory. Accepting that reality will help you get through it a little more easily.

Prescriptions for Health and Healing

The lifestyle prescriptions for cancer patients are the same ones offered for non-cancer patients. They encourage healthier living in all areas of your life. They are all the ones we already know about and strive toward in the ideal, but ones with which most of us less than perfect folk struggle in our real day-to-day lives. They encourage cancer patients to eat healthier, moderate if not eliminate alcohol use, exercise regularly, seek out fun times with others, enjoy warm loving relationships, and get a good night's sleep. Got that formula everyone? Go at it then!

I imagine that you are in total agreement with this prescription but wondering how to do all that when you are vomiting, weak and exhausted, experiencing the runs, in much pain, and generally feeling like crapola (to my editor's surprise that is a real word!). Obviously, during those periods you can't follow any regimen whatsoever and are just trying to hang on.

Clearly, people who are drowning are not worrying about their next meal or orgasm; they are focused on staying afloat until they can get the hell out of the water. The same is true for you. Hang on to whatever can keep you afloat, while assuming that your discomforts will be short-lived and that you will live much more comfortably for a long time. Let's assume there will be windows of opportunity to enjoy your life once again and get back to the groove of healthy living.

This, by the way, is why so many survivors say that having cancer taught them some important lessons. Cancerville wakes you up to having taken too many things for granted—especially the simple things. We all tend to take our basic functioning for granted until we don't have it anymore or lose it for a while. Then, all of a sudden, being able to a walk and talk, drive to work, put in a hard day, have a normal bowel movement, hold down a meal, not be racked with pain or be bloated by steroids, or sleep through the night become wonders to experience and for which to feel a deep sense of gratitude.

As you wait for all that to return, try to tolerate the wretched retching (or whatever unpleasant experience with which you are currently coping) in the same way a pregnant woman copes with her morning sickness while excitedly awaiting her second trimester. In her case and yours, the ultimate result is worth the suffering—the birth of a baby or the rebirth and recovery of you!

Note that there are some unique folks who somehow pump up and follow the "healthy" prescriptions to the letter. They are the Stuart Scotts of the world, able to do martial arts a few days following chemo. Please give yourself permission to do it your way. How you feel will determine how you deal, and whatever you decide to do (or not do) is okay.

There is much information available about having cancer and dealing with the basics of everyday life. I leave you to search that out in detail on your own. Let's take a brief look at each major area.

Parenting

This is by far the most difficult area for most parents wrestling with cancer. Almost all parents want to be there for their children in every way possible. They want to enjoy the good times and support their children during the not-so-good times. They want to live up to their responsibilities totally and completely. At least some of the time, you probably won't be able to be there for your children during your treatment. There is no way to drive carpool with a puke bucket, nor help with homework when you are in pain or are feeling tired and weak. Many people in Cancerville report feeling very grateful to family and friends for "pinch hitting" for them with their children during tough times.

Your "heart and soul" giver team can handle those and other tasks while you recuperate. What your children really need are hugs and kisses; an occasional bedtime story; and reassurance, when realistic, that you will be okay soon. Please don't torture yourself with guilt for what you can't do—

instead put all the emphasis on what you can do. Children above the age of eight are amazingly sensitive and supportive of your needs and will accept your being temporarily "off-duty." Younger children may not completely understand but typically adapt.

Partnering/Family Relationships

This is the second most difficult area with which you need to reckon, if you are in a committed relationship. All of the above comments pertain to this one as well. Love is all about being there for the other person when one needs to be. Your being in Cancerville demands that those who love you be there for you in every way possible—every way and then some!

Partnership means sharing, caring, and stepping up to the plate at crunch times. Illness, job problems, a car accident, and all of the other traumas and tragedies of life demand that partners support, contribute, and suck it up. That is not true of those life problems that people bring on themselves via addictions and the like. But it does apply to all of life's difficulties for which we did not volunteer and are innocent victims.

No one signs up for Cancerville, which is why all partners need to be there completely for those they love who have unwittingly stumbled into this territory. Once again, that you are temporarily "off-duty" is okay as it is par for any illness and most especially so while dealing with cancer.

I am assuming and hoping that your partner is supportive and giving and is the epitome of a "heart and soul" giver. Should that not be the case, Chapter 21, "Having a Counselor/ Support Group in Your Corner," and Chapter 22, "Communication in Cancerville," aim to help smooth out some of the rough edges. The sad truth is that some partners run away. They are the ants of Cancerville and didn't deserve your love and caring. Should that be the case for you, assume that you will find a partner who merits your love in the future. For the moment, give all of your love to yourself as well as those who are there for you now.

Sex

There are too many individual differences in Cancerville and in life to be able to generalize much about your sexual interest or activity. For most people, sex is associated with calm, quiet, relaxed, and romantic times. Those words do not describe Cancerville. Rather, it is a difficult, demanding, distracting, distressing, and disconcerting time—and that is on a good day! If you are not in the mood, I get it. I hope your partner gets it too (or perhaps lovingly tolerates not getting it). Then again, sex can be a stress reducer, love re-assurer, and peaceful interlude. However, like car-pooling, it doesn't work well with a puke bucket, pain, or the self-consciousness that cancer can initially cause.

Sex is one of the most difficult areas for couples to deal with and discuss. Most people turn into adolescents and avoid that topic as if it had germs all over it. You and your partner need to follow Dr. Ruth's encouragements about open communication and find ways to have clear discussion in that area. I think you also need to distinguish between sex and warmth. The former may not be desirable for you, but the latter sure helps at times. Set boundaries clearly so that warmth doesn't turn into sex if that is not yet comfortable for you physically, emotionally, or both. Try to see into the future when that part of your life will return, and reassure your partner by sharing those images.

If your communication fails, seek out counseling support and couple's help. In that setting people tend to be more comfortable expressing sensitive feelings. It is important that you understand your partner's feelings and he or she knows yours. Fears, self-consciousness, and other concerns need to be shared, processed, and resolved; otherwise they linger, fester, and turn toxic. I know of couples who have not been intimate since one of the partners struggled in Cancerville, even though that was several years ago. The only way to deal with your insecurities, fears, concerns, and feelings is openly and directly. That is what partnership is all about.

Work/School

I am here reminded of a cancer-related support group I facilitated for a company many years ago. Several members of a department admired the courage, but not the reality check, of one of their colleagues dealing with Cancerville. He, while going through chemo, dragged himself to work every day. If he couldn't drive, his wife did. What upset his co-workers was what happened after he got to work. He would pass out, vomit, soil himself, fall down, and the like; some days he was incoherent. They all wished he had just stayed home during those difficult times. It wasn't good for their morale and they didn't like seeing someone they cared about in such dire straits. He followed my "balls to the walls" positive encouragement a little too well and obviously missed my chapter on realistic optimism.

The lesson here is to take care of yourself during difficult times in Cancerville, and not try to function at pre-cancer levels. Bosses and teachers are usually supportive, and there are laws that aim to protect those who are seriously ill. It is not likely that you will be able to consistently perform at peak levels during your Cancerville treatments, so do the best you can—when you can. Here again, be realistic and accept the fact that cancer is your main event and all else will need to take a back seat. Nothing, and I mean nothing, is as important as your getting an A+ in Cancerville and getting promoted from patient to survivor. That said, work and studies can be a helpful distraction for many people, so when you are up to it, by all means try to strut your stuff.

Socializing

Being around people is always promoted, in and out of Cancerville, as a positive thing. I frankly think it depends upon your nature and your immune system. If you are a "recovering" introvert like I am, you may prefer to hang out with yourself, finding all kinds of pleasant diversions and distractions. If you are a social person like Ronnie, you may prefer to have lunch with a friend, whenever you can keep it down. If you are like Martin in Chapter 7, you may not have much of a choice until your immune system recovers. Do what works, feels comfortable, and is healthy for you. There are no rules, so try not to have regrets.

In addition, your feelings and moods may change on a regular basis. Some days, when you are feeling better, you may want to hang with your "hood"; other days you may want to hang yourself—"oops," I left out the word by! Though you may want to hang yourself, please don't. Remember a key phrase: "This too will pass!"

Healthy Eating and Exercise

Do your best. Do what is comfortable and what feels right. For some, the gym is an oasis of comfort and relaxation; for others, it is slow torture. I enjoy walking in the park, but hate walking on a treadmill—to each his or her own. Yet having just recovered from a "seven-day" cold, I did not walk in the park; I gave myself permission to rest and nap.

Obviously, exercise and nutrition are not guarantees. If that were the case, Lance Armstrong; Olympic Gold Medalist Shannon Miller; my daughter, Jodi; or Josh, whom we are about to meet, would not have been in Cancerville. Nor would all of the baseball/football players or other professional athletes who have developed cancer. They were all in great shape at the time of diagnosis.

Real People Facing Cancer

Josh

I met Josh through his mom, Mimi, who works at a unique school that rehabs guys and an occasional gal who are troubled and often in trouble. I have been volunteering there for twenty-five years. At the young age of twenty-three, Josh was

diagnosed with testicular cancer, Stage III, which had metastasized past his lymph nodes to his lungs with small nodules
in his brain. His doctors told him that it was ten times worse
than what Lance Armstrong had. Josh wasn't very surprised
based on how badly he felt and his repeatedly throwing up
blood. He kind of knew he had cancer.

Josh is a most unique young man with a profound faith in
his Lord. His commitment was and remains powerfully strong.
If anything, his experience in Cancerville strengthened his
faith. He says:

> I initially felt, 'God, why me?' but those thoughts
> faded pretty quickly. I knew through my faith in
> Christ that He had a plan and He was going to
> get me through this. I felt a certain peace that I
> knew came from God.

Things moved along pretty quickly for Josh and he had
little time to think or feel. He was diagnosed on a Tuesday,
admitted into the hospital on Wednesday, had surgery Thurs-
day, and started chemo on Monday. "So I didn't really have
any time to react or think about what was about to come—
but to know I was about to lose all of my hair," he says. The
chemo hit him really hard. He was in ICU for ten days as his
body functions shut down—he was connected to all sorts of
tubes and a breathing machine.

Josh went from his athletic 170-pound pre-Cancerville
body weight to 133 pounds two weeks after chemo. He
had lost all desire to eat. This football- and basketball-
playing student attending Liberty University in Virginia, a
faith-based college, was sidelined. It took him five months
to get back to playing ball. Slowly, but surely, Josh came
back to life.

Josh credits his family and friends with keeping his spirits
up during this demanding time. He has four sisters and a mom
and dad who are very caring, "so they did my crying for me,"
he says. Though he feels God gave him strength during this
ordeal, he believes his family and friends added to that signifi-

cantly. Knowing that so many people around the world were praying for him helped too.

Josh's father stayed with him the entire time, and friends and family visited him in Virginia often. His doctors felt he was much too sick to return home to Florida at that critical point. Though he took a few classes online, he was pretty much incapacitated. He says, "I think, overall, I dealt with it pretty well—with a lot of joking and smiling. I worked hard to not allow my family and friends to feel sad or down so I did my best to act strong—even when I didn't feel very well."

Josh's treatments have concluded, and the tumors in his lungs are healing on their own. He admits:

> I don't know if I will ever feel 'out' of Cancerville. I have check-ups every four months, and every time I cough I check to see if there is blood. Through Cancerville, I have been able to understand that if I die I go to heaven (awesome) and if I live I get to preach Christ (equally awesome)!

As you may have guessed, Josh has completed his biblical studies, is a teaching pastor, and wants to start a church of his own some day. I am optimistic—realistically— that he will do just that. What a great story he will have to share with his congregants to inspire faith in his and their Lord.

In Sum

Cancer can hit you hard in every life zone imaginable. For a while during treatment, nothing is quite right. Often, however, treatments conclude and life slowly returns to calmer and more comfortable levels. As a survivor you return to being able to function as you did previously, ever more aware and grateful for the little things in life. The stronger you can be emotionally, the better prepared you will be to counterbalance all of these life challenges.

This suggests that we need to better understand how our minds work and what helps them to work even better. This is a subject that I know like the back of my mind—even more clearly than that. In the next chapter, allow me to share with you how I came to understand how minds work. It is a very interesting but difficult story for me to tell. I suddenly came to learn that my doctoral degree did not come with a vaccine!

PART III

Making the Land
Your Own

CHAPTER 10

I aim to be "dam" strong at all times.

How Minds Work

The more clearly you understand how your mind works, the better able you will be to protect it in Cancerville. During my very serious emotional down many, many years ago, I came to understand the workings of my mind and what caused it to not be working so well. I realized this discovery applied to other people as well. I have used this way of describing minds in my work helping others ever since. Hopefully, you will find it useful in keeping your mind as strong as possible, not only in Cancerville, but throughout your life.

Come back with me to 1973. Much of the world was simpler then than now; there were no Internet, tweets, cell phones, or digital cameras. An apple was what you ate to keep the doctor away. The world didn't seem so money focused and neighbors actually talked to each other. That was the year after Ronnie, our two young sons, and I moved to Ft. Lauderdale, Florida. Now that I think about it, our first neighbors were anti-Semitic and didn't allow their children to play with ours. So maybe I'm glorifying things back then just a bit.

Overall, however, it was a user-friendlier world. In spite of that, it was also the year of my serious emotional down. Unfortunately, as I previously said, my psychology degree did not come with a vaccine. All of a sudden I went from calm, cool, collected, and confident to being flooded with overwhelming anxiety. I was wrestling with panic disorder and agoraphobia, but since it was 1973, these words had yet to become part of anyone's vocabulary.

I was diagnosed instead with neurasthenia, a Freudian term that has long since been removed from the *Diagnostic and Statistical Manual* that is used by today's mental health practitioners. Frankly, I still don't fully understand what Freud meant by that diagnosis. To deal with this emotional down, I reluctantly began psychoanalysis once again.

My Struggles with Siggie

My first experience with Dr. Sigmund Freud's ideology occurred in 1971. I was working as an organizational psychologist for IBM in Westchester County, New York, and attending a Freudian postgraduate psychoanalytic training institute at night in Manhattan.

One of the school's self-serving rules was that students had to engage in psychoanalysis with one of their professors. I chose to see and work with a stereotypical analyst complete with an accent and goatee. He began our "work" together by ripping me apart and then set about to put me back together, Humpty Dumpty style. But there was nothing much wrong with me at the time because I wasn't there due to a problem. I was there simply because of the requirement for us to personally experience psychoanalysis. Eventually, I dropped out of

Analysis 101 as I realized that my professor's wild interpretations were akin to mental abuse.

Paradoxically, there I was, back on the couch again in 1973 three mornings a week, reviewing every emotional "dirty diaper" of my life. I desperately hoped that it would relieve my constant anxiety. From my analyst's office, I went to mine to help other people with similar problems. Unfortunately, I struggled throughout the day with high levels of physical and emotional discomfort. I helped the people who visited my office a lot more quickly than my analyst and I were helping me.

Five years later, I emerged from that "couch potato" cocoon pretty well healed. In today's world, my colleagues or I could help someone with similar problems resolve them in once-weekly visits within five to six months, rather than years. We have come a long way in helping people with emotional issues by using much more practical cognitive tools and, when appropriate, modern medications. Cancerville has come a long way as well, in being able to save people's lives. For all the ills of our twenty-first century, it is hard to deny the progress that has been made in just about every life zone.

A Graphic Model of the Mind

While I was trapped in what I came to call Anxietyville, I searched for an explanation of what I was experiencing. I looked through every book I came across, but found none that explained my anxieties. There was nothing back then to help me understand what the people I was trying to help and I were going through. It was the dark ages of mental health knowledge.

I needed and finally found a way to explain myself to myself and help others more clearly understand the basis for their distress. It was a simple, graphic model that described the architecture of the mind. It provided a blueprint to help visualize and understand how minds work. I feel confident this model will teach and encourage you to build a stronger and more protective emotional fortress. It will also help you realize how the mind-strengthening tools I talk about later work and can make an important difference for you.

The Importance of Our History

During what I came to call my emotional down, my shrink and I concluded that historical happenings strongly contributed to my hysterical experiences. I also observed that the same was happening with the people I was helping in my office. Hard as it was to understand, old emotional news as far back as the 1940s was making painful headlines in the 1970s.

I give Freud all the credit in this area. He discovered and uncovered the unconscious (subconscious) part of our minds that store our histories, even if we can't consciously remember all the details. In many ways, he demonstrated how our unconscious both influences and, at times, distorts our day-to-day lives.

My emotional down and all my needless anxiety led me to realize that, in some neurological form, the many neurons and other "wired" connections in our brains are constantly storing information much like a computer. We all have a "save button" inside our heads. Even if we don't remember the details of what is stored or remember to press save, it happens automatically.

My unconscious was spilling all over my head with the force of a broken water main. Old lessons learned were mixing with new experiences. The "little boy" in me was freaking out about the decisions my adult self had made. My entire being overreacted and felt at risk for disaster. I was a "dam" mess.

The good news is that we can debug much of our early programming and bring those "headlines" up to date. The really neat thing is that we no longer need to clean every emotional "dirty diaper" over years of therapy time. We can now accomplish that much more quickly by using a variety of cognitive and coaching tools.

Initially, it is not easy to understand how our history can cause us emotional difficulties in the present. It seems almost ridiculous to think that what my parents did or said when I was younger could affect what I thought, felt, or did when I was older. However, strange as that may seem to you, it is exactly how our emotional system works. As I said in *Getting Back Up From an Emotional Down*, "Artists in their own unique way, our parents take the clay of our soft, impressionable minds, add some personal colorings, pour us into societal molds, and sculpt us into our personhood." Please know that it is not just our parents that leave their mark. All of our early experiences, our successes and our failures, as well as the influential people we met along the way, affect us in both positive and negative ways.

A Storage Space for Pain

To keep things simple, I suggested that we all have two major storage areas and two additional ones that feed into them. The first stores the hurts and corresponding feelings that we encounter during our journey from birth on through our years of experience. I came to realize that we all have the neurological equivalent of what I called a cesspool, located in the back of our heads.

Our cesspool stores all of the not so pleasant experiences and associated emotions. This includes times we felt or were provoked to feel sad, bad, mad, lesser than, worthless, a failure, stupid, guilty, etc. All of these less than glorious moments are stored in our cesspools. In addition, more serious trauma that includes the death of a loved one; the divorce of our parents; physical, emotional, or sexual abuse; and other difficult and damaging experiences end up occupying large spaces in our cesspools. Please understand that this is not only about our childhood. The pool is always being added to by new cess—our whole lives.

Believe me when I say you would not want to swim in your cesspool; it is, quite likely, polluted. Yet, in some ways, we can sometimes end up doing just that. It is what I was doing in 1973 and for several years thereafter. I wasn't exactly swimming—I was drowning and holding on to my "dam" raft for dear life.

Dam It!

If all we had in our heads was a cesspool, we would all live in a collective state mental hospital where we wouldn't be able to tell the difference between the patients and the doctors. Fortunately, there is another storage center that holds all of our positive experiences. I called that area the dam. This too is built over the course of our entire lives. It is possible to start with a weak dam and build it into a strong one; the opposite is also true.

In that dam of support and protection are our memories of all of the times we felt and were encouraged to feel proud, accomplished, successful, worthy, loved, and deserving. Our dam stores all of the positive, pleasant, and prideful words and images of the good times we have experienced and enjoyed. A strong and solid dam is able to prevent the cess in your pool from flooding over or through it. A person with a strong dam has high levels of self-confidence, self-esteem, and hopeful optimism that help block the cess. These qualities are needed to help you navigate your life in general, and most especially in Cancerville.

A Balance of Powers

In a nutshell, and a very nutty shell at that, we feel and function just fine as long as our dams are strong enough to contain the cess. In contrast, when our dams are weakened, we end up feeling anxious, depressed, distressed, and uncomfortable. This is due to internal or external forces that allow cess to leak through our dams onto our day-to-day functioning. When we go through an emotional down, our dams are as underwater as many mortgages these days.

What inner forces might push our dams down below the water line of our cess? Fatigue, a cold or illness, hormonal shifts, alcohol or drugs, too much sugar, or a variety of other physical events all can weaken dams and diminish our ability to cope. Or, it can occur because cess in our pools is agitated and comes at the inner walls of our dams with the fury and vengeance of a tsunami. In both cases, cess leaks through the dam and causes discomfort in our everyday lives.

All kinds of upsetting events can diminish and weaken our dams. Getting in trouble at work can trigger it; losing an important sale can too. Bankruptcy takes us there quickly, as can being caught misbehaving by our spouse. There are, unfortunately, numerous situations and circumstances that add cess to our pools; this in turn agitates us in ways that feel awful and interfere with our comfortable and effective functioning.

Certainly, being in Cancerville automatically agitates and accelerates cess while weakening your dam. That is precisely why just about every encouragement I offer is intended for you to vent cess and shore up your dam in Cancerville.

Hope, in all of its many forms, supports your dam, while pessimism weakens and puts holes in it, adding to your cess. The following is an illustration of what my mind looked like the day we received Jodi's call telling us that we were all about to enter Cancerville. Obviously, I had some "dam" work to do because my cesspool was flooding through my dam and onto my everyday life.

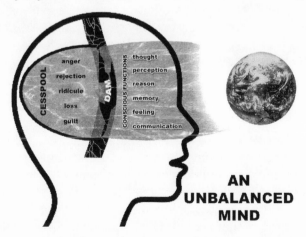

AN UNBALANCED MIND

Two Additional Storage Areas

In addition to the cesspool and dam, my belief is that we have two emotional "accounts" that keep track of the cess and dam deposits that we encounter. These are our pride banks and shame and blame accounts. When we do positive things, it adds to our pride banks, which also contributes to strengthening our dams. When we do things that we later regret, it feeds into our shame and blame accounts, which ultimately end up in our cesspools.

Taking charge of these two zones is important, especially in Cancerville. Your goal is to add consistently to your pride bank and avoid additions to your shame and blame account. Lots of visible VIPs have yet to figure this out. I hope you do. It forms such a simple charter by which to live your life and helps you to make healthy, appropriate, and self-fulfilling choices. Upon reflection, finding the bar in the men's room at Sloan-Kettering was not a great idea. Not only did alcohol feed my depression and anxiety, but it also fed my shame and blame account at the very time I needed to be feeding and filling my pride bank.

One of your many challenges in Cancerville will be to strengthen your dam by adding to your pride bank while minimizing shame and blame entries that add to your cesspool. Unfortunately, the opposite often occurs under stressful and cessful conditions. Stress can bring out your "wild child" in ways that add to your shame and blame account, thereby creating even more cess in a very vicious cycle kind of way.

Stop the Glop

The word I use for that which attracts us to self-defeating shame and blame behaviors is glop. I chose that word to discourage people from indulging; who of us wants to do glop? There is glop in alcohol, nicotine, pill bottles, street drugs, casinos, bedrooms, and even boardrooms, not to mention unhealthy foods that we eat. Glop surrounds us and calls out our name. It tempts us into self-defeating zones and is one of the most destructive forces known to humankind.

We repeatedly see it bring down the strongest, mightiest, and most successful people, as well as those who sit in the opposite position. Obviously, it is much better to go to the gym, a yoga class, or watch a funny movie while we are in Cancerville, than to get drunk, do drugs, gamble, visit porn sites, or otherwise pursue glopful activities. These hurtful behaviors are all part of what I call our "little boy" or "little girl" choices, while the former are healthy adult choices. We all drag our child/teen parts silently behind us via our cesspools, and they can jump out at any moment and make a mess of things. They operate on impulses that seek immediate satisfaction and reflect the poor judgment and risk taking of our younger ages and stages.

I encourage you to do your best to keep your "child parts" in check and stay in your adult zone in Cancerville. Wanting to throw caution to the wind is a tempting but undesirable choice. All of your energies need to be focused on keeping your dam as strong and solid as possible.

Cesspools and Dams in Cancerville

Cancerville is a factory that spews out cess, like pollution from an under-regulated industrial plant. I don't have to spell it out for you, as I'm sure you already know what I mean. So much of our added cess and weakened dams in Cancerville are based upon feeling a lack of control, fearing the unknown, thinking about dire possibilities for ourselves, and trying to overcome the stresses of a place that is neither kind nor user-friendly.

Even before Cancerville comes along, there is a deep, dark, and scary cave that contains our innermost fears. Cancerville inhabits that cave like a large, ferocious, and hungry bear. All of this combines with our old cess to make a strong and forceful partnership of hurtful, disconcerting, and terrifying emotions. This book is a counterforce to scare off the bear. If all else fails, throw it at him!

On the other hand, not everyone limps weakly into Cancerville. A unique minority seem to be surprisingly resilient and immediately optimistic. We have met people in our "Real People Facing Cancer" sections who have entered Cancerville with a strong and solid dam. This was based upon how they were raised (i.e., having Doris as a mom—Chapter 1) or their life experiences, which moulded a more positive perspective (i.e., Harvey—Chapter 2, Martin—Chapter 7, etc.). On the other hand, however, we have my less than glorious entrance into Cancerville. Let's take a closer look at why that happened.

More Than a Peek into My Pool

I want to use myself as an example to show how cess weakens our dams in general, and particularly in Cancerville. Obviously, our vulnerabilities begin before Cancerville and escalate the day we arrive there. Though I am not a psychologist who tries to needlessly blame parents and other important people in our early lives, there is no denying that they program us in both functional and dysfunctional ways. I owe both my stunning successes, as well as my dismal failures, to my parents, other family members, teachers, and friends. It is likely that you do too.

My anxiety in the 1970s was, in part, related to my very nervous and highly overprotective parents who, unwittingly, taught me that the world was a very dangerous place. My analyst dubbed me "the egg" early on because they raised me to feel as if I was fragile and could easily break. In fact, I did at age thirty, and neither all the King's horsemen, nor my psychoanalyst, could put me back together again for some time.

In my analysis, however, I discovered many examples of my being programmed by my folks to see the world as a scary place. To learn more about my experiences and find a more complete description of my model of the mind, see my book, *Getting Back Up From an Emotional Down*.

My father's fears were programmed in at sixteen, in 1926, when his father died of leukemia. This sent a clear message to Dad about just how dangerous the world could be. He was forced to leave school and find a job to support his mother and three sisters—he was Cinderfella! From his loss and all those feelings and responsibilities, all the more overwhelming because he was only a teen, came his fears and strong need to feel in control. His worries were palpable and hardly hidden from my view. I learned these "life is dangerous" lessons early, repetitiously, and well. I was an excellent student when it came to "home" schooling. These were all validated when he had a heart attack and died at a young age when I was only eighteen.

By then, my fears were firmly planted within me like weeds, waiting to grow and go wild at age thirty. My emotional down was inevitable. The brilliant psychiatrist, Theodore Isaac Rubin, said in his book, *Compassion and Self-Hate*, [16] "We are all the victims of victims of victims...." In this sense, Dad was a victim of his "scenes and genes." He, in turn, passed that along to me and I, unintentionally, passed the genes along to my sons and the scenes to all three of my children. It is important to note that they and I have successfully overcome these challenges. Hopefully, the muck stopped here!

Much more of my cess came from many loved ones dying young. From my vantage point, death was inevitably linked to youth. It certainly didn't help that I was named for my father's father, a man I never met, but whose grave I was forced to visit every year from a fairly young age. I can still remember staring at my name on his headstone as my father cried for a very long time. In so many different ways, I was taught that we all live on a very precarious perch—every day of our lives!

These experiences explain why I tape-recorded my eulogy on my thirty-fifth birthday in 1977. Can you believe that? It is, strange to say, a fact—in some way, it gave me a sense of control. Yet to do that underscored how convinced I was that I was not long for this world; no wonder I was flooded with anxiety. Perhaps it is significant that many years ago I misplaced the tape containing my eulogy. I am pleased to say that I am seventy years young!

The combination and culmination of all that cess sitting in my pool from my childhood left me vulnerable to an emotional down. Leaving a stable job and a safe and secure "perch" in New York and moving to Florida, for what quickly turned into unemployment, shouted danger to my "little boy" self, like an alarm going off in the middle of the night. I was now sitting and swaying on that very precarious "perch" I was taught to fear. My cesspool erupted like a volcano in Iceland.

Let's take it one step further to the year 2005 and my arrival, by proxy, into Cancerville. Might my less-than-positive initial entry into Cancerville have been influenced by my parents' teachings so many years ago, too many young people dying among my family and friends, and my emotional down in 1973? Could there have been a direct relationship? I certainly believe there was, but then again, I am one of those "shrink" types. Feel free to disagree if you have a clearer explanation.

My honest sharing of so many people in my family dying young is intended to help you know what is in my cesspool. Please do not allow that to raise your spotlight on catastrophe. Many of these people died of causes other than cancer; these ranged from suicide to heart disease. In all cases, in and out of Cancerville, it is likely that these people would have lived if the recent advances in medical knowledge and treatments existed at that time. In a paradoxical way, that can increase rather than decrease our optimism in today's modern medical world.

I hope this description and explanation of how minds work helps yours to work well, even in Cancerville. The formula for that is straightforward—dump your cess, strengthen your dam, fill your pride bank everyday, and avoid glop and the shame and blame entries it brings with it. Unfortunately, that is all easier said than done, which is why this isn't the last chapter of my book. I will explain more about how to accomplish all of this as we go along.

In reference to "easier said than done," let's not forget about the glopful bar this most intelligent and aware person found at Sloan-Kettering shortly after entering Cancerville. By working on dumping cess and adding pride bank deposits to strengthen my dam, I was able to lose that bar the same way I lost the tape of my eulogy. It takes time, patience, support, and effort to get back into balance, but I am confident that if you need to, you will. The following is the picture of my mind in Cancerville once I took charge of it and made the land my own. As you can see, my cess was contained by my strengthened dam and was no longer leaking onto the rest of my life.

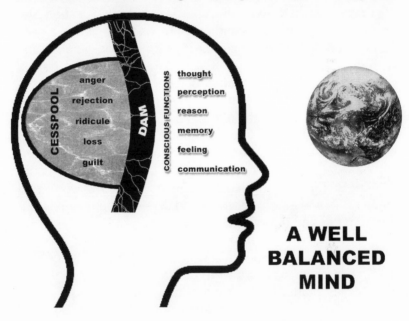

A WELL BALANCED MIND

Real People Facing Cancer

Susan

I owe Susan a debt of gratitude. Though she did not win her Cancerville battle, she did win her way by convincing me to write this book. When I first began writing *How to Cope Better When Someone You Love Has Cancer* in 2010, my goal was to help family and friends with a loved one in Cancerville. That was my only priority at that time; I was intent upon writing the book I needed to read in 2005.

I knew Susan for more than thirteen years, during which time she popped in and out of counseling, just as she pops in and out of this book many times. She was a tough Brooklyn gal who relocated to South Florida. Susan was a nurse, health care educational administrator, and nursing teacher, as well as a devoted mother and partner.

I began to help her with anxieties and other issues that occurred in her life. Over and over she had been dealt a poor hand, but she was the poster person for playing a poor hand well. Ironically, when she first visited me, Susan was having panic attacks related to her fear of dying. We spent many sessions dumping cess and adding to her dam until she was feeling much more comfortable.

She returned to visit twice weekly for quite a while when her husband was unexpectedly shot and killed. Such a tragedy definitely raises the level of one's cesspool to flood conditions. Being a strong woman, Susan waded through that messy time and emerged whole and dry—her dam ever stronger from her and our efforts.

She returned to see me once again in 2009 for Anxietyville-related issues. Her plate was a bit full from a variety of external stressors, but we were able to sort them out in a few months' time. Just as we were about to conclude our meetings—in fact, at our last scheduled meeting—she dropped the biggest bomb of all into my cesspool. Susan said, "Last weekend, when I was at the ER, I was diagnosed with ovarian cancer, Stage III-IV." OMG! One of the first things she said to me was, "Having cancer has cured me of my fear of death!" Ironically enough, as I previously said, that is exactly where we began all those years ago.

I gave Susan a copy of many of the typed chapters of my book for family and friends. She read them, offered some very helpful feedback, and said the book really enabled her to gain a much more positive perspective. Her reaction convinced me that my slightly modified and redirected words could help you, the patient, as well. Although I hadn't initially intended to write a book for patients, this quickly became my strong desire. Helping and being there for you, as well as your family and friends, became a very important goal for me and it has finally been fulfilled.

Though Susan drew strength from her dam and fought a very positive and strong battle, the odds were stacked against her from the beginning. None of the different protocols she tried worked against her aggressive cells. They were obviously from Brooklyn too—from an even tougher neighborhood! She searched for experimental trials, but all to no avail. There came a time when we had to switch from hope and optimism to the reality of her imminent passing. I will continue to tell you the rest of Susan's story in the "Real People Facing Cancer" section of Chapter 23, "No One Really Knows Where the Road Goes."

Susie

Though born and raised far from Brooklyn, Susie, originally from San Francisco, also had a strong dam. She not only inherited her mother's cancer gene, but also her strength and courage in the face of adversity. Susie's mom had a really tough life and a really rough end of life. Both of Susie's mom's sisters died from cancer at a young age.

At age forty-six, more than twenty years ago, Susie was diagnosed with ovarian cancer, despite her previously having had a partial hysterectomy. They had left her ovaries, but after her diagnosis, they were removed. She received heavy-duty chemo at a time when there were no anti-nausea meds available. She could only manage three of her four treatments, "because they were killing me!" she says.

Less than a year later, Susie was diagnosed with breast cancer and had a double mastectomy followed by more chemo. "I always took the most aggressive treatment available because I never wanted to look back and feel I should have done more," she stressed repeatedly. "I went to my daughter's wedding wearing a wig—but I went and that was what was important." Nine years later, Susie's CA125 numbers (Susan's nemesis as well) went from normal to fifty in three months. Her ovarian cancer had returned; despite having no female organs to attach itself to, it had found a spot. Surgery could not get it all, so it was back to the chemo room (or in Susie's case, chemo closet) again. "I don't do support groups or like to sit with others getting chemo, so they put me in a closet," she told me. "I don't do research. I just do what I have to do and move on!"

Then Susie went to MD Anderson Cancer Center for a few months of daily, targeted radiation. Today IMRT radiation is available locally in Florida. However, Susie says, "I had a good time in Houston. I met many nice people, my sister and friends from California came, and we made the best of it." I hope you hear the "DAM STRONG!" attitude that she has consistently shown.

Though her oncologist retired a few years ago, Susie still gets chemo every three weeks with only minor side effects. She still goes back and forth to Houston for scans and check-ups. Susie says, "My cancer is not curable, but it is livable. I am very lucky, not for getting cancer, but for living long enough for modern meds to help me survive. All in all, I feel very grateful."

Susie has never been depressed about her Cancerville struggles, but does get very tired of it—especially the doctor visits, tests, and wondering what, if anything, they will find. She goes on to say:

> I guess in my family we got used to sickness and disease early and learned to live around it and function as normally as possible. My mother taught me to do that from age ten when she was first diagnosed with breast cancer. I do that every day, in every way I can, and have been doing that for the last twenty years. I will continue to do that for as long as I can.

I truly believe that Susie's strong dam and healthy, accepting, and fighting attitude will enable her to do just that. Before we hung up from our phone conversation, I encouraged her to stay in the parking lot where she had stopped when I called, and for thirty seconds or so, fill her pride bank full. I am quite convinced that Susan and Susie would have been fast friends had their paths crossed. They both came from a similar place, even though their origins were far apart in many ways.

In Sum

I am excited that you can now speak my language. Hopefully, by understanding cesspools, dams, pride banks, shame and blame accounts, and glop, you and I have a whole new vocabulary with which to communicate. You now have a new set of ideas in your dam with which to evaluate your present choices and behaviors. I hope these contribute to your understanding of how minds work and what enables them to work better.

Use these ideas to navigate through the cess-filled streets of Cancerville, while protecting your dam at all times. These simple ideas can help you better understand yourself and guide you to work on areas where your cess is strong and your dam has some cracks and crevices. My graphic model of the mind can help you more clearly understand the value of counseling. We will discuss this in more detail in Chapter 19.

Now, as a way to keep your dam as strong as possible, let's take a look at a simple philosophy that can help you remain realistically optimistic in Cancerville.

CHAPTER 11

I will continue to strive for optimism and hope.

Embracing a Really Simple Philosophy: Realistic Optimism

I t is not easy, either in life or in Cancerville, to go forward with hopeful and optimistic feelings when they collide with difficult realities. Though our goal is to be strong and positive, the diagnosis of cancer and all that goes with it can rapidly sink our dam, flood us out, and knock the wind right out of our emotional "sails." I remember it all too well from when Jodi was diagnosed.

These choppy, cess-filled waters can throw us right off the boat without a life preserver or raft. Prepare to hold tight to the side of the rocking boat when necessary. My encouragement and plea is that whenever you can, reach out and hold onto a buoy of optimism. I am trying my best to move many of those in your direction.

Research consistently shows that positive mindsets pay multiple dividends in just about all areas of our lives. In Cancerville, we absolutely need that perspective to help get us through. We will discuss this in more depth in the following chapter, "The Power of Positive Self-Talk."

My Evolving Philosophy

When the U.S. economy tanked and people panicked a few years ago, I began to write a blog at *copewiththeeconomy.com*. My goal was to help people stay upbeat and cope better with their financial stresses. Those blogs still exist, as does the other blog it birthed, *mindlymatters.com*. The latter is still being updated to help people deal more positively with all of the stresses in their lives.

I named the philosophy underlying my brief comments in both blogs "realistic optimism." It encourages a strong, hopeful set of beliefs in line with and tempered by reality. After my family's Cancerville experience, I came to feel that we needed a philosophy that was neither shaded by rose-colored glasses nor black ones. The lenses through which you look at Cancerville need to be clear.

My philosophy encourages you to use the clear lens of reality to assess any situation and, where appropriate, add a filter of optimism. For example, in my day-to-day life, reality says that the odds of my winning the Powerball lottery are slim to none. To be optimistic here would be silly, although I might wager a few dollars with the thought that someone has to eventually win. I would not, however, give up my day job before the results were posted. Frankly, I doubt I would give up my day job completely in the unlikely event that I won, as

I really enjoy helping people. It fills my pride bank, even if the lottery eliminated my need for piggy bank deposits.

Similarly, in the popular book *The Secret*, [17] which emphasizes the importance of positive thinking, readers are encouraged to visualize checks arriving instead of bills as they walk to their mailboxes. Since there is no connection between people's thoughts and the envelopes the U.S. Postal Service delivers, this seems to be an inappropriate application of positive thinking. Reality needs to be the basis for our optimism, although some believe that, at times, unrealistic optimism has its place. This complex topic will be discussed in Chapter 26, "On Becoming Even More Empowered."

Clearly, to be optimistic that I will drive from my home to my office without getting into a car accident is realistic based on my past experience. That still won't keep me from being realistically vigilant, especially given the drivers in South Florida. The same applies to many potentially dangerous situations that we comfortably approach vigilantly, but optimistically.

Applying Realistic Optimism to Your Cancerville Experience

In Cancerville, this philosophy encourages you to be optimistic within the realistic circumstances of your situation. If treatments are proceeding on course and you are rebounding with resilience, the more optimism you can generate the better you will feel.

Try to stay in the hopeful, positive, optimistic zone until and unless there is clear information to the contrary. Unfortunately, sometimes the reality of the circumstances, right from the beginning, imposes a realistic limit on one's ability to be optimistic. My seventy-nine-year-old cousin Marilyn was diagnosed with Stage IV lung cancer several years ago and was only given weeks to live. I would not have encouraged her husband or children along the lines of optimism and would not have given them this book to read.

However, if they had called me, I might have encouraged them to hope and/or pray for a miracle. Unfortunately, lotto-like odds limited Marilyn's prognosis from having a happy ending. It was possible she could have beaten them, but not likely. That is where the realistic part comes into play. Sadly, she died in three weeks.

Yet I recently heard about a woman with the same disease who lived after participating in a clinical trial of an experimental medication. Sometimes miracles do happen, just like the story of my friend Tom, whom I previously mentioned.

Of course, there are other times when a person successfully fights back for a period of time and then begins to run out of options. Former President Bill Clinton said that when he last spoke to Steve Jobs, Steve said, "I don't think I have any weapons left, but I had a good time trying to beat it." This shows that even when reality bites hard, people can find ways to remain positive. Let us assume, if it is realistic to do so, that you will beat it for good.

Good Vibes Going Viral

Not knowing what will happen brings out the frightened, confused, and overwhelmed parts of us in all life's areas, and especially in Cancerville. The philosophy of realistic optimism seeks to offset our automatic pessimistic reactions. It strives to replace hopelessness with hopefulness because hope is the cornerstone of life. It is the energy that pushes us to set and achieve our goals, which keep us moving forward instead of standing still or going backward. Hope also enables us to encounter difficult realities and believe that we can overcome them. In my opinion, nothing of significance has been accomplished without hope and optimism.

By empowering yourself in an optimistic direction, you will also empower your family and friends. What I have learned from talking to many people in Cancerville is that positivism spreads back and forth from the patient to the family and friends and vice versa. Feeling hopeful and optimistic is infectious in a really good way. Hope and optimism spread virally like an interesting YouTube video. You can experience a supportive cycle instead of a vicious one. As positive feelings bounce back and forth like a colorful beach ball, good vibrations linger in the air and feed everyone's dam.

When you are in Cancerville, it is important for you to seek optimism and hope to counterbalance any negativity within you that may arise. The following ideas underscore why that is true:

- There are millions of cancer survivors. Assume that you will be among that group of very strong and special people.

- When you are fighting in any war zone, especially Cancerville, you need to believe you will ultimately win.

- You need to be there for yourself in both a positive and proactive way.

- Research shows that positivism boosts immune systems.

- Hope is like a flashlight in the dark. In Cancerville, it makes your journey a little easier, helps you find your way, and lightens your load.

- Hope and optimism are assumptions you can choose to make. Take a leap of faith that you will ultimately be okay.

Using Realistic Optimism When Talking with Your Family and Friends

By promoting optimism and positivism, I am not encouraging you to pretend, blow smoke, or hide concerns or other feelings from your family and friends. Authentic communication resonates better than pretense. People become annoyed and/or concerned if they are superficially given feedback that doesn't seem to fit.

Susan gave me a relevant article at the same time I was writing about realistic optimism in the book for family and friends. I read it and discovered that it was very much related to this issue of balance between optimism and realism. Sometimes serendipity seems like more than just coincidence.

The article from *Cure* magazine's 2010 Cancer Resource Guide discusses "protective buffering," a term created by James Coyne, Ph.D. He uses this to describe patients suppressing their true feelings to avoid hurting or upsetting their family and friends. The same applies to the family and friends buffering their communication to protect the patient. As is often the case, professionals are divided about whether this buffering should be done or not. Clearly, without specific details, it is hard to say; as in most complex areas, I believe there is a need for balance.

Somewhere between total denial and total disclosure, there exists a reasonable, responsible, and honest way to communicate. Saying that "everything will be fine" or that "everyone survives these days" would be taking optimism to a higher level than I am encouraging. Remember that your dialogue and your optimism always need to be based in reality; denying that reality will not help the situation.

Here are some examples of ways to talk to your family and friends that are realistically optimistic:

- I hate us being in Cancerville and dragging you through it, but I choose to believe that I will be okay. We are a strong team and will get through this together. How are you dealing with all of this?

- We will get through this together. I believe I will be okay. Let's pray every day that this will happen. What are you thinking and feeling these days?

- Cancerville is a scary place, but I have a good medical team working to get me well, and I am assuming that that is exactly what will happen. I hope you can embrace that belief as well, since it really does us no good, and much harm, to be consumed by fear and worry. How is it going on your end?

- I am so sorry to put you through this. As you know, I didn't volunteer for this assignment. I am going to fight this as hard as I can and appreciate your support and love.

- I am having a rough day so please don't take my grumpiness personally. Hopefully, tomorrow will be a better day.

- Most of me doesn't want to go to chemo tomorrow because it so wears me down, but I will go because I believe it is helping me get well.

These statements, expressions of feelings, and gentle inquiries seem to fall somewhere between saying too little and saying too much. By balancing your communication with your family and friends, you are modeling and encouraging them to be more forthright too. How you communicate with children, obviously, will depend on their age. Total honesty may not always fit with children and teens, but positive, reassuring, and realistic statements are essential.

The Ups and Downs of Cancerville

Reality in Cancerville plays with your mind while it tugs at your heart. Your slightest ache or pain can rapidly take you down dark and dreary paths. The same is true for your family and friends. Try to bring a flashlight of hope with you during these emotional jogs. Most of the time these speed bumps in your journey are the equivalent of static on a radio and have no significance whatsoever. Yet, when we are on red alert, every little "noise" becomes an alarm. I do not expect you to stay optimistic consistently, but I do encourage you to keep climbing back onto a horse named Hope whenever you fall off.

I personally experienced tumbles during Jodi's treatments in Cancerville as my mind and body fell off the Hope horse. I scrambled back to get atop as quickly as I could. I liked the stride and the strength with which she moved us forward. Let's not forget that rallying cry taught to us by the teen girl who lost a major part of her leg in a car accident—"Let's just move forward!"

Realistically, you will have ups and downs in Cancerville; they come with the territory. It is likely you will have your own personal tumbles as your cesspool overflows in response to someone's comment, a newspaper article, treatment side effects or whatever. The sooner you get back up on Hope, if that is realistic, the better you will feel and the more optimistic you will be.

Real People Facing Cancer

Jerry

I have known Jerry since I moved into my first Florida community in 1974. I know him to be a quiet person who likes to maintain a low profile. He is a devoted family man who raised three daughters with his wife and they now enjoy eight grandsons. Jerry is an astute and successful business-man who will go nine rounds with you about any financial or political topic. He also has a gentle side through which he raises orchids, bakes delicious pies that will take you right off your diet, and square dances all over the world. Jerry also plays a rough and tumble game of tennis three to four times a week. He may be as close to a Renaissance man as I have ever known.

That said, I don't really know Jerry well. So when I asked to interview him and his wife for *How to Cope Better When Someone You Love Has Cancer*, she said, "Of course," and he said, "Of course not." He wanted no part of it. Then he came to my book launch party, and something changed his mind. Jerry and I had lunch a while ago and explored his Cancerville experiences, as he had cancer twice. Not surprisingly, hardly anyone knew.

When I asked him why he didn't want to talk to me the first time around, he said: "I never thought that having cancer was so earth-shattering. I never allowed myself to be negative. I just took charge." How's that for realistic optimism?

The simple version of Jerry's experience in Cancerville began with rectal bleeding while he was on vacation in Prague. Being the quiet, stoic type, he never told his wife, completed the trip, and went for a colonoscopy when he returned. After finding he had lymphoma of the colon, Jerry had surgery and began a course of chemo. He told me:

> I took control in 1997. I called the American Cancer Society, the American Lymphoma Society, and MD Anderson Cancer Center in Houston, Texas. I researched on the Internet, limited as it was back then. I talked to different doctors. I went to Sylvester Comprehensive Cancer Center in Miami, Florida for a consult. Then I went to the world's leading lymphoma specialist, Dr. Armitage, in, of all places, Omaha, Nebraska. My doctors in Coral Springs, Florida administered Dr. Armitage's prescribed protocol.

Jerry indicated that he had no anxiety and just assumed he would be okay. He drove himself to chemo for six months, stopped at a pizza joint on the way back for lunch, worked every day, and did his best to live his typical routine.

Despite his low profile nature, Jerry is a strong advocate for support groups. He went to the one for patients, while his wife went to one for "heart and soul givers." He says:

It was sad when people didn't return and you knew they had passed, but you have to remain positive. With a negative attitude it is likely you will lose. If they tell you there is a three percent chance for survival, then assume you will be in the three percent "club.".

Not only does Jerry advocate realistic optimism, but he also embraces unrealistic optimism. We will revisit this idea in Chapter 26, "On Becoming Even More Empowered." Clearly, Jerry is as "balls to the walls" as they come!

He doesn't claim that it was always easy, as he recalls many times when the chemo side effects were a big strain. However, he pushed himself through them for the sake of his wife, family, and himself. Jerry says, "I had to live a normal life, and if that meant going to a New Year's Eve party for my wife's sake, even though I had major diarrhea, so be it. I sat in one place the whole night and held tight!"

As if to test his will and optimism again, seven years later Jerry was diagnosed with prostate cancer. In his inimitable fashion, his take charge, calm, methodical, data-based approach ruled. He looked at the options, picked the path of least resistance, and chose the radioactive seeds. They did the trick, and he is fine today. Jerry concludes:

The irony of my Cancerville experience is that all my adult life I feared dying of a heart attack. Both my parents died from that at a young age, as did many, many in my family. I never really figured on cancer taking me out, which is perhaps why I dealt with it so positively. I still think about a heart attack, but I kind of think I am done with cancer. Then again, one never knows for sure. You just have to think positively and expect the best, not the worst. That's been my philosophy in all areas of life, and it has paid multiple dividends for me.

If there ever was a poster person for realistic optimism, it is my friend Jerry, whom I still don't know well, but whom I know a little better after our lunch—the first time in all these years we ever did that. We "low profile" guys can be kind of silly sometimes!

In Sum

What I would like you to take away from this chapter is that you can and need to be optimistic and hopeful while facing Cancerville. It is important that your optimism be based upon the reality of the circumstances.

I hope you will work to embrace realistic optimism whenever you can. It will make your journey a little easier. Try your best to remain seated and balanced on the horse named Hope for as much of your journey as possible. The tools and discussions in the remaining chapters will help you to accomplish that goal.

Let's move on to discuss positive self-talk. This will give you a voice through which realistic optimism can be achieved. As you will see, I wrote it "DAM STRONG!" so you can learn to speak to yourself in an empowering way.

CHAPTER 12

I can write my inner script to be more positive.

The Power of
Positive Self-Talk

This may just be the most important chapter in this book. It is also the longest because the ideas in this chapter are central to my beliefs about facing Cancerville positively. As you are aware, the words you use to talk to yourself can have a very powerful influence on your feelings, behaviors, and outcomes in a variety of situations. Specifically, the words that form your inner dialogues can take you to dark spaces or, preferably, help you follow the realistic optimism philosophy. This will help you to sustain a more positive outlook in Cancerville.

When I was a boy growing up in the Bronx, there were a couple of people who lived in my apartment building who walked along talking to themselves. We were taught to see them as strange but harmless. At that time, I didn't realize that we all talk to ourselves throughout our waking hours. Now, I know that the difference is that we make sure that our inner chatter and self-talk are silent. This keeps the rest of the world from knowing that we are talking to ourselves.

Those Who Oppose Positivity

As I mentioned in my Opening Letter, my field is divided about the value of promoting and teaching positive programs. Some fear that encouraging patients in Cancerville to positive hopes and optimism can set them up for failure when they can't sustain those feelings. Jimmie Holland, M.D., has been a pioneer in the field of psycho-oncology since the 1970s. In an otherwise helpful book written with Sheldon Lewis, *The Human Side of Cancer*, [19] they hit this subject hard in just the second chapter, "The Tyranny of Positive Thinking." What, I wonder, is the harm in promoting, encouraging, and teaching a positive mindset when you, the patient, can find the strength and comfort to embrace those feelings?

I have talked frequently about falling off mountains in Cancerville or off a horse named Hope, as I know firsthand how those slips and falls can happen. No one expects you to stay in positive mode all of the time. The Cancerville tides, as well as your feelings, can shift with the winds of what you encounter on a day-by-day basis.

Some patients worry about sustaining positive feelings or faking them to please others. Randy Pausch in *The Last Lecture* said:

> It has not always been easy to stay positive through my cancer treatment. When you have a dire medical issue, it's tough to know how you are faring emotionally. I had wondered

whether a part of me was acting when I was
with other people. Maybe at times I forced
myself to appear strong and upbeat.

Although, as you know, I advocate authenticity and balanced communication, faking it until making it real for you is
not always negative. Josh, from Chapter 9, admits to doing
exactly that, until he could find his natural and sincere voice of
positivism. However, you need not feel obliged to fake or force
your feelings. Instead, I encourage you to go with the flow of
your feelings, shifting as need be.

Here is a practical example of what I mean. Let's assume
you had chemo a day or so ago and you are vomiting on and
off all day today. You feel awful, can't hold food down, and
are drained of energy but can't really sleep as your digestive
juices are swirling like a rolling sea. I surely don't expect you
to say, "This is wonderful. I am so happy. Life is good and I'm
great kicking cancer's butt!" Instead, here is the script I would
write for you:

I feel like crap—as low as low can feel. This
really sucks. I am hopeful that tomorrow will be
a little better. Let me see if I can put on some
peaceful music and distract myself in some
way or other. This too shall pass eventually.

I encourage you to strive toward such a mindset whenever
it is possible.

An important role of clinicians generally, and especially in
Cancerville, is to teach that glasses are sometimes half-full
and sometimes half-empty. In fact, in my view, it is not about
how full the glass is, but what the glass contains. As Martin
from Chapter 7 pointed out to me, the Buddhist teacher Thich
Nhat Han said the same thing: "When we say the glass is
empty, you have to ask 'empty of what?' It is not empty of air.
It is empty of tea, but is full of air. So the intelligent question to
ask is empty of what?"

Clinicians can and do help many people put positive feelings into their glasses. Some people can do that naturally based upon their genes and scenes, and some people need to learn to do that better. Clearly, I am in the latter group, but I adapted and learned every step of my Cancerville way. Both personally and professionally, I'll take a half-full glass of hope and optimism any day, over a half-full glass of pessimism and woe. That is my encouragement to you.

When you can, try to fill your glass with as much positivity as you can muster. Rather than seeing it as a tyranny, see it as a potentially healing symphony playing harmoniously in your head. When you are having a difficult time, allow for some off-key and discordant notes, assuming that soon it will sound harmonious and beautiful again.

This shift toward more positive views may not be easy to accomplish, but it is doable. That is why people seek psychological support and counseling in the first place, as they wrestle with their not so positive beliefs, feelings, fears, and the like. When clinicians promote a more hopeful view that encourages a transformation in our clients' thoughts, many dividends follow for them.

I personally learned early on in Cancerville that if I didn't change my way of not coping well, I—as well as my family— would be in major trouble. Martin Seligman, Ph.D., as we will see in this chapter, found that people can be taught to become more optimistic in a variety of settings including Cancerville.

Though some practitioners and patients may feel that a medical crisis is no time to work on oneself, I have found the opposite to be true. In all of my years of practice helping thousands of people and countless more whose counseling work I supervise, it is usually a crisis that brings clients to our office— people typically do not seek support during calm times.

In my experience, a crisis is a perfect time to work on strengthening and enhancing a person's cope-abilities. That is when people are motivated to work on themselves and learn to cope better. Our family's Cancerville crisis is what motivated me to work on myself. In fact, I will go so far as to say that a crisis is the most likely time to make changes in a variety of ways. That is why we often call a crisis a "wake up call!"

O. Carl Simonton, M.D., and his wife built a cancer research, counseling, and support center in the 1970s. In their book, *Getting Well Again*, [20] they say:

> Some people may be concerned that we are offering 'false hope,' that by suggesting people can influence the course of their disease we are raising unrealistic expectations.... There is always uncertainty... but hope, we feel, is an appropriate stance to take toward uncertainty.... A negative expectation will prevent the possibility of disappointment, but it may also contribute to a negative outcome that was not inevitable.

The Power of Words

As a therapist, I have always marveled at the power of words. Words are the only tools that my colleagues and I have to positively influence the people we help. That we are able to do that for the majority of those who visit us demonstrates just how powerful words—theirs and ours—can be.

A man came into my office for the first time. He was quite depressed for a variety of rational reasons. He left one hour later with a smile on his face. Did I cure him? Of course not! But I planted some helpful seeds, via my words, which will move him forward over the course of our next several meetings. Because of the advances made in my field, this is a whole lot better than my five years of psychobabble.

The positive words and actions of other people, as well as our own positive self-talk, are what build our dams. On the other hand, the negative words and actions of other people, as well as our own negative self-talk, are what fill our pools of cess. Throughout our lives, words are the building blocks that program us for better and for worse. Therefore, words are powerful tools to help us debug those programs that promote our cess or weaken our dams. The right words, at the right time, spoken by others or us, can undeniably move our minds into more positive directions. Isn't that precisely why we read books like this one?

For centuries, many philosophers, spiritual leaders, and mental health professionals, as well as everyday people, have come to realize the value of positive thinking and positive self-talk. As far back as 300 BC, Epicurus encouraged positive thinking as a vehicle toward greater happiness. More recently, in 1952, Norman Vincent Peale published his popular book, *The Power of Positive Thinking,* [21] which has sold millions of copies. The popularity of Peale's book and the many others with similar themes demonstrates the appeal of and need for learning how to be positive. Positive self-talk helps us to accomplish that goal.

There have been naysayers as well. They have preached a more negative and pessimistic set of beliefs. They can be summed up by the sad statement, "Life sucks and then you die." Sometimes, that is most unfortunately true. Then again, the more one feels that way, the more likely these self-fulfilling prophecies will come true, over and over again.

As is my nature, I am trying to strike a balance between your being overly optimistic or overly pessimistic. Realism deals with what is, and optimism deals with what can hopefully be. It accepts, at times with pain-filled disappointment, that into each life some rain will fall. It takes the good with the not-so-good and creates a more comfortable blend of how to look at the world. I hope you can relate and embrace this philosophy too. It can help buffer all the twists and turns in the road, in both life and Cancerville.

The Power of Our Thoughts

Albert Ellis, Ph.D., was an important contributor to the field of psychology and helped change our understanding of human emotion. He was a prolific writer who published many books including the popular *A Guide to Rational Living.* [22] Dr. Ellis founded the Rational Emotive Therapy (RET) school of thought in the 1950s and spent the rest of his career studying, writing, and lecturing about his beliefs, as well as helping many people as a therapist. His later works speak of Rational Emotive Behavioral Therapy (REBT). Ellis teaches us (I was fortunate to have attended one of his lectures while in college) that it is not our emotions that influence our thoughts, as other psychologists believe, but the other way around. He, along with others who founded the Cognitive-Behavioral movement, realized that our thoughts directly and powerfully influence our feelings. In my opinion, our thoughts and our self-talk are one and the same.

Dr. Seligman, whom I referenced in Chapter 2, points out that the question of whether we should talk to ourselves optimistically or not depends upon the cost of being wrong. This directly translates, in my mind, to the realistic part of realistic optimism. The example he uses considers being optimistic about driving home after drinking too much at a party. The cost for that unrealistic optimism can be injury or death to self or others, or a serious DUI. Obviously, that is much too high a cost and risk. That person needs to be realistically pessimistic and call a cab or phone a friend.

There are many other examples of overzealous and costly optimism. I read in the local newspaper about a family who took their small boat out on a stormy day. It overturned and the owner's elderly mother drowned. In this regard, I also think about the terribly tragic story of John F. Kennedy, Jr. who made the poor choice of flying his plane with his wife and her sister on a night most experienced pilots said they would not have gone up. There again, his optimism and positive "can do" self-talk sadly cost their lives. As I previously said, there are many paths to heaven, only one of which is cancer.

What is the cost of optimistic self-talk and hopeful anticipations in Cancerville? Being optimistic in Cancerville costs nothing unless it is entirely unrealistic. Even then, there are many stories like George's and Salvatore's in Chapter 8, which show that, at times, positive people are able to overcome dire predictions. If optimism is appropriate or just part of your nature, like Shelley's was in Chapter 4, it will make your journey a little easier. It is also possible that optimism may contribute to your comfort, peace of mind, hopefulness, and might even tip the scale toward your survival. On the other hand, the cost of pessimistic self-talk is very high in every possible way. It is much better to remain neutral, if you must, than be negative and pessimistic.

Dr. Ellis developed a simple ABC model to help his clients understand how their negative beliefs and self-talk created problems for themselves. A is for the adverse activating events that people encounter in life. As we know, Cancerville qualifies as an adversity generator of grand proportion. B is for the beliefs the adversity generates, sometimes automatically. These lead to C, the emotional consequences that arise from the beliefs, which greatly influence our feelings, behaviors, and choices. Ellis taught his clients to replace their negative beliefs with more positive and optimistic ones. He and his colleagues were alert for those negative beliefs that occurred automatically in response to adversity.

Let's take a look at the ABCs of Cancerville:

The pessimist says…

A:I have cancer.

B:I will not survive.

C:I feel depressed, terrified, anxious, and overwhelmed. I can't deal with this.

The optimist says …

A:I have cancer.

B:Many people survive these days.

C:Although I am not happy I am here, I am hopeful I will get through it. I will do all I need to do so I can become a survivor. I assume that will be the case. Period!

Even if your mind initially goes the way of the first ABCs, you can learn to work toward bringing it closer to the second, more optimistic view. The tools in Chapter 17, "Cognitive Tools for Taking Charge of Your Mind," will help you to accomplish that.

The Positive Influence of Positive Self-Talk

Research consistently shows that if people speak to themselves in a positive way, more successful results usually occur. For example, when people anticipate positive outcomes and speak reassuringly to themselves before surgery, a big test, giving an important speech, or the like, the results in all cases are measurably better.

Conversely, for those who speak to themselves with anxious and worrisome anticipations, the outcomes are not nearly as successful. The positive news is that Dr. Seligman and his colleagues all over the world found that people whose self-talk and beliefs are negative can be taught optimism and more positive ways of encouraging themselves forward. Seligman's latest book about positive psychology, *Flourish,* [23] as well as his other books can help you strengthen your optimism and positive self-talk.

To put their extensive findings in simple terms, people can learn to believe that there isn't a black cloud following them around. The more they can see their situation as random, temporary, and resolvable, and the more they can talk to themselves with reassuring and positive words, the more optimistic they can be about their future.

In your situation in Cancerville, when appropriate, these research findings encourage you to view your illness as temporary, treatable, and due to random external forces that, unfortunately, just happen to some people. This research confirms the work of the Simontons back in the 1970s when they promoted positive mindsets and powerful images for their patients. These findings take you right back to the self-talk mantras I encouraged previously—"Cancer can be cured. Let's just move forward!" This helps you to see it as conquerable and manageable. This healthier, more optimistic, and positive self-talk helps contain your emotional cess, while your treatments are working to contain your cancer cells.

In *Learned Optimism*, Dr. Seligman tells a story of a young boy with cancer who rapidly went from hopeful to hopeless and sadly died within a day. He says, "Such stories are told the world over, frequently enough to inspire the belief that hope is by itself life-sustaining and hopelessness life-destroying." It is not just that positive self-talk can be helpful and possibly even healing, but that negative self-talk has a profound, unwanted effect that we all would do well to avoid.

A personal example comes to mind. My cousin Alan died in Cancerville from chemo complications because the technology was so limited in the 1970s. He was in his early thirties and left behind a wife and young daughter. My Aunt Nettie, Alan's mother, fell into a deep depression. Every time I saw her over the next few years, she looked as somber and sad as she had the day of his funeral. Within that time, she developed cancer and died shortly thereafter. It was as if she willed herself to be reunited with her son. There was no doubt in my mind that her chronically depressed state, negative self-talk, and overall misery over the loss of her son lowered her immune system and allowed that to happen.

Fortunately, there are more positive stories shared by Dr. Seligman as well. One involved a research project with people dealing with colon cancer and melanoma. In addition to their regular chemotherapy and radiation treatments, patients received weekly cognitive therapy. They were taught to deal with change, recognize and dispute (remember this word for Chapter 17) automatic pessimistic thoughts, and use distraction techniques. This was supplemented with relaxation training. The goal was to see whether or not these efforts could raise patients' immune systems to help fight off their cancer cells.

These forty people were matched with a control group dealing with the same type of cancers, but who received no cognitive therapy or relaxation. The results were quite impressive. For those who received the additional therapy, their natural killer cell count (the good army) was sharply increased. For those who did not receive the therapy, there was no increase in that cell activity.

Additional research in Cancerville using larger samples also supports the idea that positive beliefs and feelings are beneficial. It makes sense, really, when you consider that the mind and body are directly connected in so many ways. As Susan said, "All of our cells communicate with each other all of the time. That is how the body and mind work together to form a whole and integrated person." She was undeniably correct in recognizing the importance of that yin and yang interaction.

Self-Talk in Cancerville

Please understand that I am not encouraging you to embrace positive self-talk because it will definitely and directly influence your outcome in Cancerville; it may or may not have that potential influence. I am, however, encouraging you in that direction because it can help make your time there a little easier and much less stressful; it will help you cope better. It will also give you increased energy, greater emotional strength, more patience, a stronger focus, and a brighter outlook.

I am very realistic about this most challenging goal of keeping your spirits up in Cancerville. Undeniably, some days will be better than others. I recall talking to Susan on a difficult day a few months into her chemo. She reminded me just how difficult it is to stay upbeat and optimistic there. She was coming undone and said:

> My CA-125 numbers are not low enough and I struggle with pain; I'm a mess for more than a week after chemo. Why am I even bothering? I'm going to die from this, I'm tired and I just don't feel good. Look how positive Gilda was, and it didn't do her any f'in' good!

It was hard to argue with Susan's misery and negativity, but I chose to do just that, while understanding and being sensitive to her angst. I spoke to her about adding to her torment by allowing these thoughts to sneak past her dam and generate even more emotional turbulence. I encouraged her to assume that she would be one of the lucky survivors and to see her aches, pain, and hair loss post-chemo as hurting the enemy cells as well. She seemed to comfortably embrace that idea.

In addition, I encouraged her to distract herself when she could to relieve some of her physical and emotional pain. We talked about her watching funny TV shows, movies, and other simple but pleasant activities. I did not discount her distress and discomfort, as it was more than understandable. I did, however, encourage her to seize some moments when she could to briefly escape Cancerville's "choke-hold."

After our meeting, I had a break and went to Morakami Japanese Gardens, not far from my Boca Raton, Florida office. It is a lush place filled with foliage, relaxing images, and an interesting history. I sat on a bench with a beautiful view of the garden's calming green landscape and pondered our meeting. As a therapist and life coach, I often have important responsibilities in areas that are far from clear. I take this responsibility very seriously. I consciously refuse to play God or overstep my boundaries. Just as my degree did not come with a vaccine, neither did it come with a crystal ball.

I asked myself if I was being fair and appropriate to encourage Susan with such a positive agenda under circumstances that were less than positive. Was I promoting unrealistic, naïve, and distorted beliefs? Was I giving her false hope and setting her up for disappointment? I weighed the issues back and forth in my mind like a college debater in a tournament. Yet I ultimately concluded that the preponderance of evidence was on the side of "balls to the walls" positivity in Cancerville, especially for this strong woman.

I felt that even if she didn't win her battle, positive self-talk would lighten her Cancerville experience just a little bit. In fact, toward the end of her journey she told me exactly that, which helped validate my decision to promote positive self-talk. Knowing what I now know, I still would have pushed that hopeful agenda until reality intervened and forced us to go in a different direction.

Part of Susan's difficulty, which applies to you as well, is that at certain times Cancerville can wear down even the strongest of us, both physically and emotionally. This is why we tumble and have to work hard to get back up on that horse named Hope. When we are drained, distraught, and distracted, working hard is not all that easy, but I believe you can do it. Simply stated, the more positive self-talk you can muster, the less worn you will be, and the more you will be able to focus on what needs to done.

I would like you to recall times in your life when you rose to a challenge. In one way or another, you have been doing that since you were old enough to walk and talk, perhaps even before. Walking and talking were no easy feats to accomplish back then. Look how far you have come since those early challenges and how many others you have taken on and overcome since then.

I am here reminded of that special little train who willed himself up that high hill by saying, "I think I can, I think I can," as he huffed and puffed himself all the way to the top. Like that little engine, your positive thoughts and self-talk will provide the fuel for you to have the energy to manage Cancerville as well as you can.

Please understand that assuming and believing that you will be a survivor helps make your journey just a little easier. Antje, who has been fighting her cancer battle for more than twenty years, says "Be strong in Cancerville, and if it all starts to get to you be even stronger!"

The Placebo Effect: Positive Expectations and Positive Results

Like Bernie Siegel, M.D., the Simontons whom I previously referenced as encouraging their patients toward positive expectations, also discuss the placebo effect, which demonstrates the power of our mind's influence on our bodies. Those who believe the "medicine" will help seem to get positive results even if the shot is filled with purified water. In the Foreword, Bernie said that patients who thought they were getting treatment but didn't due to medical errors still experienced side effects and tumor reduction.

I've seen this with psychiatric medications as well. Those who trust their psychiatrist and believe the pill will be a helpful answer for them enjoy much greater success than those who have little faith in what has been prescribed. Those in the latter group typically develop all kinds of side effect problems and stop taking the medication very quickly. Often, the side effects are more based in the patients' expectations than in the chemicals themselves.

The Simontons say:

> The placebo effect is not limited to the administration of sugar pills. Throughout medical history there have been countless practices, such as "bleeding" the patient...that have no physiological basis for curing but still frequently worked, apparently because everyone—including the physician—believed in their efficacy. Indeed, some surgical procedures that were in

vogue during the last fifty years seemed to produce remarkable results even though we now
know that, in many cases, there are serious
questions about their value.... Once again, the
results can be attributed to the patient's belief
that the treatments would work and because of
his confidence in the doctor.

They also cite a statement made by the president of the
American Cancer Society in 1959:

The importance of Dr. Pendergrass' view is not
just that it underscores the role that psychological factors play in aggravating a disease,
it also emphasizes the possibility that psychological factors, including the patient's beliefs,
may be mobilized to move toward health.

"Yeah, But..." —A Contrarian Point of View

All of these reasonable and rational words aside, I fully
understand that it is not always easy to influence a racing mind
gone wild over cells gone wild. I get it—I really do. The dips
into more negative thoughts and feelings will occur—especially when you aren't feeling particularly well, are tired and
lethargic, are on heavy pain meds or steroids, or are experiencing a physical setback of some kind. All of these whack
away and weaken you and your dam.

They also cause much worry, which agitates cesspools.
Such shifts create a river of negativity. All you can do during
these times is pick yourself up, dust off the cess, and refocus
on getting past this speed bump and back to a more positive
point of view.

Despite my strong words encouraging you to remain positive, I can almost hear some of you thinking less than positive
thoughts such as the following:

Okay, Bill. You want me to be positive in a place you have characterized as hell, a torture chamber, and a war zone. Need I say more? Okay, I will continue my rant. My life is in danger, and I am terrified. As you have said, Cancerville operates in slow motion as my mind races along at one hundred and fifty miles per hour, wondering how I got here and how/if I will ever get out. Really, Bill, you expect me to be positive? I feel really awful almost all of the time. I think I'd rather be dead already and get it over with. How's that for positivism? I know you mean well, but Buddy you're way off base! Why don't you try this regimen for a few months and let's see how positive you are Dr. Happy Smile?

Ouch, but I do understand those feelings. You have every right to feel the way you do. As your friend, companion, and supporter in Cancerville, I would like to encourage you to move beyond that kind of negative thinking for the sake of your sanity. Yes, have those negative thoughts if they come along (I know I did, and I was just there by proxy), but then allow them to pass through your mind and evaporate.

Try to see Cancerville through the more positive self-talk filters of hopefulness, not because I said so, but because that positive attitude may just help you to feel a little better. Sometimes cancer patients selfishly wish they were dead in the early times of their Cancerville arrival. "Selfishly" is definitely the key word in that sentence. In so many cases, their lives have improved since those dark days of treatment. I would like you to optimistically and positively believe that yours will too.

I am realistically optimistic that if I personally face Cancerville one day, I will be able to apply everything I am saying in this book. Will I have some off days? Absolutely! Will I get past them? I am certain that I will, and I am also confident that you will too.

More Evidence for Hopefulness

Susan not only lent me the *Cure* magazine article refer-enced in the previous chapter, but also another gem from *Forbes* magazine, March 2, 2009. I chuckled out loud when I read the headline printed boldly on the cover—" Sharon... was 24 and dying from cancer. Then her tumors melted away. What science is learning from... *Miracle Survivors*." The arti-cle describes several people with very serious forms of can-cer who were told to prepare for their lives to conclude within a few months.

In each case, they experienced an unexpected and complete recovery. Their cancer had totally disappeared. Some were spontaneous remissions, while others were from experimental medications. In all instances, some-thing empowered these patients' immune systems to take charge, tame, and eventually eliminate those ugly cells. Positive self-talk combined with new treatments and a little luck may just have the potential to turn immune systems into superheroes.

The reason for my chuckle was that the article validated the conclusion I had reached sitting on the sunny bench ear-lier that day in the gardens, while I struggled with how best to help Susan and others in Cancerville. If people sitting on a very precarious perch in Cancerville can make a comeback to solid ground, then we can't pessimistically count almost any-one out.

Accordingly, if a Cancerville doctor told me that I only had a few months to live, my most appropriate and optimistic response would be, "Maybe, maybe not! I'll wait and see what happens." Since miracles and Hail Mary passes only occur on occasion, I would hope and pray for one, while I realistically put my affairs in order and bid my farewells.

Real People Facing Cancer

Cindy S.

Cindy's story is so powerful and poignant that I considered devoting a whole chapter to it, although it probably deserves a book of its own. Then again, so many people whom I have met in Cancerville have told me amazing tales of their journeys and the strength and courage that they were able to find there.

There is no denying that Cindy was the poster person for positive self-talk and hopeful optimism. Like the inflatable, punching shmoo doll I used to play with as a young lad, she gets knocked down regularly but pops back up reliably. She doesn't just ride through Cancerville on a horse named Hope—she embodies the spirit of one!

Her story begins in 2001 when she found a tiny, pea-sized, hard lump near her breast. She knew immediately from the look on the face of the doctor who was doing the biopsy that this was serious.

As a financially struggling single mother of two young children, Cindy knew she was in major trouble. A week later when the doctor called with the results that validated her belief, she was sad but had already faced her fears.

Cindy, like so many, talks about the structured schedule of tests, doctors' visits, consults, more tests, pre-op/post-op, etc. She reports that she didn't really feel the full impact of the diagnosis, which was diluted by these distractions. She says:

> After my surgery, which was a lumpectomy, I kept on living my life. I had to make sure I was in control of it and worked very hard to balance my treatments with my children's activities. I could not allow my treatments to take me away from their lives. It was important to me not to do anything that would make them think or feel

like the cancer was so serious that they were second in my mind and actions.

Cindy's treatment consisted of two lumpectomies, removal of some lymph nodes, surgical installation of a port, chemo known as the "red devil" (Jodi's drug of "non-choice!"), and radiation for a month. Before her hair began to fall out, she had her children help her cut it off. She told them, "This is how we take control of something we can't really control." She goes on to say, "I didn't want the medicine, which will help me, to be the force to take away my hair." Together they donated four feet of her hair to Locks of Love.

Through it all, Cindy remained positive and hopeful for herself and her children. She says, "At some point, despite researching on the computer till you fall asleep there, you have to surrender and put trust in your doctors and your entire medical team. They are the experts and they care about you and your well-being."

Cindy attributes her strength, courage, determination, and toughness to having been abused as a child from age six to sixteen. This is atypical, as many who suffer such experiences go the other way and are weakened permanently. Cindy says:

> I am tough in general and handle my break-downs in life pretty well. I know how to reassure myself. Since I was a very young girl I knew I would always be okay. Even as a child being abused at my very worst moments, I kept hearing a voice in my head say that no matter what I would be okay and poof—one day I was. Early on I made up my mind that no one and nothing would ever take control of me ever again. I would find a way to manage—no matter what!

Cindy managed her way through Cancerville quite well. She managed to use her voice of reassurance to help her hold tight to its slippery slopes, while loving and raising her children who were the center of her being—her reasons for being. From that point on, things went well. She slowly but surely recovered, reestablished her life, and found warmth and friendship again. In 2004, while working as a party planner, she met Linda whose son's wedding she helped to plan. You will come to see the importance of this soon. Cindy says, "I thrived in the freedom of having my life back."

After almost ten years of being a fortunate and happy survivor, Cindy's cancer returned in 2010. She was diagnosed with Stage III in her left breast and Stage IV in the right. She owns her own self-neglect in terms of not doing follow-up checks, but her money was tight and she had no medical insurance. This also meant no treatment for her newly discovered cancers. Mark my words that Tracey, whom you will meet in Chapter 19, will wince when she reads these words. She and her staff work tirelessly at the American Cancer Society to help those in need in South Florida.

This is where Cindy's friend Linda came into the picture. They disagreed about Linda's commitment to helping Cindy by paying whatever it cost to save her friend's life. Linda had recently lost her beloved father to lung cancer and refused to lose anyone else. She helped Cindy find some insurance coverage through Broward County and gifted the rest to her along with living expenses. "She helped me keep my home and my dignity through unconditional love and unconditional financial support. She never made me feel like a pauper or beneath her. She is a walking angel here on earth," Cindy said. I know Linda and wrote about her love and loyalty to Cindy in *How to Cope Better When Someone You Love Has Cancer.* As I said in that book, "Who of us could not use a Linda in our lives?"

Cindy's saga continued, and she had a radical double mastectomy after a course of chemo in 2011. She decided not to have reconstructive surgery because, "I had to get my ego out of the way to mobilize all of my energies to fight the cancer." Linda was right there again, taking her to all doctor and chemo appointments, welcoming her into her home post-surgery for rest and recuperation, and giving her the kind of TLC only "nurse" Linda could provide. Cindy's adult daughter, Holli, was right there too, for much physical and emotional support. Holli as well as Cindy's son, Justin, wanted to quit school to be there for her, but Cindy would not allow it.

I am sure that by now, just as I was, you are thinking enough is enough for this strong but worn and weary woman. I am sorry to say that is not the case. While working at home on her computer and cell phone, Cindy became unable to focus. By the time she got to the hospital, she had seven more "seizures." Tests revealed her cancer had spread to her brain—Stage III and more tumors than they could count—which necessitated twenty-one radiation treatments, which seem to have taken care of most of the tumors. Cindy expected the rest of them to be neutralized, although she needed even more treatments, including cyberknife radiation.

When I met with Cindy in March 2012, she was trying to get help with what the doctors believed was a benign tumor of her tear duct, which would require surgery at Bascom Palmer in Miami. She was grateful to be part of a research study, thereby avoiding the costs. It just doesn't stop for Cindy and hasn't since she was a child. The good news is that her surgery was successful. Next on her seemingly never-ending "to do" list was cyberknife for the three remaining tumors in her brain. That seems to have gone well too.

Nonetheless, her resolve and voice of reassurance was strong. She said:

> I have a life to live, and this little thing called cancer isn't going to prevent it. It's just going to take me the long way around the block instead of the usual and normal path that I would rather be on. Anyone who knows me knows that I am a survivor—undeniably tough and driven and will not stop no matter how hard the times will become. I do write poetry, read uplifting books, pray, meditate, use visualizations, and talk to

myself a lot. Sometimes I just live and breathe by the look in my children's eyes; or the sound of their voices on the phone, and the angelic hope, love, and support of my siblings and friends.

Please know that up until this point I have left out many of the difficult and demanding details of Cindy's story, including the fact that after she was diagnosed in 2001, her mother and sister were in a horrific car accident, which instantly took her mother's life. I have also chosen to not go into great detail regarding the difficult side effects as well as the physical and emotional scarring she repeatedly suffered from her treatments. I completely left out any discussion of the men she jettisoned in 2001 and 2010 because they had too much on their plates and would not be able to support her needs.

Nor have I shared how ashamed and overwhelmed she was to tell her family that she had cancer again and then again. She says, "How do you tell your kids that you have cancer again, and how can you possibly upset their lives by telling them that it moved to my brain now?" She ultimately did do that, and it was possibly the most difficult pain of all that she has endured.

Nonetheless, Cindy remained positive, spiritual, and empowered. She once emailed me and said, "Open your windows and let the fresh air in." I did better than that and went for a walk in the park to let the fresh air clear my head from writing this story about the amazing and positive Cindy—the poster person for a strong voice of positive self-talk and for not letting anything control her or block her way—ever! In a recent email, she said, "As Mary Poppins said, 'Once it's begun it's half done. The hardest part is just getting started.'" Cindy knew both how to get it started and how to get it done—just call her Mary P.

But alas, Cindy's brain tumors could not be eliminated or contained. She passed peacefully in May 2013. For twelve years she fought one heck of a "DAM STRONG!" battle to be a survivor for as long as she could, for the good of her children. Her strength, optimism, and resilience can inspire and empower you in many different ways. Her positive self-talk made her journey easier for her family and friends, as well as for herself.

In Sum

I fully understand that people in Cancerville will struggle with staying in the positive zone. Like Susan, you will have periods of optimism followed by times of worry, upset, and, yes, pessimism, hopelessness, and negativity. I encourage you to increase the former and reduce the latter whenever possible. No one expects you to always be in good spirits. My hope is to help you talk to yourself in more positive ways more of the time, just like Cindy does every day.

I want you to try to do everything you can to look past the negativity of this place and believe it is only temporary, conquerable, and life-saving. You need to try your best to see yourself as a survivor. It is important to do that for your physical and emotional well-being, insuring that this yin and yang team is flowing together harmoniously.

The more you can embrace realistic optimism and its helpful sidekick, positive self-talk, the less difficult and demanding your time in Cancerville will be and the more you will be able to be there for yourself in every way possible.

Let's move on to help you use more positive self-talk to offset any depressed feelings you may encounter. There may be times you will feel temporarily debilitated, but hopefully not clinically depressed.

CHAPTER 13

I will try my hardest to bounce back emotionally.

Dealing with Depression, Debilitation, and Distress

D epressed feelings in Cancerville are like wild weeds in a garden—unwanted and unhelpful, but something that usually comes with the territory. How could it be otherwise? There is nothing positive about being in Cancerville except for receiving treatment and support once you are there. But knowing you have cancer is obviously and undeniably depressing. Having those feelings is natural and appropriate—really!

I am not trying to talk you out of experiencing those kinds of feelings. My desire is to help you vent them appropriately so you can push past them, know when you might need some professional support, and remain focused on the brighter side of your life and your future.

It is important for you to not allow the paralyzing effects of depression to set in and block your way. Those "weeds" of depression need to be pulled so that you will be free to act, move forward, and smell the fragrant flowers that are all around you.

The Many Frowning Faces of Depression

When I think about all the people with depression who have visited my office throughout the years, I realize just how complex this word and associated feelings can be. For example, I have met people whose lives suggested they would be happy, but they were miserably depressed. I have also met people whose lives gave them every reason to be miserably depressed, but they were not. I've even met people going through Cancerville who were not particularly depressed. Eileen and her family from Chapter 1 are prime examples.

To make matters even more confusing, I have observed depression take on many forms in terms of the behavior it promotes. Some can't eat when they are depressed, while others can't stop eating. The same goes for sleeping—some are up half the night, while others want to continually sleep Rip Van Winkle-style. I have even met a few people who crave sex when depressed, even though most dealing with depression are not very interested in that activity. In some people depression and glop become paired in a hard to break loop of negativity. Others take charge of their lives, like a Marine in boot camp, when depressed.

Going a step further, depression sometimes partners with anxiety or tag teams with anger—sometimes all three are present. We will discuss anxiety in the following chapter and anger in the one after that. The word depression, like the word cancer, has many dimensions and associated issues. Neither word is clear or precise, and both summarize many different conditions. The word depression relates in one way or another to a person feeling sad, down, lethargic, unhappy, and the like. People who are depressed have, for whatever complex of reasons, lost their interest, enthusiasm, and zest for life. For that person, most everything is a bummer and a downer.

The Emotional and Physical Dynamics of Depression

As we know, cess can make a depressing mess as it pours through or over our dams onto our conscious functions such as our thoughts, memories, communications, etc. Depression has the potential to distort all of these conscious functions. As I have said, Cancerville is a cess generator that stirs up existing cess while adding a whole bunch more. From issues of mortality to those that deal with the practicality of managing its unique demands, Cancerville adds gallons of cess to your already quite full pool.

As I previously described in my own situation, the combination of old and new cess joined forces and initially wiped out much of my dam, leaving anxiety and depressed feelings in its wake. It took me a while to get to "DAM STRONG!" This is why it is so very important for you to counterbalance all that cess-based pressure with venting and healthy dam-strengthening activities, which we will discuss in Part IV.

In addition, we now know that brain chemistry plays a very significant role in creating emotional agitations of all kinds, including depression. Malfunctions in the delivery of neurotransmitters such as Serotonin or Dopamine can deprive people's brains of those much-needed chemicals. Modern mind meds can be miraculous. That said, taking medications is not always a clear or simple process and requires adjustments by a psychiatrist to find the right medication(s) and the helpful dosage(s).

As a psychiatrist once told me, "Every brain is unique and reacts differently." For this reason some people swear by the very same medicine others swear at! I believe that, just as cancer treatments are becoming more precise, we will see more accurate measures for mind medications in the future. This will allow for a more scientific approach to identifying which brain type can benefit from which medicine(s).

It is important to note that the most common cause of neurotransmitter breakdowns is stress. Few events in life are as stressful as entering Cancerville, which is why it is common for people to feel depressed there. The many sources of stress and strain in Cancerville can simultaneously affect dam stability and brain chemistry.

It is important for you to be both vigilant and honest with yourself as you journey though Cancerville. Consider seeking emotional and/or medical support if you find any of the following to be happening:

- significant difficulty sleeping, eating, concentrating, and/or performing other basic life functions

- wide-ranging mood swings within short periods of time

- spending too much time in bed

- long-lasting tearfulness

- fighting constantly with everyone

- losing faith, hope, or an ability to be positive

- an inability to enjoy anything

- using glop regularly

- inability to distract yourself or find a way to relax and calm down

- thoughts of hurting yourself in any way

We will discuss the value of seeking professional help in Chapter 19, "Having a Counselor and/or Support Group in Your Corner."

Distinguishing Between Depression and Debilitation

Although subtle at times, it is important that we distinguish between being depressed in a clinically diagnosed sense and being debilitated in Cancerville. The former requires treatment and support, while the latter requires time to heal.

Just before treatment and while you are wrestling with any side effects from it, you may feel debilitated. You might experience fatigue, nausea and vomiting, difficulty eating, pain, mouth sores, and the like. These do not make for a zippity-doo-dah-day. When you feel awful physically, you tend to feel that way emotionally too. Physical discomforts weaken people's dams as if terrorists were bombing them; Cancerville treatments do just that.

An important measure is in your resilience. If the emotional symptoms lessen as your physical symptoms lessen, it is likely that you were weakened by the physical discomforts—you were temporarily debilitated. If the emotional down feelings linger after your discomforts dissipate, however, it is more likely that you are dealing with depression. Then again, if you know you will be facing yet another round of chemo, radiation, or whatever in two weeks and again and again for a while, it is not easy to distinguish between depression and debilitation. This is where a professional can help determine what is going on and, even more importantly, help you contain the cess and strengthen your dam. What we call it is not as important as actually addressing and overcoming it.

More D Words—Distress and Demoralization

We mental health folks are really good at coming up with descriptive words; put ten of us in a room and we can generate words at the same rate Cancerville generates cess and stress. If I'm in the room, many will all start with the same letter. In the September 2011 issue of *Psychiatric Annals,* the focus was on Depression and Cancer. One article was entitled "Distress, Demoralization, and Depression in Cancer Survivorship." It quotes the National Comprehensive Cancer Network that defines distress as an:

> ...unpleasant emotional experience of a psychological...social, and/or spiritual nature, that may interfere with the ability to cope effectively with cancer, its physical symptoms, and its treatments. Distress extends along a continuum ranging from common, normal feelings of vulnerability, sadness, and fear, to problems that become disabling such as depression, anxiety, panic, social isolation, and existential spiritual crises.

I think the idea of a continuum is very important as it gives us a perspective from which to evaluate your situation.

The article describes a simple Distress Thermometer that asks people to rate their level of distress from one (no distress) to ten (intense distress). The authors feel that a person with a score of four or more could benefit from additional professional evaluation, assistance, and support.

I encourage you to think about your level of distress, rate it, and write it down. Do it again next week, and if your score is higher than four both times, consider talking to someone about what you are dealing with and what you are feeling. Perhaps you are already doing that—good for you! Put that into your pride bank with everything else you are using to fight back in Cancerville.

The article goes on to talk about the paradoxes that can occur in Cancerville:

> A person can feel profoundly sad and vulnerable after a cancer diagnosis, but still appraise his or her ability to cope with cancer as optimal and therefore experience only mild distress. On the other hand, a patient could have robust resources, but still appraise his or her ability to cope as inadequate and experience a great deal of distress.

One of my many goals in writing this book was to help you cope better, and I certainly hope that is the case so far. The more you feel you are able to cope, the lower your level of distress and dis-ease. This is also self-reinforcing. The more I was able to cope with Jodi's situation, the more I felt I was more able to cope. In other words, the more you can go "balls to the walls" positive, the bigger those "balls" become. In case you are wondering, those words aren't in the *Psychiatric Annals* just yet, but you just never know what the future holds in store!

The article goes on to describe distress that creates a feeling of demoralization; this can result when the patient feels he or she is not meeting expectations. Such feelings tend to occur as people begin or conclude treatment because of the unknowns that are involved. Many of us can be very harsh and critical of ourselves, especially when the demands of a situation are unclear. Instead of giving ourselves an A+ for effort, we sometimes give ourselves a grade of D or F. Ironically, when it comes to others, we can be very generous markers. Sad to say, many of us are much harder on ourselves.

Please try hard not to be so hard on yourself. As I have said right from the beginning of our walk together, there is no right way to do Cancerville. There is no grade at the conclusion of your treatment—there is just your way of coping. No one counts how many times you fall off the mountain or the horse named Hope. What counts is that you gave Cancerville a good fight and took it on in every way you were able. What really counts is that hopefully you survived the ordeal and will for a long time to come.

Real People Facing Cancer

Patrick and Chris

Some "coincidences" are even more amazing than others. Patrick and his brother John were total strangers when they walked into our apartment in Jupiter, Florida. They had come via a very circuitous route. Pat was the creator, worker, and narrator of a TV show whose crew remodeled homes that were in need of a makeover. Our apartment definitely qualified, as it was vintage 1982.

When Pat sat down on the couch, he looked over at a book sitting on the table. It was my son's copy of *How to Cope Better When Someone You Love Has Cancer*, which he was rereading. After picking the book up and realizing I was the author, Pat looked as if he had seen a ghost. He literally turned pale and said to John, "Look at this book. Can you believe that?" Ronnie, our son Mike, and I wondered what had just happened. Patrick then said:

> I can't believe the coincidence. My best friend, Chris, has cancer and I have been supporting him emotionally every step of the way. I need your book. So does John. Our sister-in-law has been battling cancer for ten years. Our whole family needs a copy—and I am one of twelve children.

I calmly shared my "no coincidences" mantra. This led to a fast friendship between us as Cancerville brought us together with common threads and compassion as bonding agents. Of course, when I walked them downstairs, I gave them both a copy of the book. I'm still waiting for an order from their siblings!

Pat invited us to dinner one Friday evening and only he and Chris were present. Chris grilled the steaks while he shared some of the details of his situation. There was no doubt in my mind that this chapter belonged to him. When he was told four years ago that he had two years at most to live, this strong and strapping father of five fell into a "couch potato" depression. He was diagnosed with prostate cancer that had spread to his bones and his liver. The doctors did not hold out much hope. Chris said:

> I didn't do much back then. I was out of work on disability and just sat around staring into space or blankly watching TV. I also slept a lot as it was a great escape from my 'death sentence.' For my whole family and me it was a rollercoaster of emotions.

This is where Patrick jumped in. He shared that:

> Chris has been my best friend for sixteen years. He was like a brother to me even though I didn't need another sibling. His kids and mine grew up together, and we were one big happy family until this happened. There was nothing he wouldn't do for me or vice versa. I wasn't going to just let him sit there and die.

So Patrick, a tall and strong man himself, literally and figuratively lifted Chris up off the couch. He bought him a set of golf clubs and forced him to learn the game and play with him regularly. When Pat had errands to run or places to go, he had Chris go along with him. Though Chris was receiving chemo every three weeks in upstate New York where they are from, he would fly to Florida the following day to help out on the set of Pat's makeover show. Chris says:

> Pat never left my side the whole time. He wouldn't let me sit around the house. He forced me to do stuff, and it helped me to get back in the game. And here I am feeling okay and alive. It is important to stay busy, distract yourself, and focus on life—not death.

Clearly Pat was Chris' angel. Perhaps he learned from his own health issues (diabetes and heart problems) that taking action trumps taking life and death predictions too seriously. In getting Chris off the couch any way he could, he forced Chris to get in touch with the fact that he was still alive and needed to live his life, rather than waiting around for his death.

When I met Chris, there was no sign of any depression. Loving friendship and distraction had cured that and replaced it with a joy for life and a belief that his life is far from over. In fact, I believe he would say that his life is just beginning in a way that gives him a whole new spin on feeling grateful every day—for his family and for having a friend like Patrick, to whom he may very well owe his life.

In Sum

Whatever D word we choose to call it, Cancerville can easily take you down. If you sense you are drifting too low, please seek professional evaluation and support. A point I make repeatedly is that no book is a substitute for face-to-face assistance and support.

Positive self-talk and realistic optimism work against all these D words—please try to draw from them whenever you can. The tools that are still to come can help too. Try to find a variety of vents to release all the cess that comes at you in Cancerville. Try your best to be patient with and kind to yourself—you deserve that and more as you journey these difficult roads and tall mountains. Try your hardest to be just as you would be with someone you love if that person were in your situation.

Now let's turn our attention to yet another emotional hurdle in Cancerville. It is easy to feel anxious there, but our goal is to channel your energy into healthful, helpful, and hopeful directions.

CHAPTER 14

I will strengthen my voice of reassurance.

Calming Your
Fears and Anxieties

C ancer is the proverbial "monster" hiding quietly in the back of the closet until it comes out and enters your life. At that moment, it becomes an anxiety-provoking force and a source of much tension and terror. It overwhelms you because it has you in its grip.

I want to help you get a grip and assume that with your medical team leading the way, Cancerville's hold will greatly lessen over time. The power of positive self-talk, which we previously discussed, is very helpful in calming your anxieties, as it guides you toward more optimistic beliefs. Remember that little engine and jump on board as we slowly climb up the steep hills of Cancerville saying, "I know I can, I know I can!" I choose to believe that you can.

When Two Scary Places Collide

As I have openly shared with you, I entered Cancerville in a highly charged emotional state, as the parent of a patient. Just return briefly to the Introduction to get back in touch with my overwhelming angst. Frankly, I doubt you want to read that again. I certainly don't; both Ronnie and I cringed whenever it was time to edit that part of the book. For me, Cancerville started as a rough ride, which makes the Introduction a rough read. Upon arrival into Cancerville I was exploding emotionally, like a grenade. Of course, Ronnie won't let me put that word in, once again, before "exploding," but I do believe that it belongs there. Go ahead and insert it into the text on your own. You don't have to listen to Ronnie—but I do!

In Chapter 10, "How Minds Work," I also shared why my dam collapsed and my cesspool flooded over upon entering Cancerville by proxy. This was because of how I had been programmed from early on as well as the many losses I had experienced over the intervening years. Anxiety was dripping all over my mind and body and stripping me of much needed energy. I crashed into the wall surrounding Cancerville and burst into flames like an out of control racecar at the Indy 500. Like the affirmation says, I worked hard to find my voice of reassurance. In this chapter I am trying hard to encourage and help you find yours.

Like Anxietyville, Cancerville can be its own unique chamber of agitating inner torment. In Cancerville, your worries and concerns are typically based in reality. They are not ridiculous, distorted, or exaggerated, as they are in Anxietyville. Cancerville is frightening for good reason. Your challenge, however, is to keep your fears from becoming overwhelming. When that happens, your mind races and your mood rapidly declines. You can't engage comfortably in the most basic functions such as eating, sleeping, talking clearly, planning, or managing all the demands of Cancerville. If that happens, you may need some added professional help, a support group, or meds, but let's try to prevent such an overload from shutting down your emotional circuit breakers. You just can't afford to have a blackout, or even a brownout.

The way I converted from terrified to tolerant in Cancerville was by following just about all of the suggestions you will find in this book. I journaled every night, did relaxation exercises, reined in my rage, stopped the pity party, built up my voice of positivism and reassurance, and took charge of my emotional system. I also kept my sense of humor and distracted myself in helpful and healthy ways. I came to own the land in the same way I want you to strive to do. Slowly, but surely, I became "DAM STRONG!" and I want you to feel that way too.

Your goal in Cancerville is to try to manage your stresses and fears and to not get caught up in any serious or disruptive levels of anxiety, such as panic attacks and the like. The former are difficult enough to cope and deal with on a daily basis; the latter can be crippling.

Taking Care of You

Avoiding high levels of anxiety requires taking better care of you—your physical and emotional well-being are important parts of the healing equation. I have observed that when people let themselves go, their anxieties rise as their dam falls and fails to contain their cess. Surely, I was the poster boy in that department; I speak from experience! I am not bragging but just admitting that, at times, my dam was sagging and I was gagging on a mouthful of angst. I am hopeful that won't happen to you. However, if it does, I am optimistic you will be able to use my words and suggestions to strengthen your dam quickly—just as I did.

Try to take better care of you in the simplest of ways. Make sure to eat something on a regular basis if you can, even if it is light. Try to get adequate sleep to recharge your "dam" batteries. Seek out dam supports such as those that will be described in Part IV or any others that can help you to disengage or be distracted from Cancerville whenever you can. Answer your anxieties with a voice that reassures you of positive, day-at-a-time steps forward. By all means, bypass the "bars" in cancer centers or outside them and any other forms of glop. Those may temporarily reduce your anxiety, but it will then take it up a notch or three. I know this all sounds easier said than done, but try your best to get it done. Healthfully supporting yourself will help you in many ways.

Though it is not always possible, try to avoid people, places, and things that agitate your cess. That said, I fully understand that some of the people in Cancerville, the place itself, and the things that happen there are all major agitators. This is all the more reason to escape from time to time, in any healthy way that you can, and to draw upon the tools and supports that I will discuss in Part IV.

In addition, be aware of the anxiety generated when we feel "stuck" in any way. In Cancerville, the likelihood is you will feel very stuck and trapped in a place you don't want to be. Those feelings make sense, really. Reducing your feelings of being stuck is part of taking care of yourself. It will be calming and salving for you to think about your stressful time there as being temporary. In addition, picturing more pleasant and positive scenes beyond Cancerville will enable you to visualize yourself getting back to more comfortable times. The more you can see the proverbial "light at the end of the tunnel," the less you will feel stuck and trapped inside the tunnel.

Making Fear Work for You

As anyone who has experienced high levels of anxiety can attest, those uncomfortable and overwhelming feelings consume a great deal of energy and block a person from operating at full capacity. The unknown, and all that goes with it, typically pushes anxieties to all-time levels of intensity. Because Cancerville is most definitely unknown central, you may experience some of the highest levels of anxiety you have ever encountered. At the very time you need all the energy, focus, and coping you can muster, anxiety becomes a force with which you need to reckon.

Trying to reassure yourself becomes an undeniable challenge, but one that you can achieve. Dig deep inside by reminding yourself of other times in your life that your skeptical, negative voice of doubt tried to take charge. Realize that it was not an accurate voice then and isn't necessarily now. You can override it with a more realistically optimistic and reassuring voice at this time.

During times in the past when your anxiety took over, you probably compensated by increasing your effort. You studied, worked, and tried harder to do your best to prevent your anxious and negative anticipations from influencing the results. In all likelihood, most of the time you achieved your goal.

Though you don't have as much control in Cancerville, your fear can serve a similar purpose. It will motivate you to be present, focused, and on top of everything you can be for yourself. Your fear will also convert to action, which, as we have already discovered, is your trump card to override difficult emotional times. When in doubt, do something, and hope it will be helpful.

This takes us right back to Eileen's rollerblading that sunny morning. Watch a movie, phone a friend, buy yourself the equivalent of a "Pinky," or anything else you'd like and can afford. My guess is that Jake's fear motivated him to make pretty cards for the other children who were stuck in Cancerville with him. Fear pushes us to adapt, take charge, and take on Cancerville with all of our might. It is those very fearful feelings that improve our slingshot aim. Our hands may sweat and shake at times, but our aim is right on target.

Similarly, Susan's initial fears had her welcoming the surgery that would get those cells out of her ASAP. Subsequent fears about the chemo protocols not working sent her to different cancer centers to obtain additional feedback regarding trials that could help fight off her aggressive cells. Many have shared with me that their anxieties gave them the strength and courage to endure major and painful surgery, disruptive chemotherapy, and whatever else was required in their search for the cure.

I never asked Jodi, but my guess is her fears brought out the sure-footed parts that allowed her to dance the most demanding "routine" of her life with energy and grace. My fears led me to challenge my initial meltdown every step of the way and work hard to override my earlier cesspool programming. Ronnie's fears motivated her to be present at every doctor meeting, armed with her list of questions. Fears and anxieties can paralyze us if we allow them to, or they can energize us to rise to new heights. Each of us has many choices in how we overcome our fears and "power up" our voice of reassurance.

The two chapters on optimism and positivism can be drawn upon as counterforces to your anxieties. Whenever possible, use them as vaccines to insulate, inoculate, and immunize yourself so all that worry can be kept, if not completely in check, at least in balance. Talk to yourself as you would reassuringly talk to and encourage a friend in a similar position. Reassure yourself, realistically, that all will likely be well.

For those whose voice of reassurance has never been that strong, know that it can be strengthened just as optimism can be learned. I believe Dr. Seligman would agree that being able to be self-reassuring is an important part of becoming more optimistic. Start by talking positively to yourself, even if you don't believe all that you are saying. Keep talking that way, repeating the self-reassuring, positive self-talk mantras. Sooner than later, you will become more of a believer in the power and credibility of your own words.

Getting to Calmer Space

I know personally that it is definitely possible to start out in the sky is falling—Chicken Little—position and move slowly, but surely, toward soaring like an eagle. We are very adaptive, especially as we rise to take on Cancerville. Even if you catch yourself moving in a less than positive or reassuring direction, you can reverse course. You can gently bring yourself back to more neutral and reassuring thoughts and feelings.

Try to consistently flood your mind with positives. Think about the credentials of your medical team and their earnest efforts and determined, dedicated devotion to your cause. Focus on the research teams discovering new treatments and better ways to deliver them; think about the miracle cures and spontaneous remissions. I read about a man in Germany who was diagnosed with leukemia and HIV. The doctors mixed multiple treatments together, and he is now free of both diseases. He is the first person to be cured of HIV. Remind yourself that new technology is continuously entering Cancerville to shore up and expand its present artillery.

Think about all of the different heavies that you never, ever think about the way you have been thinking, worrying, and obsessing about Cancerville. Coincidently, a man who looked to be in his forties passed by where I was sitting and writing the above words. He could barely walk as he, not so easily, dragged three hundred and fifty or more pounds along. He didn't appear to be worried and anxious that he might drop in his slow tracks at any moment. Nor did he appear to be depressed to the point of missing a meal. The woman walking with him did not seem terrified or down about what appeared to be his serious risk factors either.

Some of us face far more real and present dangers to our lives every day than Cancerville poses and don't give them serious thought or concern. Even Dr. Oz admitted to dragging his tush to avoid getting his colonoscopies in a timely or protective basis. I admire his effort to get us off our butts by being so forthright.

Gaining Strength from Others and Giving it to Them Too

Another source of reassurance can come from the strength of your family and friends. Estelle, Dani's wife, said, "Our strengths played off each other. He never complained, was easygoing, proactive, and always hopeful. He gave me strength and courage and we also prayed a lot." Dani said, "Estelle was always there for me in every possible way. She took such good care of me, came to every doctor appointment, and stayed with me when I was in the hospital. She supported my survival in every way."

Shelly, my colleague for many years, told me that her husband, Mike, was diagnosed right after they were married. She said, "He was the most positive, optimistic person I knew and always believed the treatment would work. That was contagious for me and helped me through the many ordeals we experienced. He helped me become a stronger and more positive cheerleader for him."

Over and over again, I have observed people with cancer becoming even stronger than they were before. Just about all the people I've known who were diagnosed with cancer have met Cancerville squarely. Although Jodi may have cried those understandable elephant tears while walking to the operating room, overall she demonstrated a degree of strength in Cancerville that raised the bar for facing and owning its land. My daughter stared it down better than I could have!

Jodi sucked it up, rarely complained, and moved steadily forward like the beautiful and spirited dancer she has always been. She followed the chorus line of Cancerville gracefully, just as she has done in all areas of her life. The same is true of all the people going through Cancerville that I've had the privilege of knowing. People with cancer show their physical and emotional muscle over and over again in a very courageous fashion. I am confident that you are and will continue to do the same.

Real People Facing Cancer

Linda K.

Time seems to evaporate for me like a can of fizzy soda left open for too long. This is probably why I feel forty something even though I am seventy years young. So when Linda K. told me the other day that we had known each other for twenty-two years, I was surprised. We met in my office all those years ago, when she was wrestling with panic and anxiety. For reasons you now understand from Chapter 10, I have been the local panic guru all these years. Our work together and her strength helped her to get relief within three months and overcome her panic attacks within three years. Linda is one determined person. Like Susan, Linda has popped in and out over the years for a "booster shot" and/or a "battery charge."

Twelve years ago, Linda more than popped back in. She came to tell me that she had been diagnosed with breast cancer. She was understandably anxious and agitated, but that is most appropriate when facing a challenging and life-threatening illness. Panic attacks involve feeling high levels of anxiety for no reason; when first entering Cancerville, anxiety is understandable for good reasons.

But Linda did not go wild. She did what she always does by taking charge in a strong and strategic way. She identified doctors who were expert, kind, and reassuring. She phoned at least six total strangers, whom she found through friends and relatives, to gather information about their experiences with breast cancer. She also researched as thoroughly as she could back then and learned what to expect in terms of surgery and healing. This computer professor set a goal of returning to teaching in ten days after her mastectomy and she achieved it. Like many, Linda gives much credit to her family and friends for being there for her.

Linda's husband, Todd, a CPA and attorney by profession, as well as a shrewd poker player, was "all in" for her. When she came home from the doctor with her not so good news, they sat on the floor. He told her they would go through cancer together and that she and they would be okay. He was by her side all the way. He also scheduled visits with family and friends once Linda was home for a few days. In the organized way an accountant does things, a different visitor came and brought and ate dinner with them each night. In addition, Todd and Linda's best friend, Silvia, made phone calls that were too emotional for Linda to make at the time.

Linda also remembers, with a few tears of love and appreciation, the many people and professionals in Cancerville who reached out to her. Her surgeon said, "This is my expertise. Follow what I say, and you will be okay." The tech who injected a dye that checks lymph nodes yet is so excruciatingly painful that it temporarily makes you want to die, held her hand as she was prepped for surgery and reassured her that she would be fine. Her plastic surgeon literally jumped through hoops to help and be there for her, as did the stranger who saw her pain and suffering in the doctor's waiting room post-surgery and offered her turn so Linda could get checked and get home. This left a deep impression on Linda too. For many years now, Linda has been the one to say, "Go before me. I know how you feel. You will feel better soon."

Linda credits me for being there for her as well during this anxiety-provoking time and I appreciate her kind words. What I remember all these years later is her strength. She met Cancerville head-on and took charge of this strange and strained land. I also remember saying over and over the following mantra: "If you need what you call 'a slice of Klonopin' every now and again, that doesn't make you a drug addict." We anxiety and panic prone people can be so silly when it comes to meds. I don't even like to take an aspirin, and if my wife gives me two, I accuse her of going after my life insurance. Linda used her anti-anxiety/panic meds sparingly and only at critical times, but they helped her. There is absolutely nothing wrong with that, as anxiety prone people like to stay "in control" and are not likely to become abusers. Linda never did; if anything, she took too little medication to support her.

Of interest is that Linda credits having a melanoma at age twenty-five with helping her stay optimistic during her struggle with breast cancer. She still has a long scar on her leg to remind her of this earlier experience, but having beat cancer once helped her to see that she could have cancer and survive. It taught her many lessons including the one that says you just have to get back into the game of life and assume you will be fine. Such positive anticipations salve anxiety and promote calmer living. So did the massages Linda had during this time. Linda's daughter, a college student back then, also helped tremendously. Her strong and soothing presence prior to surgery kept Linda's fears and tears in check.

I think Linda would sum it up this way and you can be sure if I am off the mark, the college professor in her will be quick to correct me:

> I've been to Anxietyville and fought back with my family and friends help, including Bill's, I won that battle. Cancerville challenged me once again, but I learned from my previous experiences that you just have to summon your energy and your courage, and get emotional transfusions from those who love you.

> It has been twelve years now, and I never looked back. I may still have my anxious moments here and there, but I have tools, friends, a sliver of Klonopin, and my family and myself, and I will be okay and so, I pray, will you. If you need support, call me and I will be there for you just as others were there for me. Try not to feel anxious—feel empowered by those around you and by your own inner strength. We anxiety prone people are more powerful than we think and can rise to the occasion when we need to, over and over again.

Dani and Estelle

Dani was diagnosed with multiple myeloma twelve years ago. He was a practicing dentist in Israel when a world famous doctor at MD Anderson Cancer Center in Texas diagnosed him.

"I never panicked," he said, "because nothing really scared me. The doctor was reassuring and said I had time and that the medicines would be very helpful, and more updated ones would be coming along."

Dani was born in Iraq but his family fortunately immigrated to Israel in 1950. I believe growing up and living in Israel teaches people not to panic. There it is—a tiny sliver of a country—surrounded on all sides by enemies, winning every step of the way. It is from that very "fighting back" position that Dani entered Cancerville. He gave that advice to others when he spoke to cancer patients in Israel and offered the same to all of you:

> Survival depends on the patient. People who panic or fade will not win. You have to have the will to survive and succeed and fight this strong disease every step of the way. Cancer is not for the weak—it must bring out your strengths each and every day for as long as it takes to fight back.

Curiously, in Israel, dental students study alongside medical students for five years—then for a year or a little more, they study dentistry. Dani was accepted to med school but liked the more controlled environment of being a dentist. He also didn't want to live the lifestyle of a doctor—on call, in hospitals, life and death, and the like. Paradoxically, that is the very lifestyle he lived for the past twelve years—not as a doctor but as a patient who knew medicine.

Dani's medical training may have prolonged his life. For the first ten years of his disease, he became an avid computer searcher, studying multiple myeloma inside and out. In fact, four years into treatment in Israel, he left his doctor because the doctor couldn't answer Dani's questions regarding new treatment options. He said, "When I know more than my doctor it is time for me to find a new one." That is just what he did and saw him regularly for eight years.

Dani and his family have ridden the horse named Hope many, many times. Like so many people I have met, he did well, then not so well, then well, and then not so well. He had chemo and radiation; had his own blood cleaned, "pressed" and infused back; and received a transplant from his younger brother, who was a perfect tissue match.

Dani was the poster man for miracles over and over. He and Estelle prayed long and hard for these to occur. Each step of the way gave him more courage, which gave him the energy to keep on fighting like an Israeli soldier. They don't give up or get even, and they don't get angry—but they do stay totally focused. Of interest is that Dani's training and medical knowledge enabled him to collaborate with his doctor. He said:

> We discussed options together like two colleagues consulting on a case. He had input and I had mine and sometimes we didn't agree, but he always accepted my opinion. I have tried and rejected some meds a couple of times—and he allowed me control. We speak the same language and he respected my opinion. That is part of the chemistry between us. It has been a collaboration and a partnership. Please don't forget I rejected medicine because I wanted control of my practice and my patients. I needed control of my disease and my doctor has given me that, for which I will always be grateful.

I believe that Dani and Estelle's love for each other, and her being there for him totally and completely for their many Cancerville years, is what fueled Dani's fight. Israel taught him how to fight, and the American Estelle, whom he met in her father's pizza shop in New York, provided him with the ammunition. Let Dani and Estelle be a lesson for us all. Love, along with fearless strength, courage, and determination, can make miracles happen. Estelle and Dani made love, medicine and miracles come to life and in the process kept Dani alive much longer than the statistics they were originally given would have predicted.

Sadly, Dani passed a few months after he and I spoke. New complications had developed, and though he was tired and worn down by fatigue and pain, he did try some additional treatments. Nonetheless, he earned his stripes many times over on the Cancerville battlefield, and he and Estelle can be an inspiration to us all.

In Sum

Please work hard in all ways to prevent Cancerville from weighing you down with high levels of anxiety. I fully understand that striving to steer your mind out of fearful, anxiety-provoking space is not easy. Remember, I am the poster man for panic during my Anxietyville days, as well as anxiety during my early Cancerville-by-proxy time.

I remember how difficult it was to counterpunch and contain my cesspool, which was filled with a lifetime of anxious anticipations and pessimistic feelings—but I did. You can, too, by scoring some Rocky-esque knockout punches to that old fearful cess, as well as to those issues in Cancerville that are frightening you in the present. I am simply encouraging you to try your hardest to push your mind away from your fears and align yourself with your doctors' might as well as the strength of your family and friends. Having this team of support levels the playing field just enough to make a difference.

Now, let's take a look at yet another potentially destructive emotion that can also drain much needed energies. Let's help you rein in your rage and anger.

CHAPTER 15

I will not allow anger to drain me.

Reining in Your Rage

Everyone experiences angry feelings from time to time. Anger is a universal emotion. How we choose to express our anger and whether we manage it appropriately is a reflection of our emotional balance. When a person is screaming, cursing, or punching walls, rest assured that cess is bursting through the dam like a spring flash flood in the Midwest.

Just about everyone in Cancerville feels angry. I do not believe you can be there without periodically feeling and expressing some of that emotion. Everything about Cancerville arouses primal rage. It is an affront to your sensibilities and sensitivities, as it is contrary to all you have come to believe about fair play, especially as that applies to you. I want to explain why this is so and, as importantly, discuss what you can do to keep your anger at more manageable levels.

The Basis of Anger

Generally, people become angry and/or enraged in reaction to the following experiences:

- abuse

- insults

- inequity

- inconsideration

- irrationality

- disappointment

- hurtful consequences

- the unknown

- loss of control

We all want and expect to be treated fairly and kindly. We feel this is what we deserve. While we may all define "deserve" differently in other circumstances, it is likely that in Cancerville we are in much agreement. Just about no one deserves to be in Cancerville or be faced with all that goes with it.

In one way or another, Cancerville has the potential to create just about every issue on the above list. Those are what will fuel your anger, and those are what fueled mine regarding Jodi. Cancer is not supposed to happen to us and life is supposed to be fair. All is supposed to go smoothly and well, and we should be able to all live happily ever after.

These strong but distorted beliefs help us feel safe and secure while wrapped in our delusional blankie. That it has nothing to do with reality is beside the point. When Cancerville rips that blankie away, we react with the same fury and protest as a person who is being denied his or her basic human rights and freedom. In fact, Cancerville is not a democratic place. It is an autocratic, demanding, restricting, and, at times, even punishing place. How could we not be enraged by all of that?

The raging, righteous indignation that I felt, not only on July 8, 2005, but also throughout Jodi's treatment, was based upon a powerful but false belief. Its origin is reflected clearly in my "This cannot be my daughter's turn!" inner scream of denial and lament. I, like most, held on to the strong but inaccurate belief that bad things happen to other people—not to me, my wife, and certainly not to any of my children or grandchildren. It took a while for me to realize the error of my thinking. Susan, as previously mentioned, raised this same issue but quickly realized it was irrational in her "Cancer happens to people, and I am a person" analysis of her situation.

In Chapter 1, I referred to these kinds of distortions as belonging to a form of healthy denial because they allow us all to move freely about the planet. As I have said, this healthy denial enables us to function in our daily lives. If we sat around and obsessively worried about car crashes, we wouldn't give our children the keys to the family car or even have one. If we sat around worrying about the next Columbine or Aurora incident, all children would be home-schooled and all movie theaters shuttered. Certainly, we would be labeled hypochondriacs if we sat around and worried about being diagnosed with cancer or any other serious disease for that matter. When our necessary but inaccurate denial is pierced with negative news of any kind, especially a cancer diagnosis, the result is raging disbelief and disapproval. How could it be otherwise?

Anger and Angst in Cancerville

How could you not be angry, or at least feel some angst from time to time, that you have been forced to enter Cancerville? How could you not resent the intrusion of all of Cancerville's worries, stresses, and cess to your already existing load? Moreover, how can you bypass the bitter and enraged feelings that you are being put through harsh treatments and have been placed in harm's way? Who wouldn't be furious that Cancerville is a reality for you? For those who like to say everything happens for a reason, I'd like them to explain the reason anyone is forced to enter Cancerville. The only reason I can fathom is the randomness of life and cancer cells. It is like hitting a lousy—a really lousy—lottery.

Beyond your initial upset that you are in Cancerville, there are so many possible happenings that will add to your anger and fuel your rage. These include the treatments (some of which may have painful or uncomfortable side effects), waiting to see the doctor, mindboggling bills (independent of whether you or insurance are paying them), medical miscues, insensitive comments by medical staff that are unwittingly made, inadequate and depressing facilities, and so much more.

The Need to Suppress and Express

Talking about insensitive and/or inappropriate comments, a few months after Jodi's surgery, I asked a receptionist a simple question. In response, she made an insensitive comment, which made no sense relative to my question. I, a quiet man, had some pretty angry thoughts. For the good of the cause, I just retreated into the sea of people in the waiting room. That there were so many people in that room was heart-wrenching enough. Sometimes a held tongue is the better option. Whatever I said would have included words Ronnie would not allow me to use in this book. So one coping strategy is just to not get into it, tempting as that might be.

Many people tend to store anger like a squirrel stores nuts. For the squirrel, that behavior gets him through a cold winter. For us, there are times when we need to store and suppress the anger to get us through a potentially cold and hurtful scene. Most if not all of the time, going nuts does more harm than good. Yet it needs to be released in some way, as storing it is unhealthy. That angry cess builds up over time and eventually we implode or explode from its weighty force.

To release the anger I had suppressed toward the receptionist, I journaled like a madman that night because I was a very mad man. It felt good to get it out of my cesspool in an appropriate rant. This helped me let go of it and just move forward! It is important for you to know that there are many avenues to release and vent, only one of which is direct confrontation.

Walking around with a nuclear chip on your shoulder is not conducive to being calm and comfortable. On the contrary, all that chip does is weigh you down and cover your day-to-day life with toxic waste. Those who do store rage regularly often end up with ulcers, high blood pressure, heart attacks, or other physical problems.

In addition to all of the above, anger and rage can too easily lead and feed into depression, which we previously discussed. Though we no longer glibly talk about depression being anger turned inward, anger is still a turbulent force with which to reckon. When that anger has no place to go, it can also turn against us; it fuels our fury and can become an excuse to do glop.

All of our angst can seek out a variety of self-destructive "vents" like a moth heading for a flame. In a counterproductive way, all this does is make everything more difficult and fill us with even more self-directed rage, as well as shame and blame feelings. It is important that we be alert and watch out for vicious cycles of any kind. In life and especially in Cancerville, we need positive cycles.

The Importance of Venting Cess

As you already know, your cesspool wasn't exactly empty before you entered Cancerville. In fact, the likelihood is that it was pretty full, if not overflowing. Adding Cancerville angst to all of that existing cess is likely to send a very strong tidal wave toward your dam, like a tsunami heading right for a slumbering village. It is important, if not imperative, that your dam stands tall during your time in Cancerville, despite the tumult going on inside you. The key to maintaining balance between your cesspool and your dam is to vent your accumulated cess in whatever healthy way is comfortable for you.

Rob raged on his blog about his son's school not allowing him to set up a videoconference so that Jake, at Sloan-Kettering, could have a chat with his chums. He knew the principal would likely see the blog, but he didn't care. But then, in his signature style, Rob took it a step further. He arranged for several of the children to come to his house and did the video chat from there. He first vented his anger and then channeled it into a constructive action that accomplished his original goal. That one-two combination is a healthy way to deal with anger. In many instances, taking action neutralizes your anger by getting something done, rather than your coming undone. Many cancer patients, like Martin from Chapter 7, have created blogs as an outlet for their angst and frustrations.

Susan was furious one day in my office. She was angry at cancer, Cancerville, her pains and fatigue, the chemo that wasn't working, and some important blood test results that were a week late. The latter was pushing her over the edge. She dumped her fury and frustrations onto the floor of my office and left with a renewed sense of taking charge of her situation in an empowered way. Dumping cess in appropriate ways helps us to reduce and better manage our anger.

Talking to a psychiatrist, psychologist, social worker, or mental health counselor is an excellent way to vent angry feelings and receive emotional support at the same time. We will talk more about this in Chapter 19, "Having a Counselor and/or Support Group in Your Corner." In addition to counseling, the following are some other examples of healthy ways to vent frustrations and angry feelings:

Verbal Vents:

- joining a support group

- talking to a close friend/relative

Written Vents:

- blogging

- emailing

- social networking

- journaling

- writing poems, articles, or a book

Artistic Vents:

- painting

- sculpting

Personal Exercise:

- working out

- doing yoga

- punching a bag

- walking, jogging, or running

- jumping rope

- swimming

- hitting golf balls

Group Sports:

- tennis

- racquetball

- basketball

Physical Releases:

- crying or laughing

- ripping newspapers

- punching a pillow

- chopping wood

- using a sauna/ steam room to sweat it out

- loudly rooting for your home sports team

Any of the above activities or others that release pent-up feelings and frustrations, which are not violent, inappropriate, or glopful, are worth drawing upon when you can during your journey through Cancerville.

My personal experience and professional observations suggest that the more we vent our angers, resentments, and frustrations in healthy ways, the more we can release them safely. This prevents them from becoming toxic and polluting us in ways that ultimately lead to self-defeating behaviors, which then convert to shame and blame deposits. This also protects your dam from being weakened by the stored-up cess.

In addition, venting keeps you from allowing your angers to spill out onto other people, most of whom are innocent bystanders. In hindsight, what would my going off on a well-meaning but harried receptionist who wasn't paying attention have accomplished? It would have attracted the attention of a room full of unhappy people. I would have been seen as and felt like a jerk!

Real People Facing Cancer

Christina

Although some survivors I have spoken to minimize the anger they felt upon entering Cancerville, I have to believe I wasn't the only one filled with righteous indignation and a red-hot rage that burned from the inside out and had nowhere to go. It took me a while to convert my useless anger to helpful actions. Christina Applegate and I shared an initial reaction of anger. Upon hearing that she had breast cancer at age thirty-six, she said, "Oh my God. I was so pissed off, so mad... I was just shaking." But then she said, "Immediately I had to go into take-care-of-business mode." This illustrates that the initial anger you might feel upon receiving a cancer diagnosis can be replaced by constructive actions as you seek treatment.

Gilda

Gilda Radner brought her sense of humor to Cancerville, but did have her angry moments. Upon learning from her doctor by phone that she needed thirty radiation treatments after already having had surgery and chemo, she lost it, panicked, and started to yell in a rage. She told her doctor, "I won't do it. Don't you get cancer from radiation? Why are you doing this to me?" She goes on to say:

> Again I was arguing with a man who was trying to save my life.... I went into my room... I slammed the doors in my room and I screamed and swore and yelled. I broke bottles of cosmetics and I threw books against the walls. I tried to pierce the universe with my anger.

How powerful is that last line? Overt or covert, remembered or repressed, or somehow sidestepped, Cancerville can cause us to scream loud and long into the night.

Gilda also talks about a bad fight with her husband, Gene Wilder. She says, "People whimpering and hovering over me made me feel like I was dying. People yelling at me made me feel alive." Interesting! She was one of a kind. It is clear from reading her excellent book, *It's Always Something,* [24] that the twists and turns in her Cancerville journey sometimes threw her into a rage.

When you go through treatments that cause you to suffer and struggle, feel like you have finally reached the "non-finish" line, and then are told "not done just yet," it pushes every button in your need-for-control console; it is not very consoling. If you start to feel rage, feel free to fling some books (even mine) against the wall. Just don't throw my book out the window or sell it on eBay. We are not quite finished just yet!

Geralyn

Geralyn Lucas, whom we met in Chapter 5, could really appear in several other chapters. In her book, she not only shares her panic and tear-filled times but also her rage. As she was leaving the strip club where she went to get in touch with the boob fads of our culture, she left saying, "It is a strange place to finally say good-bye to my right boob, but this whole situation is so fucking uncharted." I am hopeful that quoting the F-word passes Ronnie's muster! More importantly, I hear anger in them there words.

When Geralyn was in her breast surgeon's office instead of being at her news desk at *20/20*, she seethed about how all her hard work to get good grades and a really good job didn't really seem to matter anymore. She says:

> The diploma, the job, the marriage, the future, all feel like they are about to vaporize with that one word: cancer. Now I am getting angry. There is nothing I can do to change the results. This is not about studying, working hard, getting the right answer, charming the right person, or nailing the interview....

Maybe a lifetime of silly worrying could somehow have prepared me for a real catastrophe.

There is much insight in her last sentence. In many ways,
all of your life challenges and your rising to meet them will
help you to meet Cancerville and take it on. Very possibly,
reminding yourself how well you have done in the past will
help you to get past anger and keep riding that horse named
Hope. In a very real sense, anger, appropriate as it might
be, is counterproductive. There is no point in raging against
an unalterable reality; I learned that the hard way. There are
many reasons to face that reality with decisiveness, deliber-
ateness, and dignity.

I hope you will try to lose your anger as quickly as
possible. Replace it with actions, healing, love, and
acceptance, with the goal of ascendance. You, too, can
and hopefully will overcome cancer someday soon and
become a survivor.

In Sum

I hope this discussion will help you to rein in much of your
rage and anger in Cancerville. In addition, there are some
excellent books and workbooks on anger management that
can be supportive.

It is important for you to find appropriate and comfortable
ways to vent and release as much cess as possible. Most of
the time, those build-ups create a variety of unhealthy and
unhelpful consequences. As you now know, too much cess
can cause a mess and much stress.

There is yet another way to vent your anger in a healthy
way. Send me an email at bill@cancerville.com; it may help you
to release pent-up feelings. I promise I will personally respond,
not as a therapist, but as your Cancerville friend and support.

Let's move on to Part IV, which will provide some simple
and practical tools that you can use to be more successful in
achieving the emotional goals I have encouraged.

PART IV

Tools that Help You Tend the Land

CHAPTER 16

I will practice relaxing activities whenever I can.

Relaxing
Tools for Natural Healing

I wondered where I would write this chapter to fully capture the essence of my message. I found that special place in January 2011 aboard a cruise ship that was sailing through Milford Sound, New Zealand at 7 a.m. It was a pristine and peaceful place where mountains and glaciers produced sparkling water-falls and exceptionally low-lying clouds, even on that gray and chilly morning. All of my senses were awake despite the early hour. Classical music was playing softly in the background. My world seemed at peace in that quiet, mostly deserted place.

The Value of Vitaminds and Mental Floss

Although that was a special and unique place, the message of Milford Sound applies to wherever you might be in the world right now and to however you might be feeling today. This message is simply about influencing how you feel by altering your sensory experience.

If for you Cancerville is a cauldron of burning sensations amid jumbled emotions and a deep sense of dread, then the tools in this chapter offer a calmer, gentler, and more peaceful alternative. They encourage you to take a break from Cancerville for a few minutes each day and experience a taste of Tranquilityville. These tools and activities represent the emotional equivalent of vitamins (vitaminds) and dental floss (mental floss). They will strengthen your dam while clearing away the plaque-like buildup of cess from the walls of your mind. They will help lower your anxieties, reduce your feelings of depression, and limit your negative self-talk, while strengthening your voice of hopefulness and optimism. They offer very small doses of peace of mind at a time when those feelings are not easy to achieve.

Most of us are peculiarly paradoxical in a variety of ways. Though many want to feel in control, we don't always take control when those very opportunities present themselves. Hear ye, hear ye, hear ye! The tools and techniques that I am about to describe offer some simple and powerful ways to better control your body and your mind.

Yet just as with taking our vitamins or flossing our teeth, we can be lazy and self-neglecting in the silliest of ways. Many of the tools I will describe only take a few minutes a day to use. Though such a small investment of time can yield such powerful dividends in terms of soothing, calming, and healing feelings, we often shortchange ourselves by avoiding them. In our busifying, dizzifying quest to do and achieve, we can forget to just be and relax—even for just a few minutes.

For those in Cancerville, the typical everyday hustle-bustle is accelerated many times over. There is everything that previously needed to be managed, plus all of the logistical challenges of Cancerville, commingled with enough emotional hurdles to make for an Olympic-sized event. For these reasons, we need to create some powerful and positive sensory experiences. These help us offset the less than lovely images that abound and surround us in Cancerville.

That you don't have much time is clear; but that you have ten to twenty minutes a day for a vitamind or two or for mental flossing is equally undeniable. You will note, as well, that some of these tools really require no time at all for you to take advantage of their benefits.

At a time when the words green and organic have become part of our ideal lifestyle, the following tools fit those natural criteria perfectly. None involve foreign or toxic substances. All are as green as the trees and foliage that grow on the soil-less slopes of the mountains of Milford Sound.

In all of the activities that follow, the goal is to soothe, nurture, and heal the agitation of your mind and body. I am quite sure you are already aware of all of the tools I am encouraging you to try. None are profound, complex, or original. I have not discovered these tools, but I have personally and professionally discovered their multiple benefits. I sincerely hope you will too.

Rather than just list these tools, I want to describe my own experiences with them. I do not expect that all of the tools I use and enjoy will fit your needs. Your goal is not to embrace each and every one; ideally, you will find a few that work for you and will draw upon them as often as you can. You may find one or two that you can enjoy with special people in your life, which will increase its power and meaningfulness.

Passive and Peaceful Tools

This section describes relaxing sensory experiences that take no time and require little energy. They simply provide a calming background to your environs.

Music

I very much enjoy listening to soothing music, either of the spa, classical, or smooth jazz type. I play that music in my home whenever I am there and listen to it when I walk alone in the park. I also have it playing in the background in my office as well as in the waiting room, along with a relaxing DVD. I have never understood why many doctor and dental offices have CNN blaring when soothing images and sounds would be more helpful.

Most mornings, I like to start my day listening to a spa-like meditational music CD in the little library just off our bedroom. I listen while thinking about everything and nothing at the same time. Sometimes a thought may hit me, and I reach for a yellow pad; mostly, I just try to be there, quietly present in this awakening moment.

Whatever type of music relaxes you is fine. You may prefer classical, inspirational, show tunes, or the like; you might be someone who relaxes by listening to rock or rap. My concern is not which music works for you, but that you choose to use music to influence your mood and brighten your spirit.

In today's world, music is easily transportable—no more boom boxes needed! I encourage you to take some pleasant music with you and listen while you wait for doctor visits and/or undergo treatments. This will help you to remain calmer and provide a soothing backdrop to a less than soothing experience.

Other Calming Sounds

I also use fountains, both at home and at my office, for similar purposes. The sound of flowing water is universally calming. Even people who don't enjoy swimming often seek out the relaxing influence of the beach in order to hear the sound of the waves breaking at the shoreline. Brookstone and other similar stores sell machines that play a variety of calming sounds including the ocean, raindrops hitting the roof, or a babbling brook. Smart phones have apps for these as well. All these sounds can induce peacefulness and sleep.

Calming Images

In this same category of passive influences are relaxing DVDs. These show calming images such as aquariums, beaches, sunsets, snowfalls, etc., combined with peaceful music. The only effort they require is hitting the remote. They are very helpful in briefly distracting you from Cancerville and giving your mind a rest.

Candles

In the same vein, I enjoy candles and light them frequently in my office when the fire officials aren't looking. I admit that I failed inspection once because I had one burning in the waiting room. Please don't tell them I still light one on occasion. There is something very captivating about the little dancing flame and the aromatic scents that have a calming influence on our senses. You can experiment to find out which aromas are helpful for you. Please don't bring these with you to your doctor meetings or treatments, but look for ways to put these images on whatever electronic device you use. Is there an aromatic app yet? If not, I imagine it is coming soon.

Calming Environs

Finally, sometimes calm and peaceful feelings arise when we place ourselves in a soothing environment. This was the case for me as our ship made its way through Milford Sound. However, it need not be as exotic, as many opportunities exist closer to home.

I previously mentioned going to Morakami Gardens in Delray Beach, Florida, because this large Japanese garden immediately relaxes me. It is Tranquilityville central! The same is true for my time at the beach in Jupiter, Florida, where I do much of my writing while enjoying the relaxing sights and sounds.

Others report similar pleasant sensations and feelings from a sauna, aquarium visit, concert hall symphony, or spiritual sanctuary. My simple encouragement is for you to take a break from Cancerville from time to time and consciously put yourself in an environment that is relaxing for you. It really doesn't matter what places do that for you as long as you seek out safe and calming spaces whenever possible.

I hope you will try to find some passive and peaceful tools from the above examples or look into others that fit your nature and your needs. There are many vitaminds/mental floss from which you can choose to help you take a brief respite from the stressors of Cancerville.

Active Peaceful Tools

The following tools require more active involvement on your part. The good news is that they are user-friendly and very effective in providing peace of mind. The nice part about these tools is that they are portable and completely within your control.

Muscle Relaxation

Progressive/autogenic muscle relaxation is a very simple and effective tool that I first learned about when I worked at Nova University. A colleague taught me this technique in 1973. I was attached via electrodes to a biofeedback machine that measured and provided audio feedback that showed my level of muscle tension. The relaxation technique simply involves tensing and then relaxing each muscle group. It helps people reduce their bodily tensions very easily.

I have even used an abbreviated version of autogenic relaxation, without biofeedback, in large audiences, and just about everyone in the room enjoyed the experience.

The goal of this relaxation tool is to create a very calm and peaceful alpha brain state. Portable, hand-held biofeedback machines, as compared to the larger ones of old, are available these days. However, I have found that relaxation exercises work very well without the biofeedback; some people I have worked with complained that the biofeedback sound was distracting and/or anxiety provoking.

I used muscle tensing and relaxing to successfully calm my own anxiety back in the 1970s and again in 2005 when I was struggling in Cancerville. I still use it for myself, as well as with people I am currently helping. It has stood the test of time based on its simplicity and effectiveness.

Guided Imagery

Guided imagery has also been a favorite of mine as a relaxation/distraction tool. I still use it to "escape" the dentist's chair by transporting myself to a different place and time. I let the dentist do his or her thing while I visit the beach, the countryside, or some other peaceful and pleasant scene in my mind's eye. I hope you have some pleasant, peaceful scenes stored in your mind's DVR to which you can occasionally return.

The book *Getting Well Again* by Carl Simonton, M.D., an oncological radiologist, and his wife, was previously referenced and is worth reading all these years later. Their program at the cancer center they established in Texas introduced relaxation and guided imagery techniques to their patients. The guided images were all focused on different ways patients could mentally "rid" their bodies of their cancer cells. Some chose a pac-man-like image, others drew upon more aggressive attacks on their cells, while some used more peaceful and healing scenes.

The results of those who used these tools validate incorporating both relaxation and cognitive tools (which we will discuss in the following chapter) as part of your coping program. Those who followed the Simonton's encouragement of regularly using these activities lived far longer than predicted, and many lived out their natural lives, even though the medical team did not expect that to happen.

When you are in the thick of Cancerville, just before getting feedback from a doctor or while having a cancer treatment, these tools work really well. You can sit in the waiting room or treatment area looking at all the other tight and worn faces; or you can close your eyes, go someplace in your mind, and take yourself away. I believe it is important to get away, literally and figuratively, from Cancerville whenever you can. You may need to be there periodically, but you can remove yourself in many different ways whenever you are able.

There are a variety of CDs available with these types of relaxing exercises. This includes my "Zen and Now" remake of a 1980s relaxation tape that has both autogenic and guided imagery exercises. Both are in my voice. There is also a wonderfully relaxing DVD that I made after a visit to Iguassu Falls in South America with some very peaceful video of the falls. Both are available at www.cancerville.com. I am happy to send them to you for the cost of shipping.

Other Peaceful Activities

I also encourage people in Cancerville to see beyond the moment and begin to picture brighter, happier, more comfortable scenes in the future. Though it would have been impossible for me to imagine my family's own fairy tale, which I shall soon share, I did try my best to see more comfortable days ahead, instead of the difficult ones I faced during Jodi's treatment time. In relation to his daring high wire crossing over Niagara Falls, Nik Wallenda said, "Anybody that's dealing with any battle—focus on the other side." I couldn't agree with him more! Talk about a well-balanced guy!

In addition, mindfulness, meditation, yoga, Qigong, Tai chi, and self-hypnosis are all active peaceful tools. They can be mesmerizing in inducing powerful feelings of calm and peace of mind. They distract from the everyday stressors and help us to focus on the now. Many websites, books, DVDs, mental health professionals, and classes exist that can guide you through these activities. Much research on yoga has shown it to have many positive effects for cancer patients, including survivorship.

If you haven't already, I encourage you to explore these tools to see if one can be helpful for you. I do understand, however, that your stressful, task-oriented days generally, and especially in Cancerville, often allow little to no time for relaxation activities. Even though I know you are very busy, I am pushing you to push yourself, from time to time, to take a short relaxation break from Cancerville.

Despite my encouragements, I admit that I have tried several of these pleasant and relaxing activities, but like many people, have not been able to sustain consistent practice and participation. Here, I run right into the doing wall of productive accomplishments that so easily blocks my path. Often, I don't take the time to seek calmer consciousness. An example is what happened to me that morning in Milford Sound. I awoke at 7 a.m. to see and be mindful of the sights of the sound. I found the views and vistas inspiring and quickly started typing rather than just relaxing. Perhaps the answer is that relaxation comes in many different forms for many different people.

Relaxing Distractions

I believe there are times when what we are doing, even if it isn't a specific relaxation exercise or activity, can also contribute to our being calmer and more relaxed. There is no reason to be judgmental about what facilitates our relaxation. For example, isn't it likely that with its clear focus, creative flow, energizing power, and pride bank deposits, writing that morning was as calming for me as being fully mindful of the beautiful vistas?

This leads to the idea that beyond the relaxation exercises I've described, there may be many other activities that can serve a similar purpose for you. Working, working out, or simply having mindless fun can all contribute to calmer feelings. Perhaps your relaxation comes from watching NASCAR, knitting, playing cards, reading, completing a crossword puzzle, or doing something else that you enjoy. I was surprised to learn that the average age of people who play computer games is thirty-seven. In the same vein, the average American watches two and a half hours of TV on weekdays. As long as it is not glopful, it doesn't matter how you recharge your batteries. What matters, especially in Cancerville, is that you do.

Your mind needs some breaks from the tension and tedium. A part of you needs to help yourself disengage from thinking, reading, or talking about Cancerville. You may even want to put down this book and take a break for a while; I will not take it personally.

Try to see these distractions as nutrients for your mind and your dam. That you are in Cancerville may reduce your appetite, but it need not stop you from eating. Neither does it have to stop you from engaging in some emotionally nourishing distractions. Feeding both your body and your mind are very important. Bernie hits this point directly in the Foreword when his friend asks him what he does when he is hungry. Clearly the choice of distractions is yours as are the many rewards that come as a relief, such as a calming and rebuilding of worn out nerve endings, a rekindling of your spirit, and a renewal of your soul.

A Passive and Essential Inactivity

We tend to take a good night's sleep for granted until we have trouble doing it. Then we quickly realize its importance in maintaining our comfortable functioning.

Research has consistently demonstrated that rapid eye movement (REM), also known as dream sleep, helps us maintain our comfort and sanity. People deprived of that in the laboratory for a couple of days literally experience a synthetic psychosis that disappears as soon as they are allowed to dream. People wrestling with anxiety or depression report much stronger symptoms when they haven't had a good night's sleep. Even those without such problems or symptoms drag sluggishly along when their sleep is limited or interrupted.

The same is true in Cancerville. Staring at the ceiling above your bed in the middle of the night does little to recharge your batteries; it is like forgetting to plug in your cell phone. Insomnia, in any form, prevents your dam from receiving a sufficient energy boost. Let's use my model of the mind to understand the important role sleep plays in your day-to-day functioning.

When you go to sleep, so does your dam. It has been working hard all day, is damn tired, and needs to be recharged. While it sleeps, cess is released all over your head. We call the results dreaming. This is why dreams can be so confusing when remembered, as they contain pieces of yesterday and from a while ago, all connected like an abstract, avant-garde movie.

Freud called dreams "the royal road to the unconscious." He felt he could understand what was going on in his patient's unconscious mind if he could interpret the symbolic message embedded in the dream. This may be true sometimes, but in my opinion, the importance of sleep is that cess is being discharged and vented, while dams are being recharged in preparation for tomorrow. This is why when you don't sleep well, you don't feel or function very well the next day.

The various relaxation activities and exercises that I have described can all contribute to a more nourishing night's sleep. They allow your mind to wind down. They induce the kind of brain rhythms that allow you to peacefully fall off to sleep and remain asleep. They literally help turn down your mind and shut down any rumination, which is especially helpful in Cancerville.

I Can't Call This One a Tool

For many people, prayer serves as a calming, relaxing, and inspirational experience. Not only does it connect them to a power greater than themselves, but it also can induce a calming, trance-like state. The nice thing about prayer is that it is portable. You don't have to be in a church or temple to draw strength from it. One can pray anywhere, anytime, and in any way.

In addition, studies have shown that seriously ill people who had others praying for them had a higher survival rate than those for whom no prayers were offered. This was true whether or not the patients were aware that people were praying. Yet independent of those findings, if prayer helps you in calming, healing, and empowering ways, then I encourage you to do just that every day or several times a day for that matter.

In addition, if a symbol of faith or hope can help you feel more empowered, I encourage you to place it in your home, wear it, or carry it in your purse or briefcase. In Cancerville, even something as simple as a rubber band with meaningful words inscribed on it seems to help people feel more powerful and hopeful. That is why I offer a complimentary purple wristband with the statement "DAM STRONG!" with each order at www.cancerville.com.

Real People Facing Cancer

Susan

Yet another Susan who appears in Bernie Siegel's book *Faith, Hope & Healing* seems the perfect person for this chapter. She is an artist who was preparing for a November show when she received the call that she had breast cancer. On the day she was to meet with a surgeon, 9/11 happened, not far from where she lived. She says:

> Craving some perspective on what was happening to my own life and to all of us… the following Saturday I drove two miles to the ocean. A walk on the beach was, for me, a dependable way to find a wider perspective on my life. As I set out, feet in soft sand, the big sky and

steady woosh of the surf brought some calm.
I found a few small feathers. I picked them up
thinking to make myself a healing talisman.
As I walked, I came across and gathered over
three hundred feathers without ever seeing a
bird's carcass.... In a few weeks, as I healed
from the surgery and awaited the start of
chemotherapy, some artist friends would join
me in stringing the feathers for an altar we created to honor all those who died when the Twin
Towers fell.

Here we see Susan putting herself in a calming space to
escape the out of control space that surrounded her life in
Cancerville and in New York City at that time.

Susan and her family did not have an easy journey through
Cancerville. Her daughter tested BRCA gene positive and had
a double mastectomy, and both mother and daughter had preventive ovary removals. Susan, a woman who meditated, ate
healthy, practiced yoga, etc., shuttled back and forth between
her own anger and fears of her body betraying her, and the
abject betrayal of 9/11. She says:

Conflict perpetuates conflict, was my view. If
I wanted the country to respond from wisdom
instead of fear, then how could I not do the
same? I took it as a personal challenge to find
peaceful ways to respond to the inner terrorists
who had attacked my body.

Susan tells of a big old elm tree in her backyard and
describes the birds up above pecking away at the small
insects. This helped her to see her chemotherapy as the little
birds in the tree—a medical cocktail coaxing cancer cells into
early retirement. Here again, she is using powerful imagery to
empower her treatment.

Bernie's reflections on Susan's statements are equally
empowering. He says:

> We all need to develop bells of mindfulness. Like temple bells, the sound gets us to become still, breathe, and find peace…. So create your bells of mindfulness and breathe peace whenever you hear or see the symbol that connects you to a place of serenity rather than interruption and agitation…. When you are grateful for the opportunity to live, life truly becomes a gift…. A walk on the beach or to a stream can create a powerful healing environment. The feathers of fallen angels' wings helped her (Susan) to put her ordeal into perspective.

Susan's choices and experiences as well as Bernie's wonderful words put the relaxing exercises I am describing into perspective. My hope is that you will draw from them or others you come upon as you walk the difficult streets of Cancerville.

In Sum

The enormous fiord-based mountains of Milford Sound, which were warmly blanketed by layers of low-lying clouds, provided peaceful and relaxing sensory images for me. Though that day may have been steely gray, reminding me of the one at Sloan-Kettering, my feelings were lighter and brighter. This was in part because we were, literally and figuratively, distanced from Cancerville. In addition, my already relaxed feelings were significantly enhanced by the calming influence of those majestic images that I still vividly remember.

I hope that in Cancerville you will seek out calming sensory experiences from time to time. It certainly doesn't require a trip across the world. You can purchase a CD or DVD, or you can take advantage of free relaxation materials over the Internet; these can be very helpful to you at this agitating time. My biased view is that it is very important that you find that which helps you relax and/or distracts you from Cancerville and commit to engage whenever you can.

Now, let us turn to other user-friendly tools that help modify negative and uncomfortable thoughts. Negativity in Cancerville can take away from your hopefulness and positive self-talk. To tend to this demanding land, you need to be able to influence and take charge of your thoughts and resulting feelings by nudging them toward a more neutral or even positive direction.

CHAPTER 17

I will try to choose what I think about each day.

Cognitive Tools for Taking Charge of Your Mind

have stressed the importance of maintaining hopeful and positive thoughts and self-talk in the chapters dealing with realistic optimism as well as positive self-talk. The question remains how to help you get there when you are wrestling with all of the difficulties and negativity that Cancerville can present.

Most people are prone to ruminate about issues that upset them in all areas of their lives. When you are in Cancerville, all of that pressure, worry, and concern becomes a major obsessional flood; it is hard to think about anything else. Cancerville shouts at you from a "bully pulpit." I hope the cognitive tools I will share with you in this chapter, as well as everything else we discuss, will help you shout back even louder.

These simple tools will help you keep your mind stronger, balanced, and more able to support your trying Cancerville experience. They will strengthen your dam as you deal with forces that can easily weaken it. Combining these cognitive tools with the relaxation ones described in the previous chapter can make for an even more powerful and protective support net.

We All Have the Same Architecture—More or Less

When I look back over my shoulder at the many people I have talked to and helped in my office for all these years, I clearly see some patterns that have occurred over and over again. We all have the same architecture, as reflected in my model of the mind, even though we are all unique individuals. What vary from person to person are our genes and scenes. Our genome and the contents of our life experiences, which account for our individual natures, are as unique as our fingerprints.

In my opinion, magnificent as our brains and minds are, the design could have been improved upon by the addition of some more direct vents to eliminate cess. Had they asked me, I would have definitely suggested some modifications along the lines of how our bodies eliminate waste. But hey, I never got the email; I wasn't even on the committee. However, the tools in this chapter and the previous one help minimize our cess and keep it from building up.

Please understand that I did not invent the cognitive tools I will be describing, although I did rename them. Also, know that not all of these tools work for everyone and not all tools work all of the time. It is a little like going to the gym for a workout. You won't like or use every piece of equipment, but the more you use a few of these mind-muscle builders, the stronger and more resilient you and your mind will become.

Changing the Channel

Our minds are like TV screens and your challenge is to find the remote; don't even bother looking under the couch pillows. Once you do find and practice using it, you can move the channel to a calmer mental "movie" if your mind wanders into negative spaces.

A Future Movie

It is helpful to picture a time in the future when life will be better, you will be safe, and your life will be back to everyday living. Picture your hair having grown back, having put back the weight lost in Cancerville, or having lost the puffiness that some of the meds can cause.

It was in November when I encouraged Rob to anticipate and picture his son and wife being home from Sloan-Kettering for Christmas. As you already know, under the stressful conditions of Cancerville, minds can go back and forth. After my encouragement, Rob could happily picture his family being together at Christmas, but then think, "OMG, what if it doesn't happen? What if my son is still in the hospital?" This would immediately eliminate and undo the optimistic image and take him right back to negative space.

I suggested that he assume his homecoming would happen and realize that if it didn't, it would not be terrible. It might put a damper on Christmas 2010, but then his happy family homecoming image could shift to Easter and Christmas 2011. Or he could picture having Christmas in January or whenever his son came home. Many soldiers have delayed holidays, birthdays, or anniversaries, as they usually can't get home on cue. The same applies to the "soldiers" of Cancerville.

Rob's family was, in fact, back home in time for a happy and heartfelt Christmas morning. There was no greater or more meaningful gift that day than their being reunited and together. Many of the people I've coached while they were going through treatment found it helpful to visualize a lighter, brighter, more peaceful and joyous time in the future.

A Past Movie

Another useful channel changer, if your mind becomes overwhelmed with negativity, is to replay a pleasant, positive scene from your past. You can draw upon your built-in DVD or DVR player to watch it all again. I can recall "watching" happy family scenes on my personal TV during Jodi's treatment time in Cancerville. It was easy to visualize her arrival day from Korea, her Bat Mitzvah, her dance performances, and many other happy scenes. I am confident that you have many happy and inspiring "movies" that you can draw from to counterbalance the tensions and tedium of the moment.

The faster you mentally leave an unpleasant scene by creating different images, the calmer you can become. The beauty of my mind and yours is its versatility. There are more soothing images you can play on your personal TV than there are channels on deluxe cable TV. Use those to your advantage when your mind "freezes" in the cesspool of Cancerville or, for that matter, becomes stuck in any other muck life throws in your direction.

You have some choice in the pictures you play on your personal TV just as you decide which pictures to rent and watch on your home TV. When you can, try to watch some "happily ever after" movies in your head, just like the Hollywood of old regularly produced. When you need to change the channel, know that you are able to accomplish that very result when you put your mind to it.

Obviously, there will be times in Cancerville when "escaping" in this way is not advisable or possible. For example, I do not encourage you to change the channel in the middle of a tense doctor meeting. However, once it is over and you are back home, more peaceful images may just help calm your mind and move it to more positive self-talk.

Fantasies are Free

Fantasies can take changing the channel to a whole new level of creativity. You can enjoy a fantasy just about anytime or anywhere. Fantasies occur when our minds make a movie about an enjoyable but unlikely event. It is about letting your mind roam freely into any area that you like. People fantasize about being the CEO of a major corporation, the President of the United States, a lotto winner, a beauty queen, or a stud muffin. As I said, fantasies are free. This is true as long as you keep them in your mind. Once you start emailing, texting, or tweeting, watch out as they can easily become very costly.

You can be the producer, director, and star all at the same time and see whatever images you want. Reality has nothing to do with it. Your creative mind can picture anything that serves to comfort, relax, or distract you. Fantasy is a powerful tool to create prettier pictures than the ones you may be dealing with in real life.

I'm not telling you anything you don't already know. You have probably had thousands of daydreams and fantasies since you were a youngster. What I am simply encouraging you to do is go there intentionally at appropriate times when your mind is rumbling like a volcano ready to blow. Feel free to try it and see if you can make it work for you.

Whatever fantasies you create need to be dam building. For example, see yourself writing the next blockbuster book about your favorite hobby or whatever interests you. See yourself getting an award or doing something courageous or important. Picture your garden weedless and in full bloom. See yourself as a survivor who decides to help others in Cancerville.

The point is that fantasies are truly free and can occasionally free you from the heavy burdens with which you are dealing.

Sometimes fantasies can even be a source of inspiration. Remember the one I chose to use in order to write this book in a clear and strong way—"That ball is going, going, and it's gone!"

The D That Comes After ABC

In Chapter 12, "The Power of Positive Self-Talk," I spoke about the ABCs created by Dr. Ellis and his cognitive colleagues. As you recall, A is for an adverse activating event, B for beliefs triggered by the event, and C for the emotional consequences caused by the belief. In this cognitive model, D stands for disputing the belief. We previously contrasted the way pessimists and optimists approach Cancerville using the ABC model. Let's review this again:

The pessimist says...

A:I have cancer.

B:I am not going to survive.

C:I feel depressed, terrified, anxious, and over-whelmed. I can't deal with this.

The optimist says ...

A:I have cancer.

B:Many people survive these days.

C:Although I am not happy I am here, I am hopeful I will get through it. I will do all I need to so I can become a survivor. I assume that will be the case. Period!

As I have previously said, my encouragement towards optimism needs to be realistic. There is an obvious and significant difference between a pessimist and someone who has

Stage IV cancer, has cancer that has seriously metastasized, or for whom no chemo is effective. The degree to which you can dispute your negative beliefs is directly related to your situation; ultimately, those realities must be taken into account.

Of course, a miracle or Hail Mary pass, as in Jake's situation can always occur. They do happen, but unfortunately, do not come often enough. Herman Cain, a successful executive and former presidential hopeful did receive a miracle. He had Stage IV colon cancer that had metastasized to his liver and was given a thirty percent chance of survival; he is alive and seemingly well seven years later. He acted quickly and decisively, took charge, had chemo to shrink the tumors, was lucky that what remained were operable, and took advantage of many new procedures.

Similarly, actor Michael Douglas had Stage IV throat cancer and reports being cancer free at the time of my writing. So much for the sadistic statistics I spoke of earlier. In so many instances people, in and out of Cancerville, overcome seemingly insurmountable odds. These miracles are all the more reason for you to dispute your negative beliefs. We will talk about the topic of unrealistic optimism in greater detail in Chapter 26, "On Becoming Even More Empowered."

Cognitive psychologists have found that people can be taught and encouraged to dispute their automatic negative beliefs and move to more positive or at least neutral thoughts. This often demands that we replace those beliefs with ones that are more comfortable, acceptable, and tolerable. In the ABC example, the pessimist needs to dispute his or her catastrophic belief because it can rapidly cause an emotional meltdown. As soon as a shift is made to the more hopeful belief, the emotional tone and reaction change, and the person can move forward.

To dispute your negative beliefs, you need to think and act like a savvy defense attorney. Think of how the famous ones are able to spin potentially damaging evidence against their client in ways that neutralize or even reverse it. Appeal to the "jury" of your mind to allow for alternative beliefs, explanations, and rationales. Be convincing and creative in reprocessing upsetting ideas that will only take you to dark and scary places. Dispute them in every way you can to change and reframe your belief and the resulting emotions. Remember how Benje's sad story about his daughter in Chapter 4 put in perspective Jodi's situation—she had a good chance, while his daughter, most unfortunately, had none.

For example, let's dispute the pessimist's belief that "I will not survive." Here is my disputational dissertation to the jury of your mind:

> Try hard not to be pessimistic, ladies and gentlemen of the jury. We have strong and consistent evidence that, thanks to marvelous medical progress these days, many people survive their Cancerville experience—almost two-thirds become survivors. We have many reasons to be optimistic.
>
> Innovations occur regularly and reliably. For example, the many types of targeted treatments, including those delivered by interventional radiologists, are already being used in effective ways. These provide direct treatment of cancer without many of the unpleasant side effects. Genomic profiling is also allowing a much more person-specific and tumor-specific approach to treatment. Who knows what other advances will be coming soon? I am betting on more and more progress, as the science of cancer keeps being better understood. You need to try to do that as well.
>
> My belief in progress is based upon the adage that the past is often an excellent predictor of the futurefuture—oftentimes the past is prologue. We have seen devastating diseases such as smallpox, scarlet fever, and

polio completely eliminated by the scientific progress of vaccines. In 1952, the year I turned ten, over fifty thousand people were diagnosed with polio in the United States, including a teen who lived on the first floor of my apartment building. Public swimming pools were closed, people avoided large crowds, and parents—especially mine—were frantic. In 2002, the number of diagnosed cases of polio in the United States was zero! Every year, I believe, we get a little closer to eliminating cancer from our world too.

In addition, ladies and gentlemen of the jury, you already know the dedication of your medical team of doctors, nurses, and other professionals. They may keep you waiting, but not wanting. They want to win as much as you do. I dispute your assumption and choose to see things more optimistically. You need to agree and see things my way by finding in favor of your survival. I rest my case and hope it helps you "rest" just a little easier!

I hope this helps you to dispute any negativity that your mind generates and increases your hopefulness and optimism about your outcome in Cancerville.

I also believe that there is a D in my model. It stands for: "DAM STRONG!" power. As we now know, it is our cess that causes us to catastrophize and stay stuck, as if by crazy glue, to pessimistic beliefs. It is our dam that helps us dispute this negativity and reverse it, which allows for realistic optimism and positive self-talk. These, in turn, allow us much calmer and hopeful feelings.

Since no one knows or can predict the future, assume it to be a positive one for yourself; try not to allow negativity to creep into your mind. If you have a pessimistic belief, use your dam to dispute it as strongly as you can. Whether you have a law degree or not does not matter. What matters are the challenges and disputations you submit on your own behalf.

Putting it Away

This tool works for some but not for others. Hard as they might try, some people just can't put their worries away, even overnight. They tend to stick to them as if held in place by cement. Still, I encourage you to give this tool a try and see if you can make it work.

Sometimes, the best thing to do with your worries and ruminating thoughts is to shelve them. Imagine that it is 2 a.m. and you can't sleep. Your mind is running wild with fear, yet you need to get up in a few hours for your chemo appointment. Say to yourself: "Self, we are going to take all of my fears and worries and put them on a shelf in the bathroom. I can pick them up in the morning or after I get back home tomorrow, if I so choose. But for now, they will wait so I can get some sleep."

Alternately, you can try to put them into storage for a longer period of time. In this case, the self-speech is slightly different: "I'm not getting anywhere with all these annoying thoughts; I'm just making myself more 'crazy' than I already am. I am going to put these in a box on a shelf in my closet, and try my best to let them stay there. They are not helping me one bit."

In addition to these useful delays in your worries, some people draw upon their spiritual beliefs to help them cope better. They send off their concerns and worries to God instead of to a shelf, carton, or other storage area. This, no doubt, is where the expression "Let go and let God" comes from. In so doing, these people are placing their faith in a higher power and praying for a positive result. They are also delegating their worry to a spiritual force greater than themselves. They clear their mind in this way and are, hopefully, better able to get to sleep. Try to push away your worries and other negative thoughts whenever and however you can.

Using the Brake, Not the Gas

Beyond the power of positive self-talk, there is power in any self-talk that encourages your mind to stop spewing cess all over your head. This tool encourages you to talk back to your mind in ways that try to stop such disruptive thoughts and beliefs.

When these occur, just say: "Please stop now," or just "Stop" a couple of times. As you say those words, picture a red stop sign in your mind. See yourself stopping your car for that sign, and as you slowly put on the brake in this image, imagine you are doing the same thing in your mind so that your thoughts and feelings can move on to more positive and productive subjects. Some people find it helpful to wear a rubber band (with or without a message) that they can snap to remind them to shut off their negative inner thoughts that can pop up like weeds in the summer heat.

People often combine this practice with one of the other tools mentioned in this chapter or the previous one and find the blend of two or more quite helpful. For example, they get themselves into a calmer state through a relaxation exercise, and then picture the stop sign that helps them control and halt their ruminating thoughts. Or they see the stop sign, change the channel, and use a relaxation exercise to calm themselves. I encourage you to experiment and be creative. There are no hard and fast rules. There are just opportunities to take charge of your mind so that you can avoid being flooded with cess.

Wide Angle or Telephoto Lensing

Considering what our eyes choose to see and "film," they are amazing still and video cameras. Right now, I am looking at the last sentence on my computer screen and can see it completely. If I want, however, I can choose to focus on the word "cameras" and make all other words go blurry. Or I can stare at the sentence and allow my peripheral vision to see the bulletin board of pictures above my desk, the printer to my right, and the plants and sunshine on the patio to my left. My eyes and yours have quite an impressive set of lenses.

How we use these lenses is what creates the proverbial glass half full or half empty perspective. I can choose to focus on the debris and the large layers of seaweed that occasionally invade the ocean at the beach in Jupiter. Or I can focus on the blue sky, large white clouds, gentle waves as they hit the shore, and the lovely birds searching for their targets down below the waterline. These impressive images make the debris and seaweed meaningless.

I had similar choices in Cancerville, and so do you. I could have focused on the pain that Jodi was going through, but instead I pushed myself to see her gain there. For example, I could have seen and snapped a "picture" of the harsh chemicals going into her veins on those difficult days, but I fought hard to try to use my telephoto lens and see those bloody bastard cells being destroyed, hundreds at a time, like a powerful B52 bomb strike. It took me a while to adjust my zoom and my words, but I am confident that you can do that too.

As another example, I could have seen Jodi's bald head through my internal camera and felt sad and down; but I chose wide- angle and saw that she was still a beautiful young woman, even without hair. This lens enabled me to recognize that she and all of the others in Cancerville are much more than their hair or other superficial characteristics.

As I pictured all of Jodi's special qualities, I paired those images with the thought that "hair grows back," and left her baldness behind. By modifying and altering what my eyes chose to see and my mind thought, I could literally change my beliefs and move my feelings in a positive direction. In this simple but powerful way, so can you.

I am quite sure that Jodi used and many others in Cancerville use this tool to cope with their temporary but difficult circumstances such as their baldness. All of the people to whom I've spoken anticipated their hair loss from chemo with much worry and self-consciousness. That seemed to last a very short time and was followed by acceptance and/or whimsical experiences.

In all of the above, I have just skimmed the surface of possible ways to influence your thoughts and feelings. People read books, blogs, poems, etc., or watch movies, listen to talk shows, discuss issues with people who have gone through similar experiences, as well as talking to professionals and/or religious leaders. The key is to keep working hard to find ways to move your thoughts from negative to positive spaces to experience and draw from hope and optimism.

Real People Facing Cancer

Sylvia

I knew I was in trouble about a minute into fast dancing with Sylvia. I was breathing heavily and she was hardly breathing. Sylvia sat next to me at a friend's daughter's wedding. She had warned me that she took three exercise classes including Zumba seven days a week; she was in perfect shape! She was also eighty-eight years young. As we sat down, she said, "I had cancer twenty-five years ago, and it taught me to be healthy in every way I could." I heard a story here and followed up.

I just got off the phone with her after chatting about her experience in Cancerville all those years ago. Her energy level and passion were stronger than a presidential debater. She is one amazing and inspiring woman who really impressed me—and I am not that easily impressed! Sylvia seemed to come into Cancerville with her cognitive tools firmly in place.

Back when she was sixty-three, she had no symptoms and no intention of getting checked out for anything; she felt fine. Her son-in-law was an endocrinologist helping Sylvia's husband with his diabetes. When they went together to see him, her husband declared, "You need to check mom's blood, as she is always cold." Sylvia shouted, "Don't be ridiculous."

Her husband responded, "I won't test my blood if you don't check yours." "You are being a five-year-old," Sylvia shot back, but she eventually gave in for the good of the cause. As we shall see, Sylvia's husband and family defined who she was and she always caved and gave in for their causes.

Her blood test revealed that she was extremely anemic and needed five blood transfusions. Hospital tests of all kinds revealed nothing, and it appeared that she was perfectly healthy despite her blood issues. After a while, her daughter encouraged her to see a gastroenterologist and have a colonoscopy. When she finally relented and visited the doctor, he found cancer—the big C in 1987—OMG! But Sylvia remained calm. At the time she was working thirteen hours a day in the pharmacy she and her husband, a pharmacist, owned in New Jersey. Her goal was to get through this and return to her husband's side in the store.

Her doctor was kind and caring, but matter of fact. He said, "We must operate and either we will get it all or we won't. No chemo or radiation will help." Sylvia said, "I was not happy, but I did not react hysterically. My family was distraught, and I didn't want them to be any more upset. I sucked it up and moved forward."

Sylvia was able to quote verbatim to me the poem she placed in her husband's pocket right before her surgery, as he, being a sensitive guy who depended on his wife, was overwhelmed with emotion. She was gently trying to prepare him if the surgery didn't go well and used an interesting cognitive tool (a poem) to do that. That she couldn't remember the author's name reassured me that she was really eighty-eight. It goes:

> Sunset and evening star,
> and a clear call for me,
> May there be no moaning of the bar,
> When I put out to sea.

Well, Sylvia wasn't ready to put out to sea and still isn't! She remains land-locked and strong of body and mind, and has outlived her husband.

When Sylvia awoke from her surgery, her positive, cognitive, self-talk perspective was:

> I have been given an opportunity. I will not be a wimp—I will be positive. I need to get back to work. I will heal and get better. No pity party for me. I need to suck it up for my husband and my family. The harder I work, the more I will heal. I have to be strong!

With that mantra firmly planted in her mind, she pictured herself back at the store working with her husband as soon as possible.

Despite being in much pain from the metal clips across her waist, she schlepped herself forward. An optimist by nature, Sylvia automatically disputed her negative beliefs and feelings. Against her nurses' wishes, she rolled out of bed and put on makeup before her family visited. Sylvia said: "I felt horrible, but had to be strong for my family. If all I have is pain I am lucky; I am alive." Here we find her using my scale of relativity from Chapter 1.

Sylvia goes on to say:

> The essence of getting better is determination. I felt so grateful I didn't need a colostomy bag. Working in the store, I fitted many people for that and was happy I didn't need one. It is all about PMA—positive mental attitude! It still is. I just couldn't leave my husband in the lurch or let my family down. You just have to listen to your body and have your body listen to you. I was back at the store in a month or so. I chose not to be self-indulgent or feel sorry for myself. I made a decision to be strong and positive.
>
> I was in a lot of pain for a while, but I did not take pain meds. Our pharmacy was for other

people, not for me. I got the pain med prescription but never filled it. While I am talking
to you, Bill, I can feel the pain from back then
all these years later. But it is long gone, thank
god.

Who really knows why Sylvia was so staunch in her positive attitudes, beliefs, and cognitive controls. Perhaps it was
a result of her growing up during the difficult times of the
Great Depression and forgoing a bus ride to school, at times,
to save a nickel so that she could buy her father a Chunky
candy. Perhaps it all started before that and was just part of
who she was and who she is—her genes and her scenes.

Sylvia told me that when she awoke from surgery, another
favorite poem played through her mind like a broken record.
She quickly recited it, and knew the author as well. Maybe she
is not really eighty-eight, but I do believe her, unbelievable
as she may be. Here is how the poem Opportunity by Walter
Malone goes:

> They do me wrong who say I come no more,
> When once I knock and fail to find you in,
> I sit outside your door waiting to be called in.

Opportunity knocks for us all. No one knows that better or
lives more by that maxim than Sylvia! We can all take lessons
from her playbook as well as her Zumba classes. May she
live and be well, and may you, too, as you hopefully follow
Sylvia's "Positive Mental Attitude" prescription each and every
day. That is really what the relaxation and cognitive tools are
all about.

In Sum

It is not easy to avoid the challenging, and at times
mind-boggling, thoughts and feelings that come along
with Cancerville. These are, unfortunately, just part of the

nature of the territory. There are, however, many ways to let go of these negative thoughts and convert them to ones that allow for inspiration instead of perspiration. The above tools represent different strategies you can use to take charge of your mind and actively work to move it from negative to more positive thoughts and self-talk. By using these tools, you may be able to bypass cess that adds to your pool, erodes your dam, and is agitating and counter-productive.

You can experiment and try to tailor these tools to fit your needs and mindset. When it comes to matters of the mind, there is much room for your own personal creativity. Combining these tools with those of the previous chapter can make for a powerful antidote to help counter negativity.

Now, let's move on to talk about the complex territory of complementary and alternative opportunities. My goal is to help you look at a variety of options and make wise, safe, and supportive decisions for yourself. It is an area with many differing opinions and very few facts. Ultimately, I believe you will choose to do what feels comfortable and appropriate for you.

CHAPTER 18

*I will do my best to make healthy
choices on my behalf.*

Traditional and Alternative Treatments and Complementary Support Options

Though the title of this chapter is often found in the Cancerville literature and on the Internet, I want to quickly
separate these three types of cancer-related treat-

ments. This separation is necessary as they are not, in my opinion, identical triplets. In fact, they are about as opposite as three ideas can be.

Traditional treatments have their roots firmly planted in scientific soil. They are based upon rigorous research and are usually people's first choice. Almost every self-help Cancerville book I have read says: "Follow your physician's advice and treatment plan."

Alternative treatments are different from traditional ones. They involve interventions that often lack a scientific basis and are more controversial. Some promoters of alternative treatments swear by the very treatments that others swear at. It is a most confusing zone, about which there are a Heinz variety of opinions. I encourage you to explore this area, if you so choose, like a researcher—cautiously and thoroughly.

Complementary options work together with traditional and/ or alternative treatments. There are a variety of complementary choices to help you get through the rigors of Cancerville more comfortably and in a more empowered way. Though they aim, like Google's informal corporate mantra, to "Do No Evil," it is important that you first check out any complementary plans with your doctors. Some options that may seem helpful and harmless may not be.

One of your many rights as a patient in Cancerville is to make any choices you think are best for you. I totally get and respect that. I want you to do what you feel is right, helpful, and in your best interest. My goal is to encourage you to evaluate your options carefully and make healthy decisions in formulating your plans. In my opinion, it is important to allow the experts of Cancerville, your physicians, to help guide you towards wellness and wise decisions.

I also want to help you avoid being taken in by people on the outskirts of Cancerville who have personal but distorted axes to grind, misinformation, and/or profits to be made, whether or not your health profits from what they are promoting. Though I assert that it is ultimately your choice, it is mine to try to impose rational and realistic markers to guide your way.

Traditional Treatments

Since I am not a physician in or out of Cancerville, I cannot speak with great intelligence or clarity about the traditional treatments for cancer. We do know they are strong measures because cancer is a strong and formidable force. They include powerful chemicals, radiation, surgery, and, if necessary, amputation of the affected part.

The evolution of traditional treatments for cancer is brilliantly described in *The Emperor of All Maladies.* Many interesting aspects about modern traditional treatment and future goals are described in Lauren Pecorino's book, *Why Millions Survive Cancer: The Successes of Science.*[25] In the Preface Lauren says her book has three themes:

> The first is that over the last few decades we have built a far better scientific understanding of the disease and of the human body's remarkable defense against tumors; the second is that there is recent progress in our management of cancer and this is changing our view of the disease; and the last but most important is that evidence-based science informs us about lifestyle choices that reduce our risk of cancer and such changes in lifestyle save many lives.

All of the traditional treatments and protocols are subject to rigorous trials analyzed by scientists who conduct experiments that include double blinds (trials in which neither the patient nor the doctor knows who is getting the real drug and who is getting the placebo). The research also includes matched control groups to see if the effects of the treatment are statistically significant compared to a group not receiving the treatment.

In my opinion, at the end of the day, science in all areas rules the day. It helps us distinguish between true effects and artificial effects that come about through chance. It also helps separate the individual anecdotal stories from the data based results across many, many people. In the old days, in all fields of study, things were much more trial and error in a way analogous to my Grandma's recipes. She would put in a "pinch" of this and a "squeeze" of that, and then— BAM—have a pot roast or chicken dish to behold and savor. Early doctors and cancer specialists cooked their "recipes" much like Grandma did.

As science evolved and as regulations were put into effect about the Federal Drug Administration's (FDA) approval, things became much more rigorous and regimented, and results had to be demonstrated before they became standard practice. Many physicians and pharmacists in Cancerville who work behind the scenes all over the world are scientists and researchers. Todd, whom you will meet in Chapter 23, is an oncological research pharmacist. You will soon discover that his dedication to the Cancerville cause has an interesting and poignant origin.

Scientifically based results add to the belief that traditional medical approaches will be helpful. Though that doesn't guarantee that the approach your doctor recommends will work for you, it does reflect that there is a data based statistical probability for his or her recommendation. Your doctor is working under the assumption that the results backed by much careful research will generalize to you. After all, many patients benefit from these established approaches.

The importance of groundbreaking research is neverending in Cancerville. This is why you may be encouraged to participate in a trial of some newly developing approach/chemo to see if and how it works. Science and our knowledge about cancer can only grow if people agree to participate in new research. Here again, it is your choice.

Some patients and their families in Cancerville believe that drug companies could find a cure for cancer if they really wanted to. They don't, according to this theory, because a cure would cut into their profits. I have seen this statement many times on the Internet and heard or read it in books on occasion. Though I respect your right to believe that, I hope you will see the flaws in its logic. If it were possible to find a "cure," the individuals and companies able to accomplish that would earn billions of dollars, as well as earning the goodwill of the world.

In addition, drug companies spend billions of dollars conducting research that will allow them to introduce new drugs to help those in Cancerville without having any assurance that they will ever recoup their investment, let alone earn a profit. Furthermore, in my opinion, there is not one person who works in a cancer-related center of any kind who would not happily close the doors to Cancerville, and direct their efforts to other difficult and daunting diseases—"hope the heck you never come back, happy to see you go!" Not you—cancer!

Finally, and perhaps most importantly, it is unlikely that there ever will be a "cure" for cancer. This is because cancer is an umbrella term that covers many different diseases. Although all cancers involve cell mutations, the many forms the disease can take are as varied as the many different sized and shaded grains of sand that lie beneath a beach umbrella.

Even within the same type of cancer there are many different variations and further differences depending upon the age of the patient, size of the cells, and so many other factors. At a recent conference I attended, an oncologist said that there are eight different types of blood malignancies and more than twenty subsets of each. I did the math and sighed audibly.

It is all of these variations that have made the task of discovering effective treatments such a difficult one, not to mention the complex problem of metastasis when cells from one area spread to another by hitching a ride through the blood stream. In fact, considering this intricacy and complexity, it is amazing that science has come as far as it has in developing treatments that are helping millions to survive. That is the very good news about traditional treatments with more coming down the Cancerville Pike regularly.

Alternative Treatments

During my travels to Africa and Asia, the pungent aromas wafting from herbal shops fascinated me. Chinese medicine has been around for an extremely long time, and many in those regions and elsewhere swear by them.

I vividly remember being in East Africa in 1982 with a group of psychologists and others, learning about alternative medical treatments. We visited a "hospital" way out in the boonies; the resident "doctor" was an herbalist whose garden grew rich in "healing" plants. There were giant pots brewing on open fires when he proclaimed his "medicines" could cure anything, including cancer. I was most skeptical that true healing could occur in this primitive setting with straw outdoor cots. But, hey, you just never know. That said, if I were facing cancer or any other serious disease, I would not call or send smoke signals for an appointment! Because the patients and the doctor believe in these seemingly primitive remedies, they are more likely to work for them.

My skepticism applies to alternative treatments wherever they are offered. There are too many to list, but a sampling includes the controversial drug Laetrille, an extreme macrobiotic diet, black seed, hyperbaric chambers, dried green barley leaves, juicing, and the like. Though there is much chatter on the Internet about these and other alternative options, there is little to no data to support their effectiveness.

In this regard, Jimmie Holland, M.D., Shelton Lewis, and I agree. In *The Human Side of Cancer* they unequivocally say: "DON'T take an alternative therapy in place of a conventional treatment. You may be delaying the use of a proven, potentially curative treatment. DO use any of the complementary therapies that make you feel better and help you cope."

In her wonderful book *The Healing Consciousness: A Doctor's Journey to Healing,* [26] Beth DuPree, M.D., a skilled and caring surgeon who now specializes in breast cancer, says:

> My clinical approach to cancer surgery remains based in Western medicine. That means the treatment of the disease called cancer begins with surgery, chemotherapy and/or radiation to treat the physical body. In my short medical career, we have made great strides in Western medicine. Our diagnosis and treatment of can-

cer has become less invasive, more precise and targeted…. Technology is the backbone of cancer treatment, but it cannot stand alone if we aim to treat the whole patient.

She goes on to say:

After treating the cancer that is the symptom manifested by the body, the complex process of healing may require lifetimes to be completed…. A partnership is required for healing, and in the process, energy is exchanged from doctor to patient and from patient to doctor…. Although it may be that medicine treats the symptom, it is love that heals.

Scary and Mysterious Alternative Examples

Here is an extreme example of an alternative therapy, which I found on the Internet:

Dr. K, a dentist by training, used alternative cancer treatments to treat more than 33,000 cancer patients. He used special diets, proteolytic enzymes, and other natural substances. Dr. K was able to cure 90% of the cancer patients who went to him instead of using chemotherapy, radiation and surgery!! Compare Dr. K's cure rate of 90% to the overall cure rate of less than 3% of orthodox medicine.

My reaction was that the claims made about Dr. K were crazy, scary, and totally inaccurate. I wouldn't go to Dr. K for a tooth cleaning! Would you? He is a dentist and self-proclaimed "oncologist," best as I can tell.

Similar sensational and unsubstantiated claims are made for many other products and "treatments." Just the other day, I received a long-winded email complete with YouTube videos about Laminine. The treatment involves extracting the "life-essence" from a nine-day-old fertilized chicken egg and turning it into an elixir. Referring to one of the researchers, the email says, "He had theorized that an injected extract from fertilized hen eggs could be helpful for a number of his cancer patients." Yet there is no data presented to back up this statement other than to say the doctor spent a decade researching his theory.

A Potentially Harmful Alternative Example

In today's Google-driven world, one does not have to search very long to find an alternative therapy that can be very hurtful to the patient. One such example is Insulin Potentiation Therapy (IPT). A family of Mexican physicians developed this treatment in the 1930s and continues to use it to treat cancer. Some American doctors who were "specially trained" use it as well. The IPTO.org website shows a cost of approximately $16,000 for three to four weeks of intensive therapy plus $2000-$3000 per week for up to four weeks of home maintenance.

The treatment is based upon the belief that insulin "opens the pores" of cancer cells throughout the body so that doctors can use milder forms of chemotherapy to achieve positive results. Despite misleading promotions, there doesn't appear to be any serious research to back up this theory. Moreover, there is a serious risk involved because rapidly falling blood sugar levels can produce stroke, shock, coma, and even death. One web site sums up IPT as follows:

> Although IPTs proponents have been treating patients for decades, they have no tested theory and have produced at most only one properly designed study of one cancer. If you would like to bet your money and your life on their general impressions, they'll be happy to do business. However, the lack of evidence should serve as a powerful warning to stay away.

Another site says it even more succinctly:

> While insulin potentiation therapy has been used for decades in Mexico and some other countries, there is absolutely no scientific evidence that it works or is safe.

A Harmless but Meaningless Alternative Example

An alternative remedy generally believed to be healthy involves the recent craze for juicing and juice fasts. In some instances, juicing has also been touted as a way to prevent and/or treat cancer. Misleading advertisements and endorsements can muddy the waters or juices even further.

On the generic, get healthy/lose weight/etc. level, Hollywood stars have jumped on the bandwagon, as have companies producing expensive juice machines. Starbucks plans to open juice bars and build a national chain. At six bucks a pop, that can be as lucrative as a latte. Yet recent evidence suggests the general public as well as people with medical problems are being duped.

Recently, POM Wonderful pomegranate juice has been found to not be so wonderful. Claims that the drink can prevent, treat, and reduce the risk of prostate cancer, heart disease, and erectile dysfunction have been reported to be misleading and inaccurate.

A more recent article described POM Wonderful's public relations campaign to "juice" their juice! They are also appealing the FTC ruling legally, although they refused to be interviewed for the article in the *Sun-Sentinel*. A noted consumer psychology professor has said, "They're getting more free mileage fighting this than they could ever possibly spend in advertising." A noted advertising attorney has said, "What they're doing is something a lot of companies that are not happy about an FTC order would like to do, but someone sensible talks them out of it." To add confusion to controversy, the female co-owner of POM Wonderful was quoted in a 2010 article saying, "Marie Antoinette could have avoided the guillotine if she had better PR." That seems to suggest that truth has nothing to do with the company's equation of "juicy" justice.

A *Time* magazine article unrelated to POM Wonderful, which is subtitled "Juice fasting makes you feel healthy, even if it isn't," reports, "It's unclear whether juice cleansing will go down as a fad, like the macrobiotic regimens of the '70's... but the trend shows no sign of slowing." They go on to say:

> The only problem is that there is almost no medical evidence that juice is anything other than innocuous, and the universal of modern medicine is that your liver and kidneys are, when functioning, quite efficient at detoxification. Plus, the weight that comes off so easily during a juice fast tends to be water—the kind that you gain back quickly after a single meatball sandwich.

According to Dr. Bennett Roth, chief of gastroenterology at UCLA Medical Center, "The concept has no basis in scientific support."

Though the choice is truly yours, I encourage you to tread lightly and cautiously in this complex territory. My simple-minded belief is that if there truly were "miracle cures" out there, that information would be well-documented and promoted throughout Cancerville. Desperate people sometimes pursue desperate measures. I understand that quest, but in many cases I know of, this desperation led to more harm than good. I will share a few stories with you soon.

Complementary Options

Complementary supports in Cancerville are designed to help you be more comfortable and relaxed as you deal with the demanding treatments. They are intended to help you stay more positive and have more energy with which to do battle. Recall Eileen's rollerblading, which did just that on a sunny morning, and you have a clear example of a most elementary complementary activity. The same is true about a simple massage, which always leaves a simple healing message on our bodies and our minds.

The tools suggested in the previous two chapters reflect other "complementary" supports. Acupuncture, yoga, physical exercise, healthy eating, counseling and support groups, massage, Reiki, and other safe and inexpensive forms of natural healing offer positive support to many patients in Cancerville.

Notice that I did not include herbal supplements as that—along with over-the-counter meds—need to be discussed with your doctor. Some supplements can actually interfere with chemo treatments or produce other unwanted effects. Try to avoid just going to your local health food shop and consulting with the resident guru. Let your doctors guide you through this labyrinth of what is truly complementary and what is not helpful for you. I recently heard from Rob about his friend who wanted to get a "DAM STRONG!" tattoo. She had read my book for family and friends, even though she was a patient. The doctors nixed that idea and were probably concerned about the dyes used and/or the possibility of infection from unclean needles.

In addition, even prescribed meds can reduce the effectiveness of oral chemo or increase its toxic side effects. Sometimes medications prescribed by primary care doctors can interfere or make chemotherapy treatments more toxic. Obviously, communication is needed between your doctors, but in today's fast-paced world, that can fall through the cracks. Please try your best to make sure that doesn't happen in your case, especially when email can easily keep your entire medical team updated and in touch with one another.

There is a wealth of easily available information about complementary options, so I see little point in repeating the details here. I think that what you choose to try will be based upon your previous experiences. If, for example, you have used acupuncture to help with back pain or some other problem and it was successful, it is likely you will pursue it during your cancer treatment (if your physician approves). If the thought of someone poking you with needles as if you were a pincushion does not resonate with you, and you have heard multiple stories about acupuncture being ineffective, it is not likely that you will try it now.

On the other hand, if while you are at a chemo treatment you talk with someone who tells you about a wonderful healing massage or a cancer group that meets to do yoga, you may just try it and may like it. Or, like Jodi, you may not want to be part of a group like that and prefer to go to an introductory yoga class at your local gym. In this entire area, individual preferences prevail, and my encouragement is to do what is comfortable for you, while stretching just a bit to try out and experiment with some new support options that are safe and not intrusive or dangerous in any way. One of your many rights as a patient is to explore, experiment, experience, and engage or not, as you see fit.

I want to share an interesting observation that deals with the plants on my patio. Though your well-being is far more important than my plants, I believe there is a message to be learned from nature that can be applied to human nature as well. Lacking a green thumb, some plants are hail and hearty in spite of me, and some struggle because of my inattentiveness. Over time, the latter wilt and turn brown. I take those and hang them in the backyard, and from then on turn them over to Mother Nature. She takes charge and slowly these plants return to life and become green and full again. They then return to my patio, ever stronger and more able to tolerate my benign neglect. Complementary options are like turning your body and mind over, from time to time, to Mother Nature. Best as I can tell, she is one amazing life-enhancing force!

The same magic that I observe with my plants can also be true for people. Supplementing traditional treatments with medically approved natural remedies like diet, relaxation activities, yoga, exercise, etc. can be healing in and of themselves. In this sense, because traditional treatments involve "cut, poison, and burn" options (as one person expressed to me in an email this morning), they represent the war zone that requires a battle; on the other hand, approved complementary options provide the healing of mind, body, and spirit from those harsh approaches. Perhaps this way of seeing and saying it can provide a bridge upon which Bernie Siegel, M.D., and I can walk together comfortably.

Real People Facing Cancer

There are many stories that speak to the issues raised in this chapter. I want to share four that reflect my feelings and those of many others in the Cancerville field. Chef Grant's story is about finding an alternative treatment within the traditional treatment spectrum. Roger and Marilyn's experiences are about going outside the realm of traditional treatments and encountering serious difficulties and unanticipated consequences. Kris' story is about drawing from a variety of complementary options, especially when no traditional treatments were available for her.

Both individually and together they tell us a great deal about making self-protective and wise choices in this most complicated area. That said, just like Bernie Siegel, M.D., encouraged in the Foreword, I trust you to draw from your intuition and make the appropriate choices for yourself.

Chef Grant—A Traditional Alternative

I can't think of another experience that better illustrates the difference between going for extreme and unproven alternative treatments and finding an alternative treatment within the traditional treatment menu. I must admit I was touched and taken by Chef Grant Aschatz's story. It was painful for me to read parts of the perfectly titled book, *Life, on The Line.*[27] It reminded me that life can be hard enough without Cancerville.

Yet it reinforced my belief that we can slowly get up from the emotional knees that Cancerville can bring us to and stand tall once again. I hope his unique story does that for you.

Even though Chef Grant would not grant me an interview, I wanted to include his story because it is powerful, positive, and empowering. His Cancerville experience put his talent and livelihood on the line, while putting his life right on (and possibly off) the line.

After learning a great deal at the French Laundry in Napa, he went on to make a name for himself in Chicago. One of his wealthy patrons and co-author, Nick, loved Chef Grant's food so much that he helped raise the funds for a new restaurant, Aliena, which means "a break from the previous chain of thought." Nick became much more than a partner—he became a loving and caring friend. The restaurant opened and received rave reviews, but unfortunately Chef Grant soon developed a tongue ache that eventually was diagnosed as Stage IV squamous cell cancer that had metastasized to his lymph nodes. The treatment plan read like a bad meal on the menu of a greasy spoon that was behind on its rent.

Okay Chef, here is the plan, they told him. We cut out your tongue, slice your jaw, and dissect your neck like a biology class experiment. Then with a little luck and some chemo, you may live a while. If not, you're a cooked goose or perhaps duck, which, by the way, you will never taste again. You won't even taste oatmeal. And just in case you are not paying attention, if we don't do this in a few weeks, you will be dead! Can you imagine? I myself cannot begin to imagine what it must have been like for a Chef or anyone, for that matter, to hear such nasty news!

In addition, Grant had two young sons from a previous relationship and a new girlfriend. He had life by the shorthairs, until life reached a little lower and kicked him in the testicles with the force of a sledgehammer wielded by a sumo wrestler. Talk about "balls to the walls!" Fortunately, Nick persevered, when Grant pretty much gave up, and finally found a doctor and an alternative—chemo and radiation. They were still part of the traditional treatment regimen—just being studied as an alternative to the more extreme traditional slice and dice approach.

The chemo and radiation kicked his butt badly, but the good news was that they cured him. In fact, his cancer disappeared completely, much like the food he puts on his patrons' plates. He was cancer free and, best as I know, remains so. He said:

> Five months after being declared 'cancer free' I was still very much living with cancer and the aftereffects of having my cells killed from the inside out. I could barely swallow, still couldn't taste, and basic human functions were a daily trial.

Yet little by little, he returned to himself. He has recently opened a new restaurant and two nightclubs, one of which serves fifteen varieties of ice, if you can imagine that. Perhaps this explains why he didn't respond to my letter. Chefs are super busy guys who work all of the time, except the few hours they may get to sleep.

The new restaurant is called Next because its menu changes, not just in content but in type, every few months. It can go from Thai to French 1925 (whatever that is) to Italian to who knows what other than Chef Grant. Another unique feature of this restaurant is that you have to buy a ticket to eat there, much as you would for a theater performance. If you don't arrive at the scheduled date and time, you lose the price of the ticket—which is expensive. Though he didn't initially like the name Next, he came to realize it related to more than the next course or ever-changing menu. He says:

> For a long time I had worried about what was coming next. Then for a short time that felt like a very long time, I didn't think I had a future. Now, every time I was asked "What's next?" I could finally enjoy coming up with the answer. Not a bad reminder.

Roger—An Alternative That Failed

Roger Ebert is a well-known movie critic who wrote *Life Itself: A Memoir.* [28] Most of it is devoted to his impressive career and equally impressive memory of the famous people he met and interviewed and where and when that occurred. Toward the conclusion of his book, he talks about his cancer, which has left him unable to speak, eat, or drink without assistance, and facially deformed.

Roger researched a great deal and chose to undergo an alternative treatment—neutron radiation—before the surgery his doctors recommended. When Roger finally underwent the surgery, it did not work because of the residual damage from the radiation; his skin was so damaged because of it that the traditional surgery failed over and over. Roger says:

> I believe my infatuation with neutron radiation led directly to the failure of all three of my facial surgeries, the loss of my jaw, loss of the ability to eat, drink, and speak, and the surgical damage to my right shoulder and back as my poor body was plundered for still more reconstructive transplants…. Like many people, I fear pain more than death…. Now I know something I didn't know before, which is that after my surgeries failed, I could live a perfectly happy life.

Perhaps the moral of this story is that we have no choice but to cope with our choices, and that some alternatives are better than others as long as they stay within the traditional treatment model. The good news for Roger is that his wife and loving partner has been there for him every slow step of the way; he credits her for moving him forward when all his pain and suffering had him stuck.

Jack and Marilyn—An Alternative That Failed

I first met Jack (not his real name) more than ten years ago, after his wife passed away from cancer. He was seriously depressed, could barely function, and craved the dark like a bat in a cave. He truly loved his wife and saw no future other than to raise his children and then kill himself. Somehow or other, together we fought our way back to level ground in a relatively short period of time. He met a lovely woman and married her—the very picture I painted for him as I struggled to show him a brighter future despite his loss.

As I was writing this chapter, I remembered something he had said to me all those years ago. It was a passing comment about he and his wife going for an alternative treatment that was very expensive. He felt it had hastened her death, rather than prolonging it. I called him recently and asked if he would be willing to share the details and he agreed.

His wife Marilyn (not her real name) was diagnosed with a very rare Stage IV sarcoma in her breast at age fifty. It had metastasized to her lung, which had many small tumors. The first oncologist they met with lacked both bedside manner and tact, and gave her two to four years to survive. They were both understandably devastated. Another oncologist advised a mastectomy and heavy duty chemo, which they did. Marilyn was in fine shape and an athlete, but the chemo hit her hard. Meanwhile, somewhere along the line, cancer had invaded her adrenal gland.

Marilyn was mentally strong and vowed to get better; unfortunately she got worse and worse. She sought out every complementary opportunity she could find. A woman who never ate veggies or salad was now munching them like a rabbit. She also tried acupuncture, herbs, massage, and hypnotherapy that lasted four hours. She even tried a light energy treatment and met with some born again holistic healers, which didn't much appeal to this proud and strong Jewish woman. Marilyn and Jack also went to two cancer centers searching for clinical trials.

When all else failed to materialize help or hope, they went to Europe for alternative treatments. They were there for about one month. Marilyn had many colonics, more chemo than may have been appropriate for her situation according to Jack, and other treatments. She had three treatments where they boiled her blood to a temperature of 107 degrees and transfused it back into her. As a result Marilyn developed shingles, which only added to her pain and required IV meds. Frankly, it is just that kind of alternative effort that can make my own blood boil!

In addition, there were many language problems, as most of the staff did not speak English. Also, unlike the United States, they were not equipped for handicapped patients. Ramps for wheelchairs did not exist in the hospital or railroad station, and the restaurants had no restroom facilities for the handicapped.

Upon their return, Marilyn developed a nosebleed that would not stop and entered the local hospital. She had no blood platelets—a likely result of their boiling her blood. She remained in the hospital for about a month and, sadly, died the day she was released. Without hesitation, Jack said they would not have put her through that torture, or have spent tens of thousands of dollars, knowing what they knew upon their return. He feels that rather than being the magical cure, it added to her suffering and hastened her passing.

One of the things Jack commented on was the negativity of the local doctors about her situation:

> You hang on every word they say. Even a little encouragement would go a very long way to inspire hope. Why not just say you have a rare and difficult disease, but we will do our best to get you through? Having something to hold onto is important for the patient and his or her family. Granted we were going uphill all the way, but a little push of support from the doctors would have been helpful. I can't repeat it enough—you hang on every word they say—and when it is so negative and hopeless it is crushing.

I did not prompt him to say that!

Kris—A Helpful Complement to No Other Treatments Available

Yet another story relates to this discussion. Kris Carr was told she had Stage IV of a rare form of liver cancer for which there was no treatment. At the time, she was in her twenties, an aspiring actress, and pissed as hell. She could have easily appeared in the chapter on "Reining in Your Rage."

With choices limited and the clock ticking a little too fast for her, she describes in her interesting and funny book, *Crazy, Sexy Cancer Tips,* [29] how she explored all forms of treatment options. Though I like her book and recommend it, especially to women, I don't love the title. Though it is catchy branding (and she has gone on to make a documentary and a cookbook using the same words) there is nothing, in my opinion, sexy about any form of cancer. It has about as much sex appeal as a religious symbol and mocks the seriousness of having cancer. Then again, I think that is exactly what this young woman is trying to do.

Nonetheless, her book is worth a read and tells how she did yoga, colonics, and other cleansing, and became immersed in eating healthily. She recommends a 70/30 or even 80/20 split between raw veggies and fruits and more substantial food. She went from quickly eating fast food to slowly preparing healthy meals, and gives many reasons why our processed, fertilized, pesticided, meat-and-milk-based diet is killing us softly, but not so slowly, and causing cancer. Many other authors echo these sentiments and they are all probably correct. Those diet shifts toward healthier eating fall into the complementary side of the treatment equation.

Truth be known, the majority of people outside of Cancerville will not change their diet—but cancer and other health problems can be a wake up call. Yet sometimes those wake up calls do not last very long. In 2001 I had an angioplasty, became a born again healthy food believer, and lost forty something pounds. As time passed and I didn't, I still maintained a healthy diet, but gained back much of the weight. My inner child has always needed to be 190 or so pounds for reasons that I neither understand, nor approve. The problem with this candor is that when Ronnie edits this chapter, she will give me a lecture. I swear, the things I do for my readers!

The importance of Ms. Carr's story is that given the lack of traditional treatment options, she chose complementary ones and didn't go to extremes or recklessly spend money on way-out options. In fact, she probably saved money by adjusting her diet and losing the junk food. In addition, from a psychological point of view, cancer in general, especially with limited treatment options, portends a total loss of control. It is like driving on the turnpike without brakes or steering wheel fluid. HELP!

In those moments, the best thing to do is take control of what you can. Boil your brown rice in sterilized water if that makes you feel healthier. Buy organic everything. Plant your own garden if you have the space. Do roto-rooter cleansing as often as is healthy. Even if none of those actually makes a Cancerville difference, the options can give you a sense of being in control; that alone is empowering, helpful, and healthy.

In Sum

I am pretty sure that you understand why this chapter has many "Real People Facing Cancer" stories. This subject is more than complicated and I wanted to present a variety of scenarios for you to consider. Let me reiterate that this is your journey and you have the need and right to do it any way that helps you feel comfortable.

Yet we can all try to learn from other's mistakes. Many avenues are helpful, some are neutral, and a few are hurtful. I don't want you to enter hurtful space and am hoping I can help you avoid it. But once again, the choice is yours. I have no crystal ball, your doctors don't either, and neither do you. If you need to go with your gut, then so be it. I hope and pray that your gut is on target like a GPS—even better.

Now, let's move on to see and understand the value of counseling as a complementary support tool. It is also an alternative to despair, depression, anxiety, and a host of other dis-eases. Often, a mental health counselor or support group can help you learn to use and apply the tools I have described or others that are similar. This personal approach to drawing upon cognitive tools is only one of the many helpful benefits of having such support in your corner. Let's talk more about these valuable resources in the following chapter.

CHAPTER 19

I will seek support if and when I need it.

Having a Counselor and/ or Support Group in Your Corner

Much like a nutritionist promoting veggies and vitamins or a dental hygienist promoting flossing, I am
biased about the importance of mental health counseling as a worthwhile coping, balancing, and healthy living
tool. This is true in everyday life, but even more so when
dealing with Cancerville. Very few things are more powerful

than one person helping another supportively get through a difficult time. I say this based on having helped many people in my career and having been helped personally as well.

A Shrink Will Help You Grow

In my book *Getting Back Up From an Emotional Down,* one of the chapters is called "Everyone Needs a Shrink I Think." That was my belief in the late 1980s and remains so now. Generally speaking, cess builds up over time while dams erode. Thus, as time goes on, many people struggle with a variety of emotional discomforts and disorders that include anxiety, depression, low self-esteem, guilt, food-related problems, other addictions, and the like.

This is precisely why millions are on psychiatric meds and millions more need them. It is also why we have become gloppers who use a wide range of "pacifiers" to fill the voids in our lives. Too many walk weakly to the finish line, and a significant number of others crawl there on their bellies. "DAM STRONG!" is an empowering call to take better care of ourselves in and out of Cancerville.

If people can benefit from a counselor in their everyday lives, they certainly can use one while in Cancerville. The reasons are quite obvious. Cancerville's cess adds to already existing everyday cess in a way that makes for hurricane warnings, tornado watches, and major flooding. As we discussed in Part III, depression, anxieties, and anger can move rapidly into our cesspool and then to the surface of our mind, like a submarine coming up quickly from the ocean floor.

In Cancerville, your head can quickly become jammed, fogged, and almost numb with an overload of emotion. Like a boxer, you will try to shake off that shot to your head until the next left jab or right hook catches you off-guard and puts you even further off-balance. To counter this, you can benefit by having someone in your corner who can help get you through this battle. He or she can't take the journey for you, but at least that person can help wipe the emotional sweat away. A professional can also help you apply the relaxation and cognitive tools previously described and perhaps teach you some others, as well, while offering a safe place to vent feelings and receive support.

Resistance to Seeking Professional Help

Despite the value I see coming from counseling, many in Cancerville will still resist seeking out and drawing upon this type of assistance. Instead, they choose to go it alone or to rely on family and friends. Hopefully, those close to you are positive supports; however, they likely lack the skill, knowledge, expertise, or objectivity of a professional. Keep in mind that much of the advice you receive from others, well-meaning as it is intended to be, can turn out to be useless at best and hurtful at worst. This is my bias and frequent observation, but it is possible that you are fortunate and have special family members and/or friends who are good listeners and supportive people on your team.

A professionally trained psychiatrist, psychologist, therapist, social worker, or counselor may be much better positioned to be of help than a layperson. Moreover, it is helpful to take the dam supports you have been taught in your visit with you, while leaving your cess on the floor of my office or those of my colleagues.

Notwithstanding all of my encouraging endorsements of therapy and counseling, people's resistance to that help has been well known since the time of Freud. Many have told me they would rather have a root canal without nerve gas or novocaine than come to my office. It wasn't about me, and I never took it personally, as I am an easygoing, pleasant, and supportive psychologist.

Resistance is about people not wanting to face themselves and their issues. Just as we don't like to look in the mirror if our bellies are too bloated, we don't like to see the bulging mess in our cesspools. Nor do we enjoy confronting our glopful habits that result from such cess. Most of us would much rather just continue with them, unhealthy as they might be. Sometimes, as I spoke about previously, denial can be healthy and helpful; other times it can be very destructive.

Another reason many people resist counseling is that they are private and feel more comfortable maintaining a low profile. They feel threatened when imagining sitting across from a stranger and speaking honestly and openly about their lives, their problems, and themselves. People generally tend to suppress and repress embarrassing and sensitive frustrations, fears, and feelings as a way to avoid dealing with and confronting them. The same is true of our secrets; we do not like to think about them, let alone talk about them openly.

Finally, there is a popular belief that often keeps people from seeking professional assistance. Many feel that they "should" handle their lives and their problems on their own; I warned you early on about the danger of "shoulds." Though mainly prevalent among men, I have met many women who feel the same way. Usually, these people have been taught this while growing up and have this mythological belief embedded strongly in their minds. This distorted belief takes independence and self-sufficiency to a very exaggerated level. I often say to such a person that seeing a counselor is no different from seeking medical or dental help. Surely, you would not expect to fill your own cavity; why then would you expect to be able to fill the holes in your dam on your own?

Thus, for a variety of personal reasons, many avoid seeking out counseling support. Oddly enough, they are often the people who could most benefit from this experience. I am hopeful that if you need it, you will push past your resistance and participate.

Sounds of Silence

As Paul Simon and Art Garfunkel taught us many years ago, as we began to awaken from the repressive 1950s, "Silence like a cancer grows." In these simple yet wise words, they summed up everything that is wrong with suppressing one's feelings in any emotionally charged situation. Silence fills pools and weakens dams. The more people "stuff" painful feelings, the more cesspools grow and the more these feelings come back to bite in one way or another. Emotional "malignancy" is also a debilitating, dangerous, and difficult disease to treat. Simon and Garfunkel were undeniably correct.

When people visiting my office talk, they are usually venting cess and relieving themselves. In that sense, counseling has the same cathartic value as a powerful enema. When I respond as an interactive counselor, I am helping to rebuild and strengthen dams by filling in some of the cracks and crevices that have developed over time.

I hope that while you are in Cancerville, your resistance to seeking counseling support will be diminished since you are not coming for an overall emotional tune-up or treatment for a specific psychiatric disorder. The focus is primarily on present day issues; you are not signing up to inspect the "dirty diapers" of your past.

It is not your general history that I would focus on if you were visiting my office for Cancerville support as much as your present circumstances, coping skills, health history, and concerns about your journey. My goal would be to provide individualized support based on the details of your situation. I would help you embrace realistic optimism and learn to use relaxing and cognitive tools tailored to your needs and nature. It would be a practical and personalized effort to help you cope better and maintain your own health and balance during this difficult time.

Be aware that I discussed the warning signs that suggest your need for professional support in Chapter 13, "Dealing with Depression, Debilitation, and Distress." Please don't be ashamed or embarrassed to ask for help. Strong people do just that, while the weaker ones just continue to suffer and struggle emotionally. Just today, we received a call from a woman who needed to reach out to us more than a year ago, just after entering Cancerville. We can help her now, but we could have been a much more supportive influence way back then.

Choosing a Helpful Professional

As with all professions, not all mental health counselors are created equal, although the majority are caring and capable people who are committed to the good of your cause. Choosing the right mental health counselor is a very important decision that is too often based upon issues that have nothing to do with the counselor's competence or your comfort. Both are key components to a helpful match with a mental health professional.

For example, people may choose a support professional solely because of the proximity to their home or office, whether the counselor participates in their health insurance program, or someone's recommendation. These practical issues make for a good starting point to one's search. In addition, however, a brief phone conversation or first visit meeting will help to determine if you are comfortable with the rapport and fit. It is important for you to find someone with whom you feel at ease and who you see as trustworthy.

Beyond seeking out someone with specific Cancerville experience, I encourage you to initially visit with a variety of questions in mind:

- Does this person seem sincerely interested in my situation or does it feel like a recorded announcement?

- Is there more emphasis placed on billing issues than on my issues?

- Did my appointment start close to the scheduled time?

- Do I feel comfortable and free to speak openly or do I feel judged and on guard?

- Do I feel I can trust this person?

- Is the setting comfortable and appropriate or am I jammed into a room that is too small, hot, or cold?

- Am I given undivided attention or are there phone or other interruptions?

- Am I given the full time I was promised?

- Is my visit helpful in setting some goals and offering me support and understanding?

- Did what he or she say make sense?

Hopefully, your experience with a counselor or therapist will go well. If it doesn't, please don't hesitate to try someone else. Choosing the right professional for you is a very important part of the process.

Support Groups

Not all people are comfortable with or can afford a one-on-one counseling experience. As I'm sure you know, there are many support group possibilities both in person and over the Internet. I have met many people for whom support groups were very helpful and some who had less than positive experiences. In most instances, our personal preferences determine the helpfulness and value of the experience.

Though I have facilitated many types of support groups over the years, I was not eager to participate in one related to Cancerville. Ronnie "dragged" me to one meeting, but I did not like it; it did not help me, so I never went back. I probably needed to check out one or two others to see if I could find a group that was more comfortable and helpful for me.

Despite my reluctance, support groups at hospitals and at places like Gilda's Club, etc. serve a valuable role for many people. Certainly, keep your mind open to this option, and see if a support group can be worthwhile for you. Some people find it very advantageous to be able to call other group members when their feelings and moods shift with the Cancerville tides. An added advantage is that almost all support groups are free.

There are many cancer specific support groups, chat rooms, and bulletin boards on the Internet these days. They are worth a try as well, especially since they are easy and efficient to access. They also allow you to maintain your anonymity and only share that information with which you feel comfortable. In addition, you can choose to be an active or passive participant.

Support groups are also a helpful adjunct to individual counseling for some people. They report very different experiences in each and find the combination and synergy even more worthwhile.

Real People Facing Cancer

In the other chapters, all of the real people I write about had cancer. In this chapter, however, I wanted to focus on people with mental health ties to Cancerville, whether or not they had personally dealt with cancer.

In this section you are about to meet Kathleen, whose cancer experience caused her to change careers mid-life; Tracey, who chose a career in Cancerville only to learn that her destiny was to participate in the very survivor runs and dinners that she organized; Marty, whose father's death from cancer caused him to choose to help people in Cancerville; and last, but by no means least, Lori. Thankfully, she never had cancer but has been helping others deal with Cancerville for more than twenty-five years.

Each of their stories is a testimony to the sincerity and dedication of the professionals who work full-time in Cancerville—each is also a testimony to fate. Their stories reflect the fate of these professionals' independent but parallel journeys and choices. They also reflect my good fortune to have met these fine people at the very time I was looking for stories such as theirs for this chapter—there are truly no coincidences.

Kathleen

Kathleen McBeth, M.A., is my colleague. But she wasn't always, as she was a businesswoman for many years until age forty-two. You can imagine her shock when, while she and her doctor were trying to correct an anemic problem, the chest X-ray lab tech said, "You need to go back to see the doctor right now!" Kathleen was more worried that the holiday pies that she had left in the car would spoil. Little did she realize, at that very moment, that was the least of her problems.

A few days before Thanksgiving, her doctor told her that she had "serious and multiple malignancies in both of her lungs!" Needless to say, her Thanksgiving was a very quiet "celebration." She and her family were literally scared to death; being thankful didn't seem to fit their moods.

Then Kathleen developed tingling in her arm, hand and two fingers. Her doctor feared there were tumors on her spine, and an MRI validated those fears. She was hospitalized, biopsied, and four or five days later learned that she had Stage IV Hodgkin Lymphoma that stretched from her neck to her groin. This was not exactly the diagnosis she expected to hear to explain her being anemic.

Ten-and-a-half months of strong chemo later, she was physically and emotionally drained and depleted. The initial shock of her diagnosis had long worn off, as had her initial emotionally blunted state of mind. In my language, her pool was flooding and her dam underwater—she was a mess of cess.

During this process her oncologist said, "I have never had to endure what you are going through." Kathleen's calm demeanor belied her mind screaming the thought, "Find me someone who has walked in my shoes because I am drowning and need support." Unfortunately, there was no one at the rural hospital where she was being treated to provide such help, and she had to "white knuckle" it on her own the whole way; fortunately, she had a solid support net of family and friends who filled in and helped her through.

Once Kathleen concluded treatment and was in remission, she made a pledge to herself to make a difference to others going through cancer in her community. She didn't just want to be a NED (No Evident Disease). In fact, she hated the term—she wanted to be cured and, in addition, wanted to pay back that weighty and wonderful debt.

Though she had to settle for NED and has for the past fifteen years, she made a personal decision and applied to graduate school. The title of her thesis tells her tale—"The Role of a Psychologist in an Oncology Field." She received her Masters in psychology and was then licensed as a psychologist in Vermont. For the past seven years, she has worked at a hospital where her commute each way is one hour. Perhaps that is a small price to pay after her cancer and chemo experiences. At least she can listen to NPR or relaxing music, or just leave Cancerville behind her for the night on her drive home.

At times, Kathleen acknowledges that working in Cancerville after having had cancer herself can stir up some pretty heavy emotions. But she says:

> I am so passionate about being able to help others who are in the same position I was in. When I say, 'I understand,' it is from my experience and from my heart. I selectively share with some of the people I help my own journey through Cancerville. Because of that personal experience, if someone tells me what they need—no matter what that is—I will do anything and everything to make that happen. I just love what I do everyday—helping people with cancer.

Obviously, the fortunate people who have Kathleen's support must love her too. They have what she didn't—a caring, compassionate Cancerville guide to help ease their burden and show them the way. Her simple advice to those entering Cancerville is to:

> Welcome and seek out support and find what works for you. You don't have to go this route alone, as I did. There are times in our life when we need support emotionally, and cancer is one of those times that both the patient and 'heart and soul giver' (Bill's lovely term) can benefit.

Last year Kathleen was diagnosed with breast cancer. Here's what she said in the Stowe VT Weekend of Hope 2013 newsletter welcome: "This year I was diagnosed with cancer again after 16 years cancer free. This was devastating and frightening. However, this time was different. I understood the benefits of support and how to ask for it..... I learned much of that by...never losing sight of the fact that having cancer can be very lonely and I don't have to do this alone."

Kathleen's powerful story shows both how cancer can be beaten and how survivors can put their energies into helping others in meaningful ways.

Tracey

Tracey Paige, who appears to be in her forties, is not a mental health professional. She spent the bulk of her very successful career in retail. Yet her present job as Director of the Fort Lauderdale American Cancer Society (ACS) involves providing support groups for cancer patients and their families in just about every hospital in that area. In addition, from March to June, she oversees forty+ Relay For Life events in communities all across South Florida. These contribute significantly to her goal of raising many millions of dollars a year. A significant percent of every dollar raised goes to provide services and research.

Tracey was previously a senior executive who was managing a fifty million dollar retail business when her friend and colleague took a job at the ACS as regional manager. It wasn't long before her friend recruited her to be the director. She was attracted to the job because her father had passed from cancer and also because she was ready for a different type of challenge—one more emotional than product driven. Thank goodness for that because within seven months she herself was diagnosed with breast cancer.

The slowness of the diagnostic and treatment process got to her Type A nature. "I needed to know my situation, and to get it out of me if it was cancer," she says. She goes on to say:

> It really wasn't a shock. You kind of get the feeling from the doctors that it isn't SOP and biz as usual. It takes on a more serious air, and you just kind of know you are going to get a positive biopsy result. Yet I still felt as if I was kicked in the stomach.

When her surgeon, a board member for ACS, returned with the results of her biopsy, his demeanor led her to say, "I guess I will be eating at many, many survivor dinners next year."

The dinners Tracey was referring to are part of the Relay For Life Program, which is dedicated to the Cancerville journey from diagnosis to survivorship. Each part of the all night Relay for Life event honors that journey, as well as those who did not survive. It is a very special and meaningful experience for all who participate. My "DAM STRONG!" team raised almost $7000 in 2013.

Tracey shared with me that she cried at each of the survivor walks or runs the prior year, which she watched as a spectator. When she participated in them the following year as a survivor, she was numb for the first five events. It took her a while to break through her denial that now she was part of that important group.

Tracey said straight out that fate brought her to the ACS at a much-needed time. She had an army of support from family, good friends, coworkers, volunteers, etc. Her closest friends and husband gave up alcohol when her oncologist insisted that she do that during chemo. Additionally, her husband (who is bald) shaved his moustache and beard when she shaved her own head before chemo. He received the highest accolades from her for being there in any and every way. He was truly a "heart and soul giver." His mom died of breast cancer when he was eleven, which had to make it even more difficult for him. But he stayed the course with love, caring, and total support.

Tracey's commitment to Cancerville and helping in any and every way she could was there from day one. Her personal experience added even more dimensions to her job. She said that she often felt like she was on the TV show "Undercover Boss" as she sat in waiting rooms, hospitals, etc. and listened to the chatter, which ultimately helped her to improve ACS services. It also increased her advocacy for the underserved populations that need screenings and mammograms, etc. She told me:

> If I didn't have a mammogram I could have died from the delay in diagnosis. ACS just donated thirty thousand dollars to Holy Cross Hospital to give one thousand mammograms to those with no insurance and no funds. My experience helped me to see how important prevention is in the scheme of things and that we have to keep doing more for all populations.

> My job in many ways is even more rewarding now, and it was surely rewarding from day one. I will never go back to retail again. I have found my home here and am pleased that I can pay it back in this empowering way—and I get to work with the best people who were all there for me and are all there for Cancerville. What more can you ask for in life?

Marty

Marty is a caring and compassionate mental health professional who devotes himself full-time to providing oncology support. Marty Clarke, PA-C, Ph.D., is one special man. I sensed it from the moment we met. He came over to us to say hello at a conference and acted as if we were old friends. Perhaps that is the Midwest way, as he is from Missouri. We are not used to that kind of down-home-friendliness in South Florida.

I was immediately impressed when he, as a psychiatric physician assistant as well as a clinical psychologist, said, "If I have to write a script, I haven't done my job properly." He doesn't mean that literally, but he prefers to find natural and organic supports for his oncology patients before he prescribes psychiatric meds. It is certainly hard to argue with that in a world that seems all too eager to promote and push pills. He appreciates that "messing with someone's brain" is a serious responsibility. I like that very much.

Something else Marty said when we chatted the other day by phone impressed me. I have quoted it several times in just a few short days. He said, "We are all connected in one way or another. If I disrespect you, I disrespect me. If I give to you, care about you, and love you, I do the same back to myself. I too receive the gifts I give you!" What a lovely way to look at our lives, our humanness, and our connections to one another.

Marty works full-time—fifty-plus hours a week—in cancer psychiatry at a very large hospital in St. Louis. The path to this career was, to say the least, circuitous. I will let him tell where it all began:

> When I was nine years old my father was diagnosed with bladder cancer. For the next three years I watched him disappear physically and emotionally as the relentless toll of his disease, multiple surgeries, chemo, and radiation therapy consumed him. Because he died when I was just twelve years old my memories of our time together are quite powerful and very special.

Fascinated by TV shows related to medicine as a young boy, Marty decided to become a paramedic while attending college. A serious accident while he was in his emergency vehicle wiped out that career. Though he tried to go back, his PTSD at traffic accident scenes rendered him less than useful. As we already know, even we mental health professionals can experience leaking cess.

He moved on to become a physician assistant and coincidentally (we know there are none—don't we?) wound up in oncology in a VA hospital. As time went on, he burned out and detoured into the business side of medicine, working for a biotech company. His million-plus dollars of stock equity fizzled as the company went belly up after a few years.

He then went back into direct service and eventually found his way into the emotional side of oncology, where he has been working for the past ten years. When he realized that he was more passionate about helping his patients live one day better than one day longer, he went back to school. Despite serious health problems of his own, he received a Ph.D. in clinical psychology in December 2011.

Marty, like Kathleen and Tracey, is quick to say that he loves his job, despite its demands. He says, "It is a weighty, very weighty way to earn a living." But for Marty, this is much more than earning money—of that I am certain. His early exposure to the resilience of humanity as a paramedic excited him, as he observed the will and determination that people can bring to the life and death challenges they face. This has continued to impress him in his work, and he feels proud, in a very spiritual way, to bear witness to the power that people bring to their Cancerville time. "I get to see people at their very best," he says, "despite their fighting a very harsh disease that forces them to feel their very worst."

He readily admits that he is still "learning" to leave Cancerville behind him—but that he practices a variety of tools, likes to be part of and photograph nature, reads inspirational books, contemplates life and the universe, and takes care of himself in a variety of ways to avoid "compassion fatigue." He even teaches classes on that to help others in similar "always giving" positions. In response to my question about what he tells others who are dealing with cancer, he says without hesitation, "To be kind to themselves." In many different ways, Marty seems to strive to follow his own advice, though he admits it is not always easy.

In a most poignant and powerful way, Marty sums it all up by saying:

> One of the best memories are the times I ran home after school to massage my father's feet and help him out of bed for a walk. With his arm around my shoulder we walked out of his bedroom, down the short hallway into the kitchen, around the table and back into his bed. He always said, 'Thank you. Now go play.'
>
> Every time I assist one of my patients, I help my dad, one more time, to get out of bed and take a short walk—together. And that is one of the many reasons I love my job and give it my all!

Lori

I don't know why I decided to go to the award ceremony at a conference in Miami, as I usually pass on that kind of program. The conference was for mental health practitioners from all over the world who spend their time helping others in Cancerville.

The speakers accepting awards for their contributions helping those in Cancerville were interesting, but one person stood out in my mind. Lori's honesty shined, as did her prose and the beautiful pictures that she had taken "behind the lens" of her camera. Her thank-you speech came after being given the Outstanding Clinical Care Award. Her words resonated with me in a special way.

Dr. Lori Wiener, Ph.D., began by saying, "For each of us there is often a story. I choose to share my story with you." Right there I was hooked like a river bass on a line. I am a sucker for the "bait" of honesty, openness, sharing, and the telling of a meaningful tale. Early in Lori's story she shared her concern about having the knowledge and skills to provide excellent clinical care when applying for her first position in Cancerville. "Do I? Don't I? Can I? Yes? No? Maybe?" she asked herself repeatedly.

Though she got the Cancerville job she applied for, Lori initially questioned her capability and whether she would be able to tolerate such a difficult environment. She asked herself, "Am I making a difference?" as she struggled to absorb and balance the overwhelming anxiety, emotional pain, and grasping for hope that she witnessed each day in Cancerville.

It is always nice to hear that parents can give wise advice. Lori's mom gave her just that. She advised Lori to give it six months: "If… you can have the emotional energy for your life outside of work, then this work may bring you great meaning. But get professional help so that you don't have to figure this out alone."

Lori followed her mom's advice, saw a counselor, and was able to work through her Cancerville issues and the questions that plagued her mind. As we know from Chapter 10, "How Minds Work," we mental health guys and gals sometimes need our own "tune-up." Now, twenty-five plus years later, she deals with the most difficult of cases and helps them as best as she can. She managed to convert her fears into motivation to continue. She says, "I never stop being amazed by the remarkable importance of how allowing people to share their stories can bring meaning and purpose to their life regardless of the medical outcome."

Lori stated in her beautiful speech that it is important and okay for people fighting cancer "to have hope until they have no choice, and then help them channel that hope into the creation of a plan B." It is no wonder her words resonated with mine. We speak the same language—a horse named Hope and realistic optimism, until we can no longer ride that horse!

The theme of Lori's acceptance speech was about people viewing her full-time work in Cancerville as depressing. In response she says, "I can honestly say that I do not have those feelings. I have been permanently moved by the love and caring, tenacity, intimacy, self-knowledge, and wisdom provided by the children and families I have been honored to know, and I have been exhilarated by so many extraordinarily beautiful human moments."

We all have a story to tell, and Dr. Wiener tells hers with passion, grace, compassion, dignity, and the beautiful pictures that she has taken as a photographer who distances herself from Cancerville from time to time "behind the lens!" How can we not be moved to believe in Cancerville's loyal mental health supporters when people like Lori Wiener, Ph.D., exist and shine day after day and year after year—committed to helping people face and fight cancer to the very core of their being?

These are just four of countless professionals who have, for their own special reasons, dedicated themselves to helping people fight cancer by providing emotional, financial, and spiritual support. Hopefully, people like them are near you, and you will reach out to them if ever, and whenever, you need to. No one needs to go it alone these days, and there are things that professionals can help you with that even the most loving of your support team can't. I hope you will look for the Kathleens, Traceys, Martys and Loris of Cancerville, and draw from their dedication and devotion to help guide and support you through your journey.

In Sum

I strongly believe that counseling and/or a support group experience can be very helpful generally, and especially for you as you travel through Cancerville. My bias, however, need not be your command, as I understand that these experiences are not for everyone. I fully respect your right to decline.

My hope is that this book provides a valuable support to help you cope better with your Cancerville experience. As I previously said and warned you that I would repeat, no book can replace an individual, tailored, and personalized counseling experience or being part of an ongoing support group. I hope you will keep an open mind and will consider the possibility of these resources. I know individual counseling helped me personally, and I believe it can be helpful to you and many other people as well.

Crying is an important and healthy emotional vent at difficult or joyous times in our lives. Let's discuss this in more detail in the next chapter.

CHAPTER 20

Crying at times is okay.

Big Boys and Girls Do Cry

I t is likely that you will cry when you are in Cancerville, as cancer has a way of bringing even the strongest people to their emotional knees. But that is okay; crying is actually helpful. It is important, however, to always come back to a more comfortable and clear-headed position.

Most people are able to maintain a stiff upper lip until they get to a private or safe place where they feel more comfortable allowing their tears to flow. I always say that tissues are the most costly part of my overhead. That's not exactly true, but many do feel safe crying in their therapist or counselor's office. That is a really helpful vent and a place where those feelings can be left behind. Take the dam builders with you, and leave your cess under my area rug. The cleaning crew will take care of the rest later.

Often, I will ask the person I am helping what his or her tears are "saying" to gain a clearer understanding of their deeper meaning. Almost always, people are able to identify the thoughts and feelings that triggered them. In my opinion, there are many different feelings that can cause us to cry. I believe that tears are a form of wordless communication that represents a variety of emotions.

Where it All Began

From our very beginnings, crying serves a variety of useful purposes. As infants, it is our only communication device to signal discomfort. It is our emergency call as helpless babies, that shout-out to our caretakers that we are hungry, tired, have a dirty diaper, or need a big burp or an even bigger hug. An infant's tears come from irritating or painful physical sensations, since their thoughts and emotions have yet to develop.

Crying is also a vent that lasts long after infancy to both express and flush out our child or teen-based displeasures and emotional wounds. Our hurts, disappointments, social rejections, academic failures, losses, sibling assaults, and other abuses all flow out in a tantrum of tears.

As adults, we still cry from strong physical pains, but our thoughts and feelings are more likely to be the stimulus for our tears. For example, when you think about your physical and emotional pain and distress, you can rapidly feel very sad/bad/mad, and your adult self can lead you down a tearful path. There, your pained adult parts may meet up with the little boy or girl who lives within your grown and even aging self. This is precisely why big boys and girls do cry in and out of Cancerville.

For those who feel crying reflects weakness, you need only look to the many settings outside of Cancerville where it is perfectly appropriate and acceptable for adults to cry. Emotional movies, celebrations, award ceremonies, and many other situations all cause people to cry freely without being self-conscious or judged as weak. Think about the big brawny athletes whose tear-filled towels appear randomly at the conclusion of the "big game." Both the winners and the losers shed their share of tears. These tears come about from the overwhelming ecstasy of winning or the gut-wrenching agony of defeat.

In her book, *It's Always Personal,* [30] Anne Kreamer talks about the value of people crying in the workplace. She says, "Crying at work is transformative and can open the door to change." Certainly, if people can comfortably cry in these different situations without embarrassment, you can cry Cancerville tears too.

As we already know, Cancerville creates many intense feelings, some of which can trigger your tears. As I mentioned, I believe there are different types of tears that are based upon and represent different thoughts and feelings. Knowing about them will help you more clearly understand what you are feeling and dealing with when your tears flow in Cancerville.

Tears of Shock and Awful

Ronnie's phone call alerting me to Jodi's diagnosis was a tear-filled explosion. Her tears spoke the otherwise unspeakable devastation of a mom whose world had just come crashing down on her head with the terrifying and overwhelming force of an emotional earthquake. Every single word of that brief conversation was streaked, if not flooded, with her tears.

I concluded my session with the client sitting across from me in mid-sentence and came right home. That was only the second time in my practice that I did that; the previous time was also for a serious family emergency. The twenty-minute ride home seemed like an eternity and yet, much too short a time to face a pain-filled reality.

Upon arriving home, Ronnie and I both cried for a while until we could calm ourselves. Once we regained our composure, we called Jodi. Even though Ronnie and I were feeling worse than terrible, we were able to plant some small positive seeds into some pretty dark soil in our daughter's mind. Obviously, she was quite shaken after receiving a terrifying and overwhelming diagnosis.

Ultimately, those seeds took root and helped her already strong nature grow into beanstalks of hope and optimism. I believe that her positive expectations contributed to her recovery. I have always felt, both in my practice and in my life that it is never too early to plant a seed—beanstalks do take time to grow.

If "heart and soul givers" can cry upon the shock of their loved one being given a cancer diagnosis as well as the awful nature of the treatments, certainly so can the patient. Many of the people to whom I have spoken initially cried upon receiving their cancer diagnosis. Some, like Jodi, also cried right before their treatment was to begin. In all instances, their tears helped clear the way for them to face Cancerville head-on.

Tears of Inequity

Considering the stakes and pressures, as well as your suffering, you have every right to shed some tears of inequity from time to time and vent your fury at the unfairness of it all. In this context, to not do that seems less than appropriate.

When you are in Cancerville, you stand in the proverbial Job-like position asking, "Why me God?" When no clear answer comes, tears over this undeniable inequity often do. You might want to read Rabbi Harold Kushner's view on this complex subject. After his young son died of a dread disease unrelated to Cancerville, he wrote *When Bad Things Happen to Good People*.[31] You need not be Jewish to relate.

As you know from the Introduction, my "This cannot be my daughter's turn!" lament and associated tears were all about the unfairness of Cancerville. It is undeniably a difficult hand to be dealt, but as I have stressed throughout, it is all about playing a difficult hand as well as you can. Actions and distractions help you look away from the unfairness of it all.

Tears of Sadness

Cancerville is a place that promotes sadness. How can you not be sad that you are there and being forced to deal with all of its challenges and demands? Few places can be as hurtful to you as Cancerville. Fortunately, the majority will get through it and can slowly return to a calmer life. Let us assume for now that you will too.

When you are sad, your tears are a natural response and release. They wash away some of your painful feelings and allow you to return to a more comfortable position so you can focus on the progress that is being made. Being sad, in and out of Cancerville, is natural—so is crying from time to time when you are sad.

I worked very hard to shake the sad feelings that would sweep over me like a cold gust of Chicago wind in February. I kept putting on the emotional equivalent of a heavy winter coat, complete with scarf and mittens. That is definitely not easy for a guy from Fort Lauderdale. Despite drawing upon the tools I have described, feeling sad caused tears to fall from time to time. They were a helpful vent and enabled us to cope better.

Even now, all these years later, as we read and edit certain parts of this book, Ronnie and I still shed sad tears that drip slowly down our cheeks and dampen the pages. We take a break, catch our breath, and return to our work. These tears help us vent the cess related to those painful memories and allow us to just move forward! No matter how positive your outcome, Cancerville leaves a residue of sadness that doesn't really ever go away. How could it?

Tears of the Unknown

As I have previously mentioned, you probably are not comfortable with the unknown. You, like almost all people, feel much better when you think and feel you are in control. Whether you truly are in control or have just built an illusion of control is not what matters. The problem is that in Cancerville there is no way to keep the illusion going; Cancerville and certainty do not typically co-exist.

I fully understand crying about unknown possibilities, but I discourage you from dwelling on that for very long. As I repeatedly reminded myself, it is not just in Cancerville that you don't know what's coming around the corner. The unknown is scary all over the place simply because you know, all too well, that you don't know! So just as you probably don't worry and cry about other possible unknown outcomes outside of Cancerville, I urge you to cry briefly, vent your feelings, and then refocus on positive outcomes for yourself.

Tears of Commiseration

The question can be raised as to whether it is appropriate or not to cry in front of or with your family and/or friends. There is no clear answer that will fit all situations or all people. I believe the answer is similar to the one we discussed in Chapter 11 when we talked about authentic versus artificial communication. You will recall that Dr. Coyne talked about "protective buffering" and the division among professionals on this topic. The examples that I suggested were more balanced and avoided going to one extreme or the other.

I hope you can strike a balance that allows for support and hopefulness as well as expressing your genuine feelings, including tears. Your tears may or may not flow when your family and friends are present. It may occur naturally, or you may choose to suppress them. It is a very personal issue and may or may not be a conscious choice.

Would I encourage you to cry hysterically for fifteen or twenty minutes in their presence? If I could write the script, I would try to contain such scenes to a few moments of a tear-filled embrace. That said, however, there is no faucet connected to our tear ducts. I encourage you to do as you and your mind and body need.

Let's keep in mind that since crying is a healthy vent and release, modeling that is helpful. I don't recall us crying with Jodi or she in front of us other than on her walk to the OR. We all cried privately, as is our nature. Our inner programs guide us automatically, especially in our more sensitive zones. Once again, I remind you that there is no "right" way; there is only your way and what feels comfortable for you.

Invisible Tears

There is another form of tears that I discovered in Cancerville. I came to call them invisible tears. These occurred when no one knew that I was crying except me—but I was. These tears flowed silently from my heart. They poured out with the force of a flood, and yet they went nowhere. There was no evidence of their existence because they stayed hidden inside me.

These invisible tears came in a variety of settings and from a variety of triggers. It was as simple as a newspaper article or as complicated as a visit to one of Jodi's doctors. It was a totally unrelated movie or show or a fleeting thought racing through my mind to nowhere in particular. In fact, all these years later, my invisible tears still flow from time to time. As I previously said, when I reread parts of this manuscript, both visible and invisible tears come on quietly but heavily. Many references take me right back to exceptionally difficult and dark days for Jodi, our family, and for me.

The problem with invisible tears is that instead of relieving your system by venting, they clog it further by tormenting. They leave an emotional residue that remains attached to your heart like the toxins of a cigarette or fatty deposits from a delicious but unhealthy plate of pâté. This is why it is helpful to cry visible tears to vent those invisible ones that can so easily stain the lining of your heart. Such stains leave you feeling down and sapped of energy and optimism. I truly believe crying can help protect your health as well as your mind. That is one of many reasons I allowed my tears to flow the night my friend Phil emailed me about his grandson having leukemia.

You may wonder why I said that crying could protect your body. It is the stress of suppressing painful feelings that concerns me. Such stress taxes your entire system. It compromises your immune system and your important organs. It weighs heavily on your body as well as your mind. It weakens you in every way. You cannot afford to do that at this time. I simply want you to go through Cancerville as physically and emotionally strong as you possibly can. Crying from time to time will help you do just that.

Happy Tears

There are also tears of joy, happiness, and relief. These, of course, are the very best tears to experience. The winners of a sporting event or award, or people who cry at weddings and other celebrations, are feeling excited and elated. In *Getting Back Up From an Emotional Down*, I wrote, "When the dam laughs at the pool it often comes out in the form of a teardrop." Simply put, nothing feels quite so good as a prideful or joyous time when a dam deposit overrides a cess-based issue or worry.

These same happy feelings will occur when you receive good news about yourself from the not-so-grim doctors. They can smile and really do enjoy positive news too. Just ask Rob how the meeting went when they excitedly announced they were finally ready to do the bone marrow transplant from one of his twins to the other.

Your tears after such a happening will be of a "thank goodness" kind. Such moments tenderly reinforce the positive thinking that I am encouraging. Savor these high-five moments and the tears that may flow because they are so very special.

Real People Facing Cancer

Betty

Betty Rollin's book *First, You Cry* was published in 1976,[32] a time when words like "cancer" and "breast" were not commonly said out loud or printed. Our "sounds of silence" world was just amping up to openness.

Betty describes her Cancerville experiences in vivid detail. I read it just after Jodi was diagnosed and, just as Betty did, first I cried! Because of an initial misdiagnosis, Betty's treatment was delayed for an entire year. She met up with distanced doctors and disconcerting interactions and interventions that included a modified radical mastectomy, which removed her breast and auxiliary lymph nodes. Her emotional experience was similar to Eileen's surreal feelings, which were described in Chapter 1. While in the hospital, Betty said: "I don't feel sick. How come this is happening? How come this is happening to me? Is it happening?"

As I read her book, my anxieties increased as hers did. Our minds simultaneously unraveled as I read about and felt her anguish. I shared Betty's tears about not wanting to look at her body post-surgery, not feeling comfortable having sex with her husband, feeling damaged, unattractive, awkward, and self-conscious. She had many other more than understandable awful feelings. These became immediately unacceptable to me as I imagined my daughter experiencing these same emotions.

What did help me was being able to observe the slow but steady process of her recovery and resilience—she slowly went from tears and jeers to cheers. She mourned her loss and ultimately accepted it and herself. She left her husband for reasons that were a bit unclear but ultimately found love. She opted not to become pregnant because of the risks, and ultimately lost her other breast to cancer in 1984. She then found saline reconstruction a plus, though a less than perfect solution.

She took the hits back then, found her way through the Cancerville maze, and survived the ordeal—not once, but twice. Her book, describing her tear-filled journey, reached out in a sincere, serious, and supportive way to women dealing with breast cancer at a time when silence was the norm. In the Epilogue, added to the book twenty-five years later, Betty writes:

> Losing a breast is not so bad. It just seemed that way at the time.... I have a lot of company—other women who have been struck, who also keep waking up each morning. We're a grateful bunch.... It's funny how lucky cancer makes you feel. Not at first, but later.... That's because death is more real to me and so I appreciate not dying.

Gilda

Gilda Radner, a comedienne extraordinaire, cried a lot both before and during her Cancerville journey. In her funny and sad book previously referenced, *It's Always Something*, she describes her experience. After a miscarriage, she says:

> I cried right through Christmas and into 1985.... When I had to leave my dog Sparkle temporarily to go to England to shoot a movie...I broke into such a gush of tears that Sparkle's head got wet. I stood weeping until I saw the plane take off. Sparkle never even looked back.

Then she was unexpectedly pregnant in England and cried on the set one day, seemingly flooding with emotion. But when she miscarried again a week later, she didn't cry as much as she expected. Gilda knew something was not right in her body, and when the doctors told her there was a malignancy, she grabbed her husband's face and sobbed. This wonderfully talented woman, who made us all laugh, struggled through Cancerville and cried a great deal. At least she let it out in between jokes. She says:

> It's all a process. And change takes time. Some days I really understand the need for kindness and self-compassion. Other days I frantically try to push against the river, or I just break down and sob.... Poking fun at cancer helped me to cope with it.

In Sum

Simply said, it is okay for adults to cry. Cancerville is an experience that absolutely demands tear-filled releases. These releases will help ease the emotional and physical pressures that build up on a daily basis.

I want you to feel comfortable with crying because, contrary to the popular belief that adults should just suck it up, big boys and girls do cry for a variety of reasons throughout their lives. My sincere hope is that the majority of your tears will be of the happy kind and will be commingled with laughter.

Laughter is the subject of the next chapter. Your immediate reaction may be that laughter and Cancerville do not belong in the same sentence. That was Ronnie's initial reaction too.

CHAPTER 21

I will find reasons to laugh from time to time.

Laughter in Cancerville

My goal in the previous chapter was to explain the importance of crying, at times, in Cancerville. I am hopeful that you will give yourself permission to do just that. I now want to encourage you to laugh there too.

I have included this chapter despite Ronnie's initial discouragement. She felt that the words cancer and laughter did not belong in the same sentence. You, like Ronnie, may wonder why I have included a chapter on laughter in a book about coping in Cancerville.

While I agree that cancer and Cancerville are not laughing matters, laughing matters a great deal when dealing with any serious illness or major life problem. Let me help you understand why I believe this is true. I hope that this will make it easier for you to see and believe in the potential helpfulness of laughter.

Obviously, Cancerville is a very serious place. That being said, funny and laughable things will happen there. Try not to be afraid of laughing at them, and don't stop yourself from cracking a joke or cracking up. You can benefit from the tension release and venting power of laughter. As we shall soon see, the benefits can be richly rewarding.

Why Laughing Matters

I understand that laughing in Cancerville does not seem to fit the scene anymore than doing that in church or temple. Truth be known, it is acceptable to laugh in solemn places; the key is all in the timing and appropriateness. I was once at a Catholic funeral where the priest said several humorous things about the deceased. We all laughed and enjoyed the pleasant memories as well as the tension release.

Making people laugh, especially those with heavy hearts, is a definite pride bank deposit for me. It is also a strategic part of my treatment plan. Yet it is always a judgment call, especially in Cancerville. These are sensitive times and your humor needs to be appropriate. Think about the fact that the late night comedians didn't air for a while post 9/11. Nothing they could have said would have worked, so they were smart enough to take a step back. We need to be that savvy and sensitive in Cancerville as well. When you are in doubt, leave it out. Some of the "tumor humor" I have read isn't all that funny to me.

Ronnie's memories of being in Cancerville are sad, pain-filled, and grim, as are mine. I also, however, remember laughing there at certain times. We sought out lighthearted and humorous plays and movies while in New York with Jodi and Zev. Being the good-humored man that I am, I continued, appropriately and respectfully, to facilitate laughter within my family, just as I do in my office. Jodi appears to have "inherited" my sense of humor and drew upon it frequently while going through Cancerville. Her lighter side definitely contributed to our brighter side; in fact, it still does! Whenever she and Zev arrive for a visit, her texts have us laughing even before we reach the airport to pick them up. We are, unfortunately, reliably late!

Rob saw and chuckled at the humor of his inadvertently getting into a Jewish Sabbath elevator at Sloan-Kettering on a Saturday morning. Eager to see his son, he was frustrated that the elevator stopped on each floor. Being an Italian Catholic, it took him a moment to realize that very religious Jews don't "work" on the Sabbath, which includes not pressing buttons or turning on lights. So the elevator is programmed on Friday nights and Saturdays to stop at every floor. Laughing in that circumstance was much better than screaming, cursing, or calling himself or the elevator names.

Because of the value of a smile, giggle, chuckle, or belly laugh, I have tried to inject some humor into this less than funny book; I wanted to try to counterbalance the more difficult parts. I believe that humor is a salve that soothes raw nerve endings and minds flooded with cess.

Personal Experiences with Laughter

Much evidence, both anecdotal and research based, has shown the positive influences of laughter. I need look no further than my Mom who laughed her way to over one hundred years of age. She validated all of the research studies that show a link between laughter and longevity. In a family not known for living longer than their early sixties, that was quite an accomplishment.

Mom laughed all the time at things she herself said. Many didn't seem humorous to me, but they must have tickled her funny bone in some magical way. Even when experiencing serious dementia toward the end of her life, she managed to laugh at different times. Though her life was pockmarked with tragedies and losses of all kinds, she counterbalanced that pain-filled cess with giggling and laughing dam supports.

I previously quoted Norman Cousins' groundbreaking book, *Anatomy of an Illness as Perceived by the Patient*. He described how he faced a serious, life-threatening disease, a degenerative condition of the spine that I can't even pronounce, let alone spell. He was told that his chances for a full recovery were one in five hundred. Upon hearing these long shot odds, Cousins stated, "It seemed clear to me that if I was to be that one in five hundred I had better be something more than a passive observer." These are obviously good words for people in Cancerville too.

Cousins took a variety of actions, any one of which could have made the ultimate difference, as he did eventually recover. He moved out of a hospital and into a hotel. He hired round the clock nurses to help him. He exposed himself to laughter by intentionally watching funny TV shows and movies and having his nurses read humorous books to him.

In addition, he had his doctor do blood work after his laughing sessions to measure his body's ability to fight off infection. The results confirmed that laughing did strengthen his immune system. He states, "I was greatly elated by the discovery that there is a physiologic basis for the ancient theory that laughter is good medicine." No one, including Cousins himself, would argue that laughter saved him; but it didn't hurt either. It relieved some of his pain and helped him sleep better.

There are many more anecdotal stories of the positive influence of laughter. As you may recall from Chapter 1, Roberta laughed and kept others doing the same during her long ride through Cancerville treatments. Many concentration camp survivors said that laughing and a sense of humor kept them going, enabling them to survive during those horribly difficult times. Another example is that for many years the popular magazine *Reader's Digest* told funny anecdotal tales under the banner of "Laughter is the Best Medicine." Just yesterday, I saw someone wearing a tee shirt that proclaimed those very words. In the same vein, throughout the years, comedians have been the hosts of late night TV shows. People like to conclude their stressful day with laughter.

Please don't laugh (although you can if you like) when I tell you that there are laughing groups that people attend for the sole purpose of enjoying the benefits of laughing. There are also laughing yoga classes for the same purpose. Laughter Yoga International says there are over 600 clubs in sixty countries. Sebastian Gendry, founder and executive director of the American School of Laughter Yoga says, "Laughter yoga just wants you to be happy.... We simulate to stimulate. We go through the emotions of joy to create the chemistry of joy." I like his words very much.

Funny enough, according to Madeline Vann, a writer on women's health, the first Sunday in May is World Laughter Day. I encourage you to laugh every day, but even more on that one. If you are interested in learning more about the benefits of laughter, check out *Laughter Therapy* by Dr. Goodheart, [33] (great name by the way) *Laughter: A Scientific Investigation* by Robert Provine, [34] and *The Healing Power of Humor* by Allen Klein, [35] to name just a few books on this subject.

Klein's book begins with his wife in the hospital with a terminal illness. She playfully hung a male nude centerfold from *Playgirl* above her bed and covered his privates with a plant leaf. As the leaf began to shrivel, they laughed about it. He says:

> Now, Ellen's long illness was hardly a fun time; there were many tense and tearful moments, but there were also periods of laughter. Frequently she would poke me in the ribs and admonish, 'Hey, stop being so morose. I'm still here. We can still laugh together.'

That story reflects why, precisely why, I have included this chapter in my book. Laughing can help you in beneficial ways. It can serve to make your experience in Cancerville just a little bit lighter.

Physical Benefits of Laughter

I can't promise that laughing your way through Cancerville will heal or even help all that ails you. I won't tell you that it will be good for your head, heart, mind, or soul. I resist the temptation to say it can be a powerful force with preventive and curative value. You must admit that I did sneak it all in though. All of the above may be true or may apply only in certain situations or just for certain people.

What laughter definitely can do is help you release, vent, relax, and dump some of the cess and upset feelings you carry with you in Cancerville. It is a physical and emotional release of energy. Susan made this important point:

> There are also physiological benefits to laughter. It increases oxygenation to the cells and releases those good old endorphins. Also, the activities involved in laughing such as watching a funny movie or show, reading jokes, and the like, help distract us from the pain and the angst, even for a brief time.

Some research studies on laughter suggest that it may be a gentle form of aerobic exercise. Robert Provine, whose book was previously mentioned, is a neuroscientist and laughter researcher. He describes work done by William Fry, who found that it took ten minutes of rowing on his home exercise machine to reach the very same heart rate produced by one minute of hearty laughing. Provine states, "Laughter is the kind of powerful, body-wide act that really shakes up our physiology, a fact that has motivated speculations about its medicinal and exercise benefits since antiquity."

These observations help explain why medical research has found that laughter can actually reduce stress hormones such as cortisol, dopamine, and adrenaline. These hormones are released when we are frightened, worried, or upset. Cancerville certainly promotes high levels of these, and hearty laughter can lower them.

Laughter also increases endorphins and other relaxing and pain-reducing neurotransmitters. In addition, a recent study showed that laughter lowers blood pressure as significantly as when people seriously reduce their salt intake. These findings are no joke. Taken together, they clearly reflect the positive influence laughter can have on our bodies.

In addition, laughter is a nonverbal statement that speaks to the lighter side of life. In its simplest form, it counterbalances the heavies or at least reduces them just a bit. The funny part about laughter is that you don't have to be happy to engage in it. You just need to be willing to see the humor in life events and experiences, despite your unhappiness and worry.

Please don't misinterpret my message. I don't expect you to be happy while you are in Cancerville. I am, however, encouraging you and your family and friends to laugh there every once in a while. In truth, you just need to be willing to expose yourself to funny situations. Laughing is usually an involuntary response that occurs automatically. It is both a personal and natural response to whatever tickles your fancy.

Every so often, even in Cancerville, the opportunity presents itself for a humorous comment. It doesn't have to be a major joke— just a giggle or chuckle will do. Recuperating from surgery on a summer day at Sloan-Kettering, Jodi was mobile enough for us all to go to the roof garden to get some fresh air. I immediately noticed all the sad, gray, drained faces sitting and standing all around. I also noticed the elaborate, extra-high fencing. My quip was, "I can't imagine why they feel it necessary to fence in the roof garden." We all chuckled, knowing exactly my meaning. "Darn, we can't jump now," would not have been at all funny. Please, in all instances, know the difference.

Real People Facing Cancer

Joyce

I wondered long and hard about whom I would find to represent this chapter; it was not an easy spot to fill until Joyce appeared. I was at a Gilda's Club all-day workshop—the very same one where I met Martin's wife (Chapter 7). I found myself standing next to a smiling lady and asked what she was doing there. She said, "I'm the keynote speaker, and I'm here to make people laugh." I responded, "After four serious doctor presentations, we can all use a good laugh."

Joyce Saltman, Ed.D., calls herself the Guru of Laughter and did a great job rallying the audience into raucous laughter. She even dropped the F-bomb at the conclusion of her talk. Good thing Ronnie wasn't there or there might have been trouble—though not really. I'm the only one not allowed to use that word—at least not in my writings.

I called Joyce later that day and left a complimentary message. To make a long story short, she agreed to be in this chapter and invited Ronnie and me to brunch—that's how warm and welcoming she is. We visited her lovely Florida home, enjoyed wonderful food and the company of her husband Sol, and had many laughs. I also found my story there.

Joyce is an educator who long ago decided to incorporate humor into her teaching and talks. Her avocation as a humorist began in the early 1980s when she was between husbands and needed to laugh and help others do that as well. Throughout all this time, she has given more than one hundred talks a year and even gets paid for some, which has enabled her to donate...drum roll...over one million dollars to her charities. These range from a small Jewish temple, which she paid to heat during the winter, to contributing to Paul Newman's Hole in the Wall camp, as well as many other donations.

What qualifies Joyce for this section, beyond her laughter-inducing sense of humor, is that she had uterine cancer in 2002. Like Eileen from Chapter 1, Joyce had surgery and was done. She is quick to say that she didn't think she would die. Rather, she believed she would get rid of those cells and continue on. The really good news is that she did just that.

Sadly and unfortunately, her husband of fifteen years at the time did not do the same. He was diagnosed with Stage IV colon cancer a few months after she was diagnosed, and he survived five years before passing. So Joyce knows Cancerville—and because of that, she seeks to lighten its inhabitants' loads through laughter.

I asked Joyce if cancer helped her to live a healthier lifestyle. Her immediate response was: "NO!" She said, "My mother was a fatalist and believed when you arrived in this world it was written when you would leave." Her mother also taught her that God put us here to enjoy life, which included good food, ice cream, cakes, and chocolates. Believe me when I say that Joyce's scrumptious brunch was neither a meal for dieters nor diabetics.

Joyce concluded by saying that making others laugh keeps her happy and healthy. Who could really ask for more? The day we visited, she was being given an award for dedicated teaching service to her Delray Beach, Florida community. Then she was heading back to her home in Connecticut for the next six months. She invited us to stay there whenever we were in town. That's Joyce—a humorist who loves to make people laugh; a *balabusta* (Yiddish for homemaker extraordinaire); a cancer survivor; and a warm, kind, and loving person. We are proud to count Joyce and Sol as newfound friends.

In Sum

Some people I help in Cancerville, or with other medical problems, intentionally expose themselves, like Norman Cousins, to comedy. They watch "I Love Lucy" reruns and other funny sitcoms. They listen to funny CDs, go to a comedy club, or watch a cute movie. They tell me that their laughter not only provides an alternative to their tears but also offers a happier vent for their pent-up feelings.

Perhaps laughing and joking have multiple medical and emotional benefits for all. It certainly serves well as a tension release, icebreaker, lightener, and stimulant to our minds and bodies. It generally can reduce people's physical and emotional pain and serve as yet another vent to let go of cess.

In addition, it allows us to get in touch with some of the absurdities of life and Cancerville, as we do our best to dodge their bullets. There is a Jewish saying that translates, "People plan and God laughs." In my humble opinion, we have the right, in and out of Cancerville, to laugh back!

In the next chapter we will talk about communicating in Cancerville. It is a place where words and communication can quickly become as tangled and knotted as a fishing line on a windy day. My goal is to help you prevent such tangles and wrangles from draining your energy.

CHAPTER 22

I will communicate kindly and sensitively.

Communication in Cancerville

Of all the people-related problems in life, communication is certainly the most common. In fact, most problems faced by couples, families, friends, co-workers, and even strangers involve communication breakdowns and failures.

What I observe, both in and out of my office, is that people become defensive and blind to their contributions in communication breakdowns. This can cause even the simplest of topics to turn into heated disagreements and conflicts. The purpose of this chapter is to help you limit, if not avoid, wasting time and energy on these communication snafus.

In Cancerville, communication needs to be clear and sensitive at all times. It is better for all involved when it comes from a cooperative and supportive mindset. In all instances, your goal is to avoid harsh words, needless tension, and conflicts. Speaking through a filter of loving-kindness and seeking a common ground of understanding can make all the difference.

Stress and Cess Can Make a Mess

Despite these goals, communication in any emotionally charged area, especially in Cancerville, can quickly deteriorate in destructive ways. With stress and cess flowing forcefully in Cancerville, communication can easily come undone. Under these pressures and upsets, communication with medical personnel, family, friends, work associates, and even strangers can quickly go off-track like a model train going at too high a speed. Fighting in one war zone is more than enough for you to handle. Let's work together to prevent creating any other combative areas.

I fully understand that it is not always easy to leave squabbles and bickering out of Cancerville. Despite our many years together, our love for each other, and our general compatibility, Ronnie and I had our fair share of hot spots, even though neither of us was the patient. She talked too much in my eyes, I too little in hers. She needed to discuss all of her fears, while I needed not to go there. Her superstitions grated against my attempt to keep my mind rational. My unwillingness to support them made her angry. In my view, a grown man should not have to bite his tongue. Then again, in retrospect, that is so much simpler than fighting about it.

Fortunately, we were able to work through those difficulties and keep moving forward with our eyes on the goal of helping our daughter. To address and reduce our conflicts, I ultimately sought counseling. I needed a female therapist from Venus to help me not be such a Martian.

The purpose of this chapter is to try to help you avoid the traps that distort communication. By doing that, you can prevent the upheaval that can result from hurtful ways of communicating. Both emotionally and practically, you and your team need to be strong and united in order to avoid adding stress to an already stressful scene. Appropriate communication will contribute to that kind of healthy functioning and enhance everyone's ability to be there for each other.

A Tower of Babel

Though we may all speak the same language, the interpretation of words can often seem like an inkblot test. Everyone perceives and interprets things differently. The "telephone" exercise used in Communication 101 classes demonstrates the distortions that can occur, even in simple interactions. The teacher gives a message to the first student in line and asks that it be whispered to the next student and so on. By the time it gets passed along by six or more students, the message has usually changed in many ways. Sometimes, the last summary sounds nothing like the first. It is both a humorous and telling exercise that shows how easily the heard message can be distorted. When this occurs in real life, feelings can be hurt and sparks may fly.

Many forces combine to cause communication misunderstandings and conflicts. First, we may know what we mean, but that doesn't ensure that we say it in a way that others will clearly understand. I wonder how many times a day someone says to another person, "Oh, I thought you meant...."

A second issue is that we tend to process words differently. In this case we may say what we mean clearly, but the other person misunderstands the message. Yet another miscue is not caused by the words themselves but by the tone in which the words are delivered. If the person's tone sounds critical, sarcastic, upset, etc., it will influence the interpretation of the words themselves. The same is true of facial expressions and body language. Sometimes, they are inconsistent with the message, which then lacks credibility and is confusing.

In addition, convenient communication tools like emails and texts can easily ignite sparks of conflict. Because they lack body language, facial expressions, intonation, and other observable cues, they are easy to misinterpret. Compounding the lack of cues is that, at times, we press send prematurely without ensuring that we have expressed ourselves in a kind, understanding, and caring way. In those instances, communication can ping-pong back and forth, causing upset and upheaval to those involved. Yet another problem I have observed and experienced is that it is easier to convey harsh messages when shielded from face-to-face or even phone interaction.

One of the surest ways to create tension and angst is to talk or write to another adult in the tone of a parent-to-child command or criticism. This guarantees that cess will be flowing fast and furiously. We may love our parents, but we didn't always love some of the times they were being our parents. I said that in Speech 101 in 1963, and Professor Bednar said, "Penzer, there is hope for you yet!" I'd like to believe he was both perceptive and predictive.

Our past experiences, and our cess in particular, affect both how we deliver communication directed toward others and how we view those that are directed towards us. Let's not forget that all of our encounters with others (e.g., a history with an angry father, bossy older sister, unreliable ex-spouse, etc.) are stored in our cesspools and that area occupies quite a large space. All of this can become magnified under the stressful and agitating conditions of Cancerville.

Adult-to-Adult Communication

Authoritative communication, where one person has more clout and power than the other, may work in some organizations such as the military, but it doesn't usually work or sit well in terms of our family and friends. This is precisely why people generally, and especially in Cancerville, need to stay in their adult voice and communicate clearly from that position. This is true in Cancerville whether you are talking to the medical team, your family and/or friends, or others. When you speak to others kindly, it is usually reciprocated—perhaps not always, but often enough.

The ultimate in communication breakdown comes in the form of an argument. Once that starts, the communication often deteriorates to child-like levels. Very quickly, the "adults" leave the scene and are replaced by their "junior" counterparts. Hurtful comments and insults can pile one on top of another. Nothing gets resolved, and both parties come away feeling hurt, angry, and unhappy.

In Cancerville, your goal is to stay in your adult position so as not to distract or drain yourself needlessly. Your energies need to be channeled into fighting the cancer enemy, rather than fighting other people. Try to catch yourself when losing control of your communication and move quickly back to adult-to-adult interaction. Keep in mind that when you are feeling drained, sick, or in pain, it is not always easy to stay calm and focused on your choice of words—try anyway.

Should someone else bait you into a downhill slide of conflict, try your best not to bite that sharp hook. Even bickering over simple things (e.g., what time to leave for the doctor appointment, who should pick up the prescription, when you will call with an update, etc.) can trigger needless battles. Your goal is to work cooperatively as a team in all areas of Cancerville.

Please Don't Hurt the Ones You Love

It is ironic that we are often more able to remain adult in our communications with strangers or relatively unimportant people than with our most important family and close friends. Most of us are polite, respectful, and considerate of people we hardly know. Women often complain that their husbands are kind and supportive to a secretary, customer, or co-worker, and yet so blunt and insensitive to them. By the same token, some men have this same complaint about their wives.

I will admit that there have been times when Ronnie requested a discussion "session" with me in my office to get past communication blocks or miscues. The obvious message was that I was kinder, more understanding, and a better communicator at work than at home after a long day of talking to others. Her request woke me up to my need for an attitude adjustment, as it was less expensive than paying my fee!

As the song goes, we often, unintentionally, hurt the ones we love. We don't do this consciously, but somehow learned that we can get away with it. People who love us often forgive us, but I don't encourage you to push your luck; sometimes it can catch up with us. Over time, repeated frustrations and hurts can cause our closest allies to become our enemies. This is why the divorce rate is high and why family members and good friends stop talking to each other for long periods of time, or sometimes forever. Make up your mind to do your best to not allow that to happen. Then again, many say you really don't know who your friends are until you face a serious life challenge.

Few things create tension between people like the stress and strain of Cancerville. This is even more likely in relationships where there have been previous issues and struggles. If communication breaks down, seek help and support from a counselor who specializes in relationships—preferably someone who also has experience helping people dealing with Cancerville. Work hard to get things resolved as quickly as possible. Think about ways to prevent issues from becoming conflicted. Plan ahead to avoid blow-ups. That is exactly what this couple needed to do in order to avoid a brief but very destructive fight:

Wife: What if I die from this? I can't bear
               the thought of leaving you and the
               kids.

Husband: I've asked you not to say that to me. I don't want to hear that crap. Shut up.

Wife: Don't tell me to shut up. What if I do? Don't you even care? Are you just burying your head in the sand like you always do?

Husband: I'll bury my head, but not you. You need to stop your crazy talk.

Wife: I'm not crazy. You are. People die from cancer every day.

Husband: Stop being so damn negative. If you don't stop, I'm walking out the door.

Wife: Go right ahead asshole. You can't even be there for me when I need you.

Obviously, this form of communication serves no purpose and hurts both people at a time when they are already hurting. Think about how you might change the dialogue to make the outcome different. We will look at another version soon.

In the above interaction, the issue of the patient's prognosis is not trivial, but it is unknown. The feeling of despair versus hope flies in the face of just about everything I have encouraged. However, I fully understand that Cancerville is about scary and unknown outcomes. This ailing patient is realistically worried.

On the flipside, her husband is angry with her for expressing her frightened feelings and going with the darker side of her thoughts. She was begging for reassurance, but his words came across as derogatory and demeaning, and he threatened to walk out and abandon her at a difficult time. In my opinion, this man from Mars takes the prize for insensitivity and mental abuse. He needed to respond differently.

Yet they both contributed to this insensitive outburst. She bit the bait and responded in kind. Knowing her husband's nature and sensitivities from previous talks, she needed to discuss her understandable fears with someone else, even though it was perfectly natural for her to want to share her worst fears with her life partner. Unfortunately, that doesn't always work out well.

Directing harsh and hurtful words towards a person one loves is never helpful. This couple went immediately into their child-based voices, rather than staying in their adult selves. I hope they both apologized to each other within five minutes. There are certain times when the best communicators can have a major meltdown. That is when "I'm sorry dear" can be a very helpful salve.

Here is a redo of this not-so-nice communication with a few changes that make a huge difference. Hopefully, you can use it as a model for calmer and more caring communication:

Wife: I know you don't want to think about this, but what if I don't make it?

Husband: You are right. I don't want to think about that possibility. I am sorry you are thinking that way. Let's try to assume that everything will be okay and that you will be a survivor, just like the many millions who are doing well.

Wife: But you never know.

Husband: Look dear, such speculations are about as helpful as wondering if we will get into a head-on collision on the way to your chemo appointment at the hospital today. Please let it go. You are bringing me down at a time I need to be strong and hopeful. If you need to talk about this, please find someone who can handle it. You could call a counselor or talk to the social worker at the hospital.

Wife: Okay, I will. Sorry. Thanks for not getting angry. You are right. Let's go to the hospital. Drive carefully!

That communication is adult-to-adult conversation personified. It took some respectfulness, caring, and self-restraint, but the result was worth it. In this new version of the conversation, the husband short-circuited the discussion without being hurtful or abusive and pointed his wife in a better direction. Her last comment shows that she understood and appreciated his gentle and supportive response.

I understand that it may seem to you as if no one talks like that. So be the first to communicate in that way, though I doubt that you will be. Some people actually do talk that way, as taking this gentler approach is a win/win for all. I am realistically optimistic you will do your level best to be clear, concise, calm, and caring as you communicate with your Cancerville team of support.

As we observed, there can be tense times and communication issues between you and those who love you. Your and their fears, discouraged feelings, and moody moments, as well as a variety of other emotions, can all get in the way of adult-based communication. All of this and more can make for a less than ideal communication experience—especially when dams are frayed and everyone is stressed.

Let's look at another example of a hurtful scene—this one between a mother and adult daughter with cancer. Once again, it shows how even those who love you can wander off into some pretty hurtful and upsetting communication. This exchange is a bit extreme, but an encounter that actually happened. It was a communication breakdown of grand proportion. Ronnie has asked me to reassure you that it wasn't a dialogue between her and Jodi. Personally, I feel you clearly know that already:

Mother: I hate what chemo does to you.

Daughter: Me too. I feel like crap.

Mother: Maybe you shouldn't have any more? It's poison.

Daughter: Mom, we've been through this before. The doctors say it is important.

Mother: But look what it does to you. It breaks my heart to see you like this.

Daughter: Then go home. I don't need your negativity on top of what I am already dealing with.

Mother: I guess I can't do anything right in your eyes. I might as well be dead.

Daughter: How the hell did this all of a sudden become about you? I hate when you do that.

Mother: Oh, so now you hate me. That chemo is affecting your mind as well as your body. It kills people, you know.

Daughter: Thank you very much for that news bulletin. I thought mothers were supposed to help their children.

Mother: I'm going to kill myself.

Daughter: Me too (her bedroom door is slammed loudly shut as both begin to cry).

This mother needed to voice her fears and feelings to someone/anyone other than her daughter. It was an outrageously unfair rant made worse by the daughter feeling weak after her round of chemo. The best thing the daughter could have done was to go to her room as soon as the topic came up and say, "Mom, I'm going to lie down now. Thanks for coming over." Even better would be if mom could stop herself from putting her worries on her daughter.

Being patient and understanding, staying in your adult mindset and voice, and/or removing yourself from a provocative scene will help limit these cess-based bursts from becoming burning battles. As I have previously said, sometimes the best form of communication is a wordless hug. Other times, you may just cry together and give each other support. Of course, there are times when words can work and when you can, by example, encourage adult-based conversation.

Your Right to Protect Yourself

Marty Clarke, P.A.-C, Ph.D., whom you met in Chapter 19, gives his cancer patients the following five rules for dealing with family and friends:

1) **Don't tell me to have a positive attitude.** Just because I don't feel good, cry, express unhappiness, anger or confusion about having cancer doesn't mean that I have an attitude problem. When you tell me to have a positive attitude I feel alone with my fears, concerns, and confusions.
2) **Don't tell me to eat.** If I don't eat enough, it's only because I can't. I understand that I need food to recover. I promise to eat as much as I can.
3) **Please don't ask me how I feel or how I'm doing**. All day long, I work very hard at forgetting how I feel and how I am doing. I just want to enjoy being with you, doing the things I can and finding something, anything, that reconnects me with "normal life."
4) **Don't give me your advice**. Everyone gives me advice. I find this overwhelming and disturbing. I don't know what to do with all this advice, much of which is contradictory. It feels like I am in a room with twenty different radios tuned to different stations broadcasting bits and pieces of irritating and senseless information. So, if I want your advice, and I might, I will ask for it.
5) **I have the right to remind you of these rules.**

You might wonder about number one above, as it seems to contradict my message of positivism. Though I encourage people in Cancerville to try to be positive, I don't demand it or naively think it is something that can be continuously maintained. Throughout, I have talked about falling off the mountain or the horse named Hope and allowing time to heal and get back on stride.

Beyond the specifics, Dr. Clarke is encouraging his patients to set clear boundaries in an adult-to-adult fashion with well-intended but not always well-done interactions by those around you. Feel free to add any other anti-irritant issues to your list that will help you to be more comfortable in Cancerville. Clearly, this is your journey and you have every right to manage it your way. The better able you are to set boundaries in an adult-to-adult way, the more energy you will have to try your best to maintain a positive attitude.

Lori Hope not only has a lovely name but also wrote an interesting book to which I previously referred. *Help Me Live: 20 Things People with Cancer Want You to Know* is a guide for your family and friends in how to be helpful and supportive—without being annoying and/or hurtful.

Communicating Feelings

Most of us do a pretty superficial job when it comes to expressing and sharing our feelings about how we are feeling. "How do you feel today?" is typically answered by "Okay," "Good," "Fine," etc., even when we feel awful. I would encourage you to go a little deeper and try to express yourself in ways that reflect your actual feelings.

As we discussed before, "buffering" in some instances is important, but too much of that can be artificial and numbing. We don't want you and your family and friends to be playing a guessing game of charades or going through the motions of communication while suppressing almost all of your emotions. Should you always tell it just like it is? No. Should you always just suck it up for the good of the cause? No. Do you need to try to strike a balance to more clearly express your feelings? Definitely. For example, here are more complete responses to someone's inquiry about how you are feeling:

> Actually, I am in a great deal of pain, and I'm quite dizzy, which may just be my anxiety kicking in. I am going to do some deep breathing and relaxation exercises and hopefully will feel better later. If not, I can always take a pain pill. Thanks for asking.

Much better than yesterday when my head was foggy and I was in a great deal of pain. Today I feel almost like myself. It is a wonderful blessing to finally get some relief.

Clear and meaningful statements about how you are feeling are important for a few reasons. First, as we have talked about, Cancerville is a cess-generating factory—every day can add new issues, worries, concerns, questions, and discomforts. The more you can express your feelings, the more you can let go of some of that cess and make a little more room in your pool for tomorrow and the next day.

Second, we would like the communications between you and your team, including your doctors, to be authentic. This allows for clear communications and lets those trying to be helpful to you know how to better do that. Finally, by modeling open communication you are encouraging your family and friends to do the same. This allows for a clearer and, hopefully, more harmonious interaction that helps to avoid the kind of conflicts we have illustrated.

Coping with Provocative Staff in Cancerville

I hope that most of the time you will interact with pleasant, caring caregivers and their staff in Cancerville. Let's remember though that many of the people who provide support in Cancerville are, well, just people. They, too, have moods, attitudes, off-days, menstrual cramps (or the male equivalent), fatigue, relationship problems, money challenges, and a myriad of other issues that affect them. They may not always be "Jolly Rogers"—sometimes they may be short, curt, rude, and otherwise insensitive. They may act as if you are just another "salami" in the factory of uncaring health care.

Please try your best not to bite their bait either. Best to not stoop to their level of disrespect. Better to report them to a superior if the issue is serious enough, or just give them the benefit of the doubt if it is not that serious. Here is an example:

Patient:	Hi. I am Tom Smith. I have an appointment with Dr. Jones today at 2 p.m.
Receptionist:	No you don't.
Patient:	What do you mean? The appointment is very important. I was told to come here at 2 p.m. today.
Receptionist:	Who told you that? (said very sarcastically).
Patient:	Whoever called me last week. I don't recall the name. What is the problem?
Receptionist:	The problem is your appointment was for 2 p.m. yesterday. You missed it and the doctor was upset. He can't see you till three weeks from now, and you better show up!

When I say, "Don't bite the bait," I simply mean don't say what you would like to say at this delicate and provocative moment. It will do you no good given the receptionist's attitude problem. It may very well make things worse. Here is what I suggest but of course, use your own words:

I am quite sure that the person I spoke with told me my appointment was for today. I wrote it down while we were speaking, but should have written her name down as well. I have been eager to meet with the doctor given his reputation about my situation and would have been here yesterday if that is what I was told. Perhaps it was not entered correctly in the computer. Please apologize to Dr. Jones, and explain what happened so that he can squeeze me in this week. I will come any day at any time. I cannot wait three weeks for an appointment. Thank you very much.

At the conclusion of Tom's appointment with the doctor, I would have him say something like the following if he felt it was appropriate:

I just want to let you know that my initial interaction with your receptionist the other day was rude and insulting. I don't know if she was having a bad day or if that is how she represents you. If it is the latter, you may want to check with a few other patients, as you seem very kind, caring, and knowledgeable, and she is not doing your image any good. Thank you for seeing me. When will we begin the treatment?

Differences Between Men and Women

There is yet another issue with which we all need to reckon. Men and women have different natures. As John Gray taught us years ago, *Men are From Mars, Women are From Venus.*[36] Once we understand this framework, it's not terribly hard to understand why we encounter challenges as we all try to live together on Planet Earth. This is what got Adam and Eve in so much trouble way back when, and it has been strained between men and women ever since.

Dr. Gray has repeatedly said that men and women have different coping strategies, especially under stressful conditions. Men, he has suggested, cope by solving problems; they are frustrated when that is not easy to do. Clearly, men's frustrations in Cancerville are at very high levels. This is one of the many reasons men get very agitated and depressed there. Their will and problem solving efforts are thwarted in Cancerville in so many ways. Yet, as we previously saw, there are many things they can do there to be helpful.

In contrast, women, as Gray has pointed out, want to talk about the source of their stress. They just need to vent and seek support and understanding. They often get upset when their man rushes in to try to fix things. Many women have said to me, "I did not ask him for solutions. I just wanted him to listen, understand, and support me. All I needed was a kind word and a hug." We foolish Martians rush in to "fix it" and if that fails, try our hardest to forget it as fast as we can. There are times, in and out of Cancerville, when we Martians just need to be patient listeners, kind-hearted friends, and sources of strength and support.

My hope is that you and your spouse or other team members can have a meeting of the mind. The key is talking it out together in an adult-to-adult manner and finding points of compromise. You can also avoid arguing about trivial issues or having debates about that which is unknown. Try to pay attention to repetitive hurtful themes so you can catch your communication drifting in that direction and intervene preventively.

When things are coming at you quickly in Cancerville, reason and rationality tend to be the first to go. I hope you can blow a whistle, call a time-out, calm yourself, cooperate, and work together with those closest to you. If all else fails, you can learn or relearn the art of apology. Sometimes a simple "sorry dear" is all that it takes to get your communication and camaraderie back on track. And if your partner needs you to knock on wood, bite your tongue, or whatever it takes to ward off the evil spirits, indulge him or her. Who knows, maybe those actually work—poo, poo, poo!

Giving Yourself Permission to Avoid Toxic People

In some instances, the best option is to limit or avoid communicating with some people. Most everyone means well, but not everyone does well. Try to avoid or limit your interactions with people whose influence becomes toxic in a variety of ways. Watch out for the hysterics and the pessimists and especially the ones that combine both. Also, be sure to avoid the narcissists who insist in one way or another that "it" is all about them. Be watchful of those who think they are doctors and know it all or those who believe they can predict the future. All of this can twist your mind into a pretzel of pessimism at a time when you need to try your hardest to stay positive.

You will know you have encountered a toxic person by how you feel when you conclude the conversation; you will feel as if you were a cartoon character just run over by a bulldozer. You will also feel drained, upset, angry, and perhaps even hurt. You will wish the encounter never happened.

If you realize you are with a toxic person, try not to be mean, but do be assertively self-protective. Toxic people add cess to your pool while simultaneously kicking holes in your dam. The strange thing is that they think they have been oh so helpful in which case you need to be oh so unavailable. Encouraging permission for this self-protection is a very important piece of advice.

What should you do if the toxic person is a family member, close friend, or even life partner? You can ask them nicely to be more sensitive to your needs at this difficult time. Calmly discuss your feelings, citing examples of times they added to your upset or were otherwise insensitive. If they cannot change their communication, you will need to find ways to block their toxic intrusions. In a couple of instances, Ronnie and I discontinued communicating with people close to us whose toxicity added to our burden in Cancerville. No one, and I mean no one, has the right to add to your cess and stress— especially not while you are dealing with cancer!

The Value of a Support Net

If you find that, despite my suggestions and words of encouragement, your communication is not working well, consider getting feedback from a counselor. As previously discussed in Chapter 19, "Having a Counselor and/or Support Group in Your Corner," sometimes, smart as we may be, we need some feedback and guidance from others. No one has perfect communication skills. That is why Ronnie edits my writings. This happens after I have edited a chapter several times. We work on it again, and often again and again, until it feels right, is clear, and flows well. Then Kerri comes in, like the sweepers at the end of a parade, and cleans up what we missed and left behind.

A counselor is to the mind what an editor is to written communication. In day-to-day interactions, though, no one has the lag time of the writer's luxury. When we talk, we basically shoot from the hip. A counselor can help us learn how to do that better and avoid shooting ourselves in the foot. He or she can help us find the "delete key" in our mind, so we can use it when necessary, and also help us find a more caring voice with which to communicate. Both counselors and editors are word teachers who help refine, refresh, rephrase, and redo our messages. My "editor" wife, Ronnie, my editor, Kerri, and my therapist, Karen, have all been extremely helpful to me.

Real People Facing Cancer

Jodi S.

I learned about Jodi S. from Kris Carr's book *Crazy, Sexy Cancer.* In 2002, Jodi, a successful attorney in Los Angeles, was shocked to learn she had colon cancer; she was thirty-seven years old. Her doctors said it was inoperable and spoke about palliative care. Fortunately for her, she did not know what that meant. She says, "There have been a few bumps along the way, and I certainly don't feel terrific, but I no longer have cancer."

After losing patience with her complaining clients, she founded New York lifelabs, which is an unusual thing for an L.A. attorney to do. Her goal was to help others like herself "learn how to live without cancer, after having learned to live with it." Her goal was all about communication.

As part of her company, she created the "re: Writing Project" through which professional writers teach survivors how to better express themselves. There are classes on poetry and prose as well as group and take home exercises. In addition, editors from major publishing houses visit to mentor those who want to write a book about their experiences. At the conclusion of this class, they publish a literary journal and have a launch party. There is also an intermediate class that runs like a grad school workshop.

From my point of view, Jodi makes an intriguing statement:

> The goal of the class was to offer people tools to become writers, but it turned out to be a huge help emotionally to participants, and really enabled them to process some difficult stuff. People were able to write about things in ways they were not able to talk about.

In my language, what they were teaching survivors was how to vent their Cancerville cesspools in excellent literary style, and that is a wonderful thing, whether their books get published or not.

Randy

There is no way I can do justice to Randy Pausch's previously referenced, poignant and empowering book, *The Last Lecture*. Within academia, there is a tradition of professors giving last lectures to their students. In these lectures, professors impart the wisdom they have acquired over the years. They are asked to consider their eventual demise and talk about what matters most to them.

It was very important to Randy to share his beliefs with his students and colleagues at Carnegie Mellon University—so much so that he left his home on his wife's birthday to be there, knowing this would be the last one he would spend with her; they celebrated her birthday the day before. They had already moved to a home near her family in anticipation of his passing. Sadly, at age forty-six, this strong, sensitive, and loving father of three young children had only a few months to live. Fortunately, he and his wife sought counseling support and worked through many problems together, including the last lecture issue.

Much more than just academic tradition, Randy's last lecture was meant as a legacy for his children. The video and book became a way for him to leave them his imprint and try to teach them the life lessons he would have rather shared in person as a loyal and loving parent. Knowing that was not likely meant to be, he chose this path upon which to leave his footprints. Oh my goodness, did he ever succeed—magnificently, marvelously, and miraculously!

Randy decided not to focus on death in his last lecture. Rather, he focused on life. He called his last lecture, "Really Achieving Your Childhood Dreams," and went on to describe all of the goals of his youth that he had accomplished. It was his way of telling his audience and his children his favorite Walt Disney line: "If you can dream it, you can do it." Randy did both over and over throughout his life.

I liked when he talked about optimism because, as you know, that is a subject near and dear to me. He said:

> My personal take on optimism is that as a mental state, it can enable you to do tangible things to improve your physical state. If you're optimistic, you're better able to endure brutal chemo, or keep searching for late-breaking medical treatments. Dr. Zeh calls me his poster

boy for 'the healthy balance between optimism and realism.' He sees me trying to embrace my cancer as another life experience.

Randy concluded by saying:

> My hour on stage had taught me something. (At least I was still learning!) I did have things inside me that desperately needed to come out. I didn't give the lecture just because I wanted to. I gave the lecture because I had to.... If you lead your life the right way, the karma will take care of itself. The dreams will come to you.... The talk wasn't just for those in the room. It was for my kids.

With that, he clicked to the very last photo of the several hundred he had displayed in his powerful PowerPoint presentation. It was a picture of him with his three children: two of them were nestling comfortably in his arms while the third was sitting on his shoulders. Randy stood tall to his last lecture's bitter end, and his legacy communication was perfect.

In Sum

In most conflicts, both parties could have made different choices if they were in their rational, healthy adult mindsets. When you're fatigued, stressed, and overwhelmed in Cancerville, it's hard not to regress to a more combative state. Yet a little awareness and effort to control that can go a long way. Having read this chapter, you can now tune into those moments when you start to move toward negative communication and stop yourself, even in mid-sentence, before the conversation gets too out of control.

People in Cancerville need to speak in a way that fortifies rather than vilifies. I am hopeful that you can find a voice that will communicate your messages accurately and appropriately. I am also hopeful that those around you will do the same. In all of life, and particularly in Cancerville, our healthy adult choices and voices need to prevail. I am confident that you agree and will work toward that difficult but doable goal.

Let's now move on to talk about leaving Cancerville behind. This is not easy to do, as it follows us in one way or another. Perhaps the best we can expect is to just put some distance between Cancerville and ourselves.

PART V:

Putting Distance Between Yourself and the Land

CHAPTER 23

I will be able to get through this.

No One Really Knows Where the Road Goes

I n the book *How to Cope Better When Someone You Love Has Cancer,* I was initially reluctant to talk about death. It seemed to be such a rash and harsh departure from the positive thinking and self-talk I was encouraging. In many ways it was, but that doesn't mean we should exclude it from our thoughts or our conversation.

In the Foreword to this book, Bernie says: "Don't be afraid to discuss death. Let it teach you about life and be comfortable with the word so you can speak freely to friends, family, and physicians." I am pleased that well before I had any communication with Bernie, I was able to get past my discomfort and help guide people through this complex territory. Though it is not easy for me to confront your death potentials or mine, it is important that I do so. We all need to make peace with this inevitable last piece of our journey.

I have thought about death ever since I was old enough to know about death. My curiosity, as well as my early terror, began because, as I previously said, I was taken to the cemetery once a year to visit the grave of the person I was named after, my father's father, who died of leukemia in 1926. Imagine that from the age of ten on I visited a grave whose headstone had my name on it. This was very heavy for a young lad living in a "sounds of silence" era. We just didn't talk about it—any of it.

My focus on death did not begin because of neuroses, but it did eventually become that. It was because of having to face death over and over again, from age ten until the present. Ernest Becker's brilliant book *The Denial of Death* [37] rightfully won a Pulitzer Prize—but there was never denial for me. Death hovered all around me like a stalker in the night. It's no wonder that on my thirty-fifth birthday I taped my own eulogy. That is true, though I am happy to say I lost the tape years ago.

My focus on and experiences with death led me to write a brief commentary called *On Life and Death* in 1964. I was twenty-two at the time and recently married. If you are curious and want to read this brief discourse, it can be found on my mom's memorial website at sadiethelady.me, **or in** *I'm Not Only a Cancer Patient I'm a Survivor: A Workbook for Adults.*

In a strange twist of fate, mom more than doubled my father's life and lived to the age of one hundred. I would love to get some feedback from my gene pool as to where I stand, but they want nothing to do with me. "Let them live and be well!" I always say.

I am hopeful that despite cancer, you are living your life strong, tough, and determined, and are trying to enjoy it as best you can. I hope that my words have helped you to do that. Even if your emotional "face" is bruised and battered, keep giving your opponent hell until you just can't swing anymore. Be Rocky to the finish and you can hopefully win this next round. By now, you surely know I am rooting for you.

Another Family Loss in Cancerville

Cancerville came and smacked us upside the head once again when Ronnie and I were on our cruise in New Zealand. We learned via email that my first cousin Debra died less than six weeks after being diagnosed with cancer. She was a dedicated mother to her adult twin children, Naomi and Alan, as well as a dedicated physician. My cousin was largely responsible for my mom living so long. Debra had been her personal, "still made house calls," doctor for more than twenty years. Ironically, Mom outlived her by sixteen days, never knowing that her niece had passed away at age sixty-two.

A common feeling that many have, and one I had momentarily after reading the email, was that all my cousin's treatments for six weeks were a painful waste of her time and energy. She had major surgery and two other related surgeries, causing her needless suffering. My initial reaction was that it was all for naught. The trouble is that once we know of a loss, we are easily led to that incorrect conclusion.

The truth is that neither the medical team nor you know the outcome before it occurs. No one can predict the future. No one knows how a person's Cancerville story will turn out. In my cousin's case, hindsight tells us that much of what occurred in the name of treatment served no purpose. At the time, however, the surgeries were essential to try and save her life. It would be like stopping CPR prematurely because the person was taking "too long" to respond. There is a sign in my office that reads, "Never, Never, Never Give Up!" I hope you are doing just that and being "balls to the walls" positive. My simple belief about fighting any life and death battle is that we should never give up unless and until we have no choice but to accept a very sad reality.

Hope for the Future

Coincidently (as we already know there are none), on the last day of our New Zealand cruise, we learned that Holland America Line sponsors an "On Deck for the Cure" 5K walk and donates the proceeds to the Susan G. Komen organization. We learned that in the past few years Holland America has presented the foundation with over two million dollars. They have this walk on every one of their ships on every cruise. Well done and bravo! Nancy Brinker has been a master at having major corporations join her fundraising efforts.

Each participant, after making a donation, receives a tee shirt, a pink rubber bracelet, and an opportunity to walk ten times around the deck in a "race" for the cure. This was a formidable challenge after eating and drinking for a couple of weeks on the cruise. Both Ronnie and I joined in and completed all ten laps around the ship. We were one of the last to finish, just before a couple of eighty-year-olds, but that we finished was what was important to us.

Though this experience did not lessen the pain of losing my cousin prematurely, it did rekindle the flame of our hopes for the future. It made us think about those whose burdens will be eased because of people's generous contributions, new protocols and their targeted delivery, more efficient and effective treatments, and leaps of knowledge forward. We went from loss and deep sadness back to hope filled with love. This powerful emotional experience, coming just at the time we needed it, helped start the healing process that allowed us over time to accept our loss in Cancerville.

Meant to Be—Moving Forward Hopefully

Those for whom the fork in the Cancerville road turns toward life are very, very fortunate indeed, but unfortunately still do not have an easy time. It is, undeniably, a long and winding road with many hairpin turns, speed bumps, and detours. Being a Cancerville survivor is a Pyrrhic victory. If you Google that or search for it in your old-fashioned Webster's, you will find that a Pyrrhic victory refers to a battle won despite many significant costs and losses. No one leaves Cancerville unscathed by the experience. You and your family and friends are all wounded warriors on its battlefield.

There is never certainty in Cancerville, no matter how long after the initial diagnosis was made. No doubt, like almost all other survivors, you begin to feel an agitated discomfort a day or two before you go for your annual, semiannual, or quarterly checkup. It is a worrisome, anxiously anticipatory time analogous to a jury returning to the courtroom for a critical verdict. In Cancerville, there are no double-jeopardy rules. You are on trial each time for the crime cancer has perpetrated on you. It is natural for it to prey on your mind and for you to pray for no significant changes in the results from your last checkup.

Though I continue to encourage you to take an "all will be well" position, I fully understand that checkups may not be comfortable times for you. Each test becomes a measure of hope potentials. That critical day is a "too high staked poker game" for most. Having been already worn down by Cancerville, and having learned enough to know that cancer can reoccur, those test days become a foot-tapping, finger-rapping, mind-trapping time. Hopefully, you will be able to draw from the tools we previously discussed to calm and support you through these stressful times.

It is my sincere hope that those times pass quickly for you and the results continue to be favorable. May the verdict be a reprieve for you, so you can go on and continue to enjoy your life. Assume that will be the case with every checkup.

You Really Never Leave Cancerville Behind

These uneasy times and the nature of the territory are why you don't ever really leave Cancerville. You can put distance between yourself and Cancerville, but it follows along like slow-moving gray clouds overhead no matter how many years have passed. What were once minor problems, such as having a headache, stomach upset, rash, fatigue, or bloody nose, etc., can all take on more worrisome dimensions for survivors and their families. When these are confirmed to be what they appear, and not signs of anything more serious, your mind can return to a calmer place.

In addition, every time you hear about a famous person or anyone else being diagnosed with or passing from cancer, your own personal Cancerville experience will flit through your mind like a black cat in a dark alley. Imagine what Elizabeth Edwards losing her long, strongly fought battle did to survivors and their families. Cancerville stories of the rich and famous, as well as the not-so-well-known, appear to be rising like the price of gas.

Then again, you can choose to focus on positive outcomes. Former First Lady Betty Ford passed from natural causes at the age of 93. She was diagnosed with breast cancer in 1974, a time when the word "breast" was hardly spoken in public, especially by someone in a prominent position. She was a courageous and outspoken "balls to the walls" woman who openly declared her disease. She later dealt directly with her addiction and subsequently opened the Betty Ford Center to help others with drug and alcohol-related problems. She was truly a first lady who made a difference. Clearly, you can choose to focus on the fact that she was treated for cancer at a time when little was known and managed to live thirty-seven years post-diagnosis.

It is, however, likely that relevant news, magazine articles, or TV programs will now take on a special significance for you. Cancer breakthroughs will be silently applauded, while sad news will likely hit you in a sensitive spot. As Ronnie and I did the 5K walk on the ship, we felt very differently about the experience from those who were just being Good Samaritans. We were survivors by proxy and, if we had to, would have finished that walk on our knees.

In addition, October, which is Breast Cancer Awareness Month, is not an easy one for us. We are aware—much too aware! All of the media focus brings it all back for millions of people as well as for us. Though we support pink in every way, we can't deny our feelings that it all really, really stinks! Here again, feel free to insert the word before stinks that Ronnie doesn't allow me to include.

Fortunately, as time goes by, your Cancerville-related thoughts will lessen, and slowly, but surely, life will return to greater and greater normalcy for you and your support team. Will you still think about it from time to time? Absolutely. Will it dominate your waking moments to the extent it once did? Not likely. All things considered, however, despite it being a Pyrrhic victory, I am confident that you appreciate and feel grateful for your continued survival.

As a result of that appreciation, many survivors or family members set their sights on helping those still in or who will be coming into Cancerville. They may volunteer at a hospital, donate money, organize or participate in fundraisers, and do special things for the good of the cause.

Real People Facing Cancer

Todd

I met Todd at a conference in Miami. As the forces of fate would have it, his display table and ours were across from one another. I wandered over to see what they were promoting and came away both impressed and with a story that shows how sometimes personal losses can be converted into multiple gains and contributions.

Todd openly shared that his mother died of liver cancer when he was an infant—the time between her diagnosis and death was only about six months. Todd already knew of his loss by the age of five or six because he visited his mom's parents and saw pictures of her. His father remarried within a couple of years and his step mom and Todd have enjoyed a positive relationship. He also gained a stepbrother as well.

His mother's death has had a profound and paradoxically positive influence on his life. Though she did not leave him a legacy in the form of letters, videos, etc., her passing guided his life's journey in many ways. As a teen he wrote papers about cancer and decided on a career in health care early on; he chose pharmacy and obtained an advanced degree. Todd now works as a researcher developing oncology medications—there are no coincidences, only opportunities—but you must be tired of hearing me say that by now.

Here is where the story becomes interesting. Two years ago Todd's uncle gave him a box filled with various family memorabilia. There were pictures of his mom that he had already seen as well as some other interesting items—one in particular caught his eye. It was a handwritten note from his mom to her brother and sister-in-law written from the cancer center in which she was being treated. She thanked them for helping take care of Todd while she was away. Todd says:

> Seeing her handwriting was powerful for me. I had never seen it before. Even though the note was not to me, it reached me deeply in a way I can't easily explain. It was as if my mother was guiding me along a path I had never been down before. It gave me a vision that I needed to explore and hopefully fulfill.

Todd's vision was to use technology to help people like his mom create an online legacy. At a pharmaceutical conference in California, Todd discussed his idea with his friend Diptesh, a fellow pharmacologist who researches HIV medicines, whose family also had cancer-related experiences. Although Todd and Diptesh live in opposite ends of the United States, they both believed in the importance of this project.

As such, they began to research companies that could create a website that would serve as a legacy project for people wrestling with cancer or other life-threatening diseases. One hundred plus thousand dollars later, most of it their personal funds, their user-friendly website can now be accessed at ZarpZ.com. It allows anyone to upload videos, pictures, notes, and letters to be delivered at a specified date sometime in the future—at no charge whatsoever. Please check it out. Here is a man who lost his mom without ever really knowing her, who decided to help others who are in the same position his mom was in.

I came to realize just how influential Todd's mom was in his life—she shaped both his vocation and avocation. Look at the influence a son's love for his lost mom can have in guiding his journey. What a blessed story for all.

Even though we don't really know where the road goes, we can make our own roads through Cancerville and beyond—forever. Come to think of it, that is exactly what I have done, too, and I will spend the rest of my days helping others in Cancerville and promoting Todd and Diptesh's loving project as well.

Susan

I have talked about Susan throughout *How to Cope Better When Someone You Love Has Cancer* and this book as well. She also appeared in the "Real People Facing Cancer" section of Chapter 10, "How Minds Work." Susan played a very important role in both shaping my ideas about coping in Cancerville and encouraging me to write this book; for that I owe her a debt of gratitude. At a point in our journey together, we sadly, painfully, and reluctantly accepted that there would be no cure and that Susan would not survive.

She and I had worked hard to embrace positive, optimistic beliefs until reality knocked on her door and caused us to open it and our minds to other more difficult alternatives. It eventually became apparent that all options had been explored—all to no avail.

The very same questions that I asked myself at Morakami Gardens that sunny afternoon about promoting positivism for Susan, midway through her journey, reappeared the day of her funeral last year. As I listened to the loving tributes by her family and friends, I once again debated my decision and I remained unwavering in my opinion. Being positive and hopeful is not about life and death; it is about easing the demands and challenges of Cancerville until the outcome is determined.

Paraphrasing the previously cited words of Bernie Siegel, M.D., it's not about dying because we all will die. It is about how we meet life's challenges and how committed we are to overcoming them and healing ourselves. In this regard, I believe Bernie would give Susan an A+, not only for how she handled herself, but also because they were both originally from Brooklyn.

Once we realized her survival was not meant to be, we switched from optimistic to realistic, but still held out hope for a miracle. She prepared herself and her affairs for her passing with the same strength and determination that she showed all through her difficult life. She planned her funeral, including where she would be laid to rest, what she would wear, who was to speak at the service, the type of casket, and everything else that was possible for her to decide. She told me she left three pages of instructions for her family and had her lawyer come to her home to make sure her will was updated.

Her will to live remained strong to the end, but sometimes it takes more than strength to defeat cancer; it takes viable treatment options, and it takes some luck as well. The miracle we prayed for never arrived. We had a concluding meeting which was not a "counseling" session as much as it was a tribute to her difficult life and our long-term professional relationship. We talked about her struggles and triumphs, her cancer and how she dealt with it, and her imminent passing. She believed in rebirth and assumed her difficulties throughout her life this go-around would make her next one all the easier. I sincerely hoped she was right and I wished her well.

She thanked me for being there for her over so many years, and I thanked her for all she taught me about facing challenges strongly, persistently, and without flinching. The boy from the Bronx and the girl from Brooklyn bid an emotional farewell. Such is life and death in all areas—we never, never give up until we have no other choice. As I drove out of her driveway for the last time, I must admit I felt a tinge of defeat, but that is the price one pays for unfulfilled optimism—and, when seen in perspective, it is a small price indeed!

Susan wanted to leave a legacy for newcomers to Cancerville. I believe you will agree with me that through my books she has! The book for family and friends as well as this one will preserve Susan's wise words and inspiring efforts for a long time to come.

In Sum

The subject of death is complicated, but it is something we need to come to grips with in all ways. Denial is natural, but unhelpful; accepting our eventual fate and destiny will help us to find inner peace as well as to prioritize "living it" every day. Try to do your best to assume you will become a survivor and that you will do your best to live your life fully, peacefully, and positively. In its infinite wisdom, the American Cancer Society calls people "survivors" the day they receive a cancer diagnosis. Ultimately and sorrowfully, we shall all take our rightful place in heaven. That is just the way it is—always has been and always will be.

Though those who have entered Cancerville are never quite the same, winning any battle in these trenches is huge. It is David finally slaying the mighty Goliath with his small but powerful "slingshot." Many say that they are even stronger from the life lessons they learned in Cancerville. I myself feel that way because of Jodi and all the other courageous Cancerville people I have met. The minor aches, pains, and irritants life throws at me pale in comparison to the cancer experiences I have witnessed.

Despite its hardships, Cancerville does teach many life lessons. Let us turn our attention to them as we continue to heal and begin to slowly conclude our journey together. We have come a long way walking side-by-side, and by now I am hopeful my words have helped you in many ways.

CHAPTER 24

I will focus on what I learned in Cancerville.

Helpful Life Lessons You Can
Learn from Your
Cancerville Experience

L ife teaches us lessons in many ways and from many different places. Beyond formal education, much is learned from the streets of our life's journey. It is important that we pay attention and take in new information wherever we go. Such is the case in Cancerville. Much as we hate being there, we can learn a great deal from this experience. That its streets are dark, scary, and mean doesn't mean that we can't learn from them.

Even though you may be worn, weary, and wounded from Cancerville, you can still come away with some heightened awareness and new perspectives. Lance Armstrong concludes his previously referenced book by saying, "Cancer no longer consumes my life, my thoughts, or my behavior, but the changes it wrought are there in me, unalterable."

We have spent enough time on the painful lessons we learn in Cancerville and how to combat all that negativity. I hope that some of my words have helped you to salve that pain and come at your experience from a different angle. I would like for us to begin to wind down our journey by looking at the more positive lessons you may have learned—ones that I know I did. Most if not all of the positive lessons were not new bits of information as much as pearls of wisdom that can easily get lost in the hustle-bustle of everyday life.

Gratitude Helps Your Attitude

Strange as it may sound, I feel grateful for rediscovering gratitude while in Cancerville. Of all I took away, this stands out as very significant. Gratitude nourishes our attitude and many other feelings. I have come to believe that gratitude is milk for our minds. Got gratitude? I can't quite figure out what to smear above my upper lip or how to do that because I have a moustache, but that isn't important.

Too often in our quest for more, we forget to acknowledge and appreciate what we already have. I am not only talking about appreciating our food, clothing, and shelter, given that many around the world lack those very basics. I am also referring to having our physical and emotional health, support from loved ones, opportunities to stretch and grow, goals that have been achieved and are in process, and occasional times that are fun, happy, and warm.

I am also talking about waking up in the morning and having something worthwhile to occupy our time, having our faculties and mobility, and even enjoying simple things such as a pleasant meal with a special person. In a spiritually oriented book, *Turn My Mourning into Dancing*, [38] Henri Nouwen quotes a friend who, upon moving away, said:

> We are thankful for all the good things that have happened, for all the friendships we have developed, for all the hopes that have been realized. We simply have to try to accept the painful moments.

The reason Cancerville reminded me to get back to gratitude was how ungrateful I felt about being there. From the vantage point of Cancerville, I could look back on everything I had in my life before that time and appreciate it in a whole new way. I took much too much for granted before we entered Cancerville, and I didn't want to keep doing that. With this new perspective, my gratitude bank, like my pride bank, now runs over with thanks for the most basic blessings in my life. I hope the same is true for you.

I also realize that it may take a while for those still enmeshed in Cancerville to feel comfortable or grateful. I understand how easy it is in Cancerville to feel that you have nothing for which to be thankful. Try to use the wide-angle lens we discussed in Chapter 17 to take in more than the difficult Cancerville scene. From that view, it is likely you will find some things for which to feel grateful, despite your present situation. If you can do that, it will help offset some of the painful times through which you are now living. I speak from experience when I repeat that gratitude is milk for your mind. Get gratitude and don't worry about your upper lip—just keep it stiff for the moment.

Everything is Truly Relative

If you go back to the first chapter of this book, you can see the scale that shows my "theory of relativity." An important life lesson that Cancerville teaches us is to be better able to see the difference between that which is truly important and that which is relatively not. All of a sudden, Cancerville provides a new yardstick by which to measure life and what happens to us. I am hopeful that you will no longer exaggerate the more minor issues that you face if, in fact, you are prone to doing that.

After Cancerville, it is not easy to go back to the magnifying glasses in your mind that enlarge the less important problems that come along. Whatever measuring instruments we carry inside our heads have the potential to automatically adjust and recalibrate as a result of having been to Cancerville.

A clear example occurred during one of our visits to New York for one of Jodi's chemo treatments. While we were there, Hurricane Wilma visited our neighborhood and home in South Florida. When it rains it pours, especially during a hurricane— and most especially in Cancerville. Flights were cancelled, and we stayed in New York for a few extra days, which gave us more time with Jodi and Zev.

We asked our friends Esther and Alex to drive by our house and report back to us. The downed trees and lack of working traffic lights convinced Alex that such an undertaking was too dangerous—so Esther went alone. Had we been more aware of the conditions we would not have asked her to go. Fortunately, she made it safely to our home and back to hers. She reported that our home had taken a major hit. Our swimming pool had morphed into an overflowing cesspool filled with trees, leaves, assorted debris, and even a patio chair—better our swimming pool than our minds!

To give you a sense of the extensive damage, we paid $11,000 just to have the downed trees in our backyard cut up, removed from our roof, pool deck, and pool, and moved to the front yard. The other estimate was $18,000. Believe me when I say that the homes in our neighborhood are not mansions and the lots are pretty small.

How much did the hurricane damage upset us? Not one bit! Even Ronnie, who tends to get more upset about those kinds of things than I do, took it in stride. It was all just stuff that could be repaired or replaced.

I could finally fully embrace a sign that has been on a shelf in our library for many years. The sign says: "Les choses importantes de la vie ne sont pas des choses." That translates to: "The important things in life are not things." This statement is undeniably true in all ways, but it feels especially true after one has been to Cancerville.

Cancerville helped us both realize that the damage to our home was not significant compared to the damage to our daughter and ourselves. Few things in life are actually more serious or significant than cancer; that lesson is learned the day you arrive in Cancerville. Actually, even before that day, I used to say to myself: "If it ain't chemo, it ain't nothin'!" as a way to keep whatever issue I was facing in my life relative and in perspective. I understand that my English teachers would not have been impressed.

Priority of the Minority

Just as your yardstick shifts after being in Cancerville, so do your priorities. What once was so important comes down a peg or two or more. Similarly, what may have once been unimportant now takes on much more significance. Working hard, earning a living, and setting and achieving goals are still important, but people often have an epiphany after being in Cancerville. That experience expands our awareness of the dangers that lurk about and of the importance of taking better care of ourselves.

Time in Cancerville can push us to find balance and to strive to hold that course. This experience leans heavily on us to prioritize setting healthy goals and sticking to them. It helps us appreciate each day and use it to our advantage. While work is important, other priorities that are often neglected can be added to our personal equation.

Of course, there are no guarantees that taking better care of you will always make a difference. There are many well-known examples of people who were very fit, yet took a major health hit. Not too many people were as fit as Lance

Armstrong, multi-winner of the Tour de France, when he was diagnosed with metastasized testicular cancer at age twenty-five. Two-time Olympic gold medal winning gymnast, Shannon Miller, was also fit when she was diagnosed with a form of ovarian cancer at age thirty-three.

Similarly, Jodi was the healthiest member of our family; her diet and exercise regimen were solid. At the time she entered Cancerville, she was a gyrotonic personal fitness trainer who taught others to use that interesting technology to work out. Go figure! What we try to do to help ourselves be healthier doesn't always work, but hopefully it does increase our odds.

As we know, life offers no guarantees. But Darwin did get it right—the odds generally favor the survival of the fittest. Lance, Shannon, and Jodi's in-shape fitness did not prevent or protect them from Cancerville, but perhaps it did help them become survivors.

A Stitch in Time Allows for a Switch in Lifestyle

One of the many shifts people often experience after having been to Cancerville is how they allocate their time. All of a sudden, as part of the changes in perspective and priority, time is made for many things that may have previously been given less importance. This includes fitting in family visits, fun times, that elusive though relaxing yoga class, or whatever else is on your "taking care of self" list.

As an observer of people, I have come to realize that many of us are self-sacrificing to a fault. We cater to others, our jobs, community, church or temple, and to a host of causes other than ourselves. Somewhere in the maze of life we get lost. There is not enough time to go around, and our piece of the proverbial pie gets smaller and smaller.

Oftentimes, we just get some occasional crumbs, and that is a crummy way to live. It assumes that we will go on forever and ever and eventually play catch-up. It is based on the belief that eventually we will take that class or whatever it is that we have no time to do now. As Cancerville reminds us, there is no catch-up in life; there is only now. So *carpe diem*! (Seize the moment!) No one's future, in or out of Cancerville, is certain.

Though in theory it should not take a trip to Cancerville to cure the problem of not allotting more time for you, your having been there can be a mighty motivator. As a result of your experience there, you realize that your time is not infinite. You come to know that no alarm will be sounded to warn you of an impending problem or to give you time to squeeze in what's important to you just before the crisis hits.

Hopefully, you have come to realize that you have worth, are special, and deserve a fairer slice of that tasty, glop-free pie. I sincerely hope that you will come away from your Cancerville experience with a sense of entitlement to more than you might have allowed yourself in the past. In my opinion, you have earned the right to calmer experiences and will hopefully choose to steer some of your time in that direction. At the very least, I hope you will draw upon the relaxing, natural tools for healing that I have encouraged.

Strengthening of Character

As we headed into Cancerville, I told Jodi that she would become an even stronger person by having to deal with all of the challenges. Did she believe me at the time? Was this statement even encouraging to her in the midst of all that was going on? Maybe she believed me or maybe not. But I truly believed that prediction at the time and still feel that it came true.

We all became stronger from this challenging experience and I am hopeful that you did too. We learned that we could take on Cancerville and make the land our own in the same ways I have encouraged you to do. We learned how to stare it down and take charge. We found that little got in our way or blocked our path. If it did, we knocked it over—if not with a flick of our wrists, with a kick to its groin. We were, in fact, "balls to the walls," and rose to the challenges like strong athletes.

My friend Rob also showed his character and strength in his journey in all the many things he was able to accomplish for his family and for Cancerville. He, like Jodi, is an even stronger person today. Of that I am certain. So are his sons!

Like Rob was for his family, Jodi was our team captain, just as she was for her Taravella High School drill team. She helped us keep marching strongly and gracefully along as she led the way. Nothing was too much for her or, as a result, for us. There was no stretch that she or we couldn't handle.

Our game plan was definitely in effect as we slowly adapted to a new world order of disorder. I grew stronger as we went along although chemo days were always rough around the edges for me. Just like Jodi, we silently and stoically accepted what came her way. We looked Goliath in the face, and every single time we needed to, we whipped out our "slingshots" and hit him squarely between the eyes. "Take that you…!" Ronnie is one tough editor. I am optimistic that your sling shot aim was similar.

Ties that Bind and are Kind

Cancerville fosters closeness in all directions. As your support team forms and grows, I hope you will all work together for the good of your cause. Over time, winning teams develop winning ways and closer feelings. Family members and friends, some who have not been close in the past, come to the fore like a racehorse on steroids. It is not only the time spent together that forges these ties, but also the combined energy spent climbing challenging Cancerville mountains.

Jodi and Zev are closer with each other and with us as well. Ronnie and I are as close as we have ever been, fostered by our Cancerville experience as well as her editing both books with me. In fact, our whole family seems to be closer since our Cancerville experience. Positive, cooperative energies flow even more now, and family gatherings take on a special meaning. These gatherings usually now include the adult twin children of my cousin Debra.

Remember way back when I said I didn't really know Rob and that he was my friend's son? Rob and I are now buddies for life, united by Cancerville's common cause. We are two fathers who have walked the mean streets of Cancerville together, like those tough cops I mentioned in a crime-infested neighborhood. We kicked some butt together and didn't allow ours to get too bruised!

Rob invited us to come to Rye, New York last November to participate in the Leukemia and Lymphoma Society fundraising Light The Night Walk. Jake and Chase led the way for their team with Jake carrying a white survivor balloon while Chase, as his strongest supporter, carried a red one. We were there in a happy heartbeat. Unrelated to our being there, many months later that same organization purchased seventy-five copies of *How to Cope Better When Someone You Love Has Cancer* to place in every one of their libraries in the United States and Canada.

Trauma seems to bind people to one another as much as happy times do. Perhaps it is as simple as wanting to savor every moment of togetherness, having come to realize that it is far from guaranteed. I hope you, too, will experience this unique form of bonding with your family and friends. It is also why I said early on that while you and I may never meet face-to-face, there might be a special chemistry that forms between us. I hope it has been that way for you.

Real People Facing Cancer

I asked some of the people who made up the "Real People Facing Cancer" sections to tell me what they learned from their Cancerville journeys. Of interest is that though Cancerville is a trying place, they all had learned some very positive lessons from their experiences.

Eileen (Chapter 1):

> I learned to tune into whatever I am sensing in my second Chakra, which I have come to learn

is my authentic self. When I do that I am truly genuine without any filters.

Harvey (**Chapter 2**):

Not to agonize over the past or worry about the future. And the realization that life is finite and should not be taken for granted. Because of this we should make the most out of every moment.

Frank (**Chapter 5**):

Before Cancerville, I had taken a lot for granted. Now I cherish every day—and just about every moment. And to cherish my 'heart and soul' giver—she has been wonderful!

Martin (**Chapter 7**):

Cancer has given me much insight into life that I hope to apply once I am freed from its prison. I believe I will be more compassionate to others as well as to myself, have more patience, and feel stronger than I have ever felt. I believe its lessons will permanently remain stored within me, just like a photograph on my cell phone.

Cindy (**Chapter 12**):

I learned many life lessons. Cancerville reaffirmed my belief in angels, bonded me even closer to my wonderful children, and taught me that I could try my best control both my life and my destiny. When it is my turn, I will move on to be an angel, but I will not go easily!

Chris (Chapter 13):

I learned how valuable my family and friends are, how really small life's challenges are compared to Cancerville, and to be much more patient with everyday irritants.

My wife and I decided that this cancer journey was something we needed to navigate through but it didn't have to be the focal point of our lives—everything else did! That is not to say we take the journey lightly, but we make a conscious effort to enjoy our time together whenever possible. I've learned that it's possible to make the best of a bad situation, that staying positive is key, and that it is okay to need support.

Linda K. (Chapter 14):

I learned that each day is important, not to sweat the small stuff, to take even better care of my body, and to reach out to help others dealing with cancer.

Sylvia (Chapter 17):

I feel so blessed to have overcome this and to be able to share time with my children, grandchildren, family and friends. I learned that my future was up to me. If I believed in myself I could conquer the obstacles when they presented themselves. I had the strength, stamina, and self-motivation to get healthy and stay that way for as long as I could.

I, myself, am not the same person who entered Cancerville by proxy in 2005. Not only did I learn to cope, adapt, and face its challenges, but it changed me. Though the trauma of that experience remains sensitively stuck in my head, I can push it aside most of the time. Occasionally, I well up over a memory, thought, or paragraph in my books or someone else's; it's that feeling when your stomach and throat seem to merge and become one, when a throbbing heaviness swells right beneath your eyes, along with an almost invisible quiver in your lip.

Mostly, though, the changes have been for the better. Like the real people above, I feel grateful every day for every moment of the day. I am far more optimistic than ever before, even in medical settings—my dam no longer caves in under pressure from my cess. Realistic as well as sometimes unrealistic optimism guides my way and strengthens my dam.

In addition, I am far more friendly and outgoing, even with strangers. I now reach out whereas before I usually stayed silently stuck within. I guess when faced with all of the possibilities of Cancerville, there is no longer much risk in saying, "Hi, my name is..." or "What brings you here?" or "How is it going?"

In the final analysis, Cancerville gives us a new perspective from which to evaluate everything else in life. It truly adjusts that scale of relativity described in Chapter 1. It gives us a new set of lenses with which to see our world and ourselves. It mellows us out, helps us mature, and strengthens our mind—not necessarily right from the beginning, but as time goes on.

In Sum

There are probably many more positive life lessons to be learned from your Cancerville experience than those I have described here. In fact, I am sure you will discover more along the way. I have certainly worked less and played more in the past seven years: "If not now, when?" I asked myself.

Some people, after their Cancerville experience, decide to volunteer in some way. I increased that part of my life as well. I have committed to helping people in Cancerville in any way that I can for the rest of my life. Such good deeds often come back to reward us in many ways, not the least of which are pride bank deposits. In the final analysis, those are even better than piggy bank ones. Research consistently shows that people who do good deeds and help others feel happier. There may be some other positive lessons, too, which will be unique to you. Feel free to share them with me at bill@cancerville.com.

I am finally eager and excited to share the amazing fairy tale experience Jodi, Zev, Ronnie, and I had and enjoyed so much as we gratefully but cautiously distanced ourselves from Cancerville. This tale is forever tattooed in my brain just like July 8, 2005. But it is a much more beautiful image—it has love and joy written all over it!

Never in our wildest imaginations could we have anticipated in 2005 that in 2009 we would be... Please keep reading to find out how we went from the outhouse of Cancerville to the penthouse of life. Our story shows that we just never know what the future has in store for any of us. I am sure you will find our fairy tale uplifting and inspirational, which is one reason I saved it for the conclusion of our walk together.

CHAPTER 25

I hope for happier, calmer, and better times.

A Modern Day Fairy Tale

I want to finally share the magical fairy tale dream trip we took a few years after my family's nightmarish times in Cancerville. I assure you that it is completely true without embellishment or exaggeration.

In 2008, we were finally feeling a little better. Although Jodi was still taking Tamoxifen, she was past the heavy-duty chemo and, though a bit tired, feeling much better. As I had previously assured myself, her hair had grown back. Her relationship with her partner, Zev, was very positive. They were starting to enjoy life again, and so were Ronnie and I.

A Seed is Planted

Our son Michael called around that time and told us he was going to an annual breast cancer fundraiser within his industry. He described a trip they were auctioning for four people. Much as he would have liked to go with us, he thought it would be more fitting for us to take Jodi and Zev "as a reward for what all of you have been through." The trip included roundtrip business class airfare for four to South Africa and a first class private safari for four in Kenya and Tanzania, East Africa. The safari was being organized by Abercrombie and Kent (A&K)—an upscale tour company.

I told Mike that the trip sounded wonderful, especially since the money would all go to breast cancer research. In fact, it all seemed to fit together perfectly until I asked him the list price. He told me it was a whopping $86,000. I chuckled and watched the developing fantasy in my mind quickly dissolve like an aspirin dropped into a glass of water. I knew that the people who attended this fundraiser were high rollers from the cruise industry who sometimes overbid the list price. As I told my son, we were in no position to bid on this trip, not even close.

Mike, being the shrewd poker player he is, simply said, "What do you have to lose? It doesn't cost anything to bid." It was hard to argue with his logic, but I feared getting caught up in something we could not afford. I told him we would sleep on it. Ronnie, a former travel agent, did some research and learned that the airfare alone was close to $9,000 per person. In that context, we authorized Mike to bid up to $40,000 for the trip, thinking and half-hoping that it would never happen. Even that number was a big stretch for our budget, especially when all of the extras were added into the mix. Still, something made us just go for it.

Maybe it was all we had been through in Cancerville and the opportunity to do something healing as a family. Maybe the extra push was the knowledge that we'd be contributing to breast cancer research. Maybe it was what I said about priorities and taking better care of us—perhaps it was all of the above. In any case, we gave Mike permission to bid.

The Seed Takes Root

Mike called the next night while at the event and excitedly said, "We got the trip!" I said, "Really, it went for forty grand?" feeling both happy and worried. He said, "Nope," baiting me in his inimitable style. I said, "I told you not to go any higher." "I didn't," he said. "We got it for $26,000!"

With this information, I breathed a sigh of relief as our budget could handle that amount. It was expensive but doable for us. I realized that it was all meant to be. *Bashert* is the Yiddish expression for that type of experience. From that moment on, we began to call it our "trip of a lifetime." As it turned out, it was, in every possible way.

We called Jodi and Zev, who were unaware of any of this, and told them of our good fortune. We presented the trip to them as an early wedding gift (no pressure), if and whenever they decided to marry. As it turned out, Zev was already planning on asking Jodi to marry him; he had even begun looking for a ring. That romantic engaging moment took place in Napa Valley shortly thereafter. Jodi said she didn't want a big wedding and there was some talk of their eloping. Our only condition was that we be present. No specific plans ever materialized before our trip to Africa.

The Beanstalk Starts to Grow Taller

We arrived in Franschhoek, South Africa, on New Year's Eve at about 11:15 p.m. just as 2009 was coming into view there. Since 2005, we had welcomed every New Year as a further step away from Cancerville.

As Jodi, Zev, Ronnie, and I began to enjoy our time in Africa together, Sloan-Kettering and our experiences there seemed very far away, not only geographically but also emotionally. It became clear that Mike's idea had been nothing less than brilliant. At some point early in our trip, Jodi and Zev, with perhaps a little prompting from Ronnie (again, no pressure), decided that they wanted to get married in East

Africa. They called Duncan, our contact person from A&K, who had planned our safari. He said he would see what he could arrange, and Jodi and Zev eagerly awaited his call.

Each time we arrived at a new lodge in Kenya and Tanzania, Jodi and Zev would excitedly inquire as to a plan, but no one had heard a word about it. Calls to Duncan were met with voicemail or immediate disconnects, as cell service in East Africa has quite a few gaps. Thus, suspense lingered in the air, but we were all so distracted by the amazing sights of being in the wild that the uncertainty about the potential wedding wasn't an irritant to our trip. I think we all quietly adopted a *bashert* attitude. Cancerville teaches patience and tolerance for ambiguity better than any other place I have ever been. If it was meant to be, it would happen.

The Beanstalk Starts to Sway

With only two nights left on our trip, we arrived at the Ngorongoro Crater Lodge where we all simultaneously had the same thought. This magnificent place with an absolutely gorgeous and glorious view overlooking the crater would be an idyllic setting for a wedding. It would be a scene out of a very special movie. We held our breath as Jodi asked, "Have you heard anything about our wedding?" "No Ma'am," came the brief reply, "but I will check into it." The odds of this wedding happening seemed to be approaching zero, but we decided to wait and see. Cancerville taught us not to pay too much attention to the odds, one way or the other.

That night before dinner, the answer finally arrived. The wedding was scheduled for tomorrow. It was set to take place at four o'clock, our last day on safari. "Oh, by the way," we were told, "it will be at the Maasai Village. You will all be dressed in traditional clothing, and the whole tribe will participate." We looked at each other in shocked amazement and excitement. This was due in part to it really happening and in part to where it would be held. Zev broke the tension by saying to Jodi, "Don't worry honey, it will be like Halloween."

I couldn't help but silently remember that Halloween-like feeling I had on that fateful day at Sloan-Kettering when I was struggling to deal with what was going on in the OR. This plan for Jodi and Zev's costumed wedding sounded like a whole lot more fun; no tricky treatments this time around!

Climbing the Beanstalk Together

At the wedding, something out of *National Geographic*, Jodi looked like a beautiful tribal princess while the rest of us looked like mere trick-or-treaters. The ceremony itself involved both Jodi and Zev being adopted by tribal parents whose job it was to convince the chief to allow and bless the marriage. Thus, Jodi may be one of the few people adopted twice in her life.

The ceremony took place in the native language of the Maasai, with an English-speaking translator provided. To honor our Jewish tradition, we bought and brought along a Maasai blanket attached to spears to serve as the *chuppah* (canopy) that was held up by four people from the tribe. We also brought an expensive crystal glass wrapped in a linen napkin (please don't report this to the lodge), which Zev stepped on repeatedly and finally broke at the conclusion of the ceremony, much to the confusion of the tribe. Our Muslim driver and guide, Shofino, brought one with him, too, just in case we forgot to bring one. I had explained our custom of breaking a glass to him the day before. His remembering and caring showed the potential for us to all live together peacefully.

They Really Raised the Bar

On the way back from the village to the lodge, we were driven to a special area where a bar overlooking the crater was set up by the hotel just for us. It was oh so much better than the BYOB one in the men's room of Sloan-Kettering.

I didn't need a drink at that moment as I was on a natural high. Notwithstanding, I had one anyway to toast the bride and groom. Tradition!

When we returned to the lodge, the staff of fifteen or so Tanzanians was waiting outside to sing and dance with us, which added to the magic of the moment. Then, we spontaneously organized a *hora,* a traditional Jewish dance, only a short distance away from a giant buffalo that decided to join in on the merriment. No, the buffalo didn't dance, nor did his size keep us from celebrating.

The entire staff joined us in this traditional dance and the party was officially on. It was a long time coming, but here it was. It was a YES, tears of joy moment in every way! I could write many more pages about this trip and my daughter's magical fairy tale wedding, but I don't have to. You can see the video, professionally prepared by Zev's video company, Milk and Honey Productions, by going to www.cancerville.com. I assure you it is worth your time. I hope it will help you to start picturing happier and more wholesome images for you and your family.

Real People Facing Cancer

Jodi and Zev: Another Seed is Planted

Clearly, there are only two people who fit this chapter, and they are our wonderful daughter, Jodi, and her loving husband, Zev. But I have already told you about her strength, courage, and determination, from which I learned to better cope with Cancerville. In many respects, this book and the previous one are testimony to Jodi's graceful dance to the complex and challenging "routines" of Cancerville's face the music times. I have also told you of Zev's devotion, love, and support as a "heart and soul giver" to Jodi and to us throughout our Cancerville journey.

Nonetheless, I have a good story to tell which really relates to this and the following chapter. It probably relates in one way or another to every chapter—particularly those parts that speak to coping with and defusing dire predictions.

This piece of their journey took Jodi and Zev from the outhouse of Cancerville, through the Penthouse of their amazing wedding in the Maasai Village, to the Pinnacle of Miracles.

After Jodi completed her heavy-duty chemotherapy, she was told that the likelihood of her becoming pregnant was low; chemo can age reproductive organs by as much as ten years, and she still had five years of Tamoxifen before they could try to conceive.

Nonetheless, Jodi gave birth to their beautiful daughter, symbolically enough, a week before Thanksgiving. It was truly a miracle. This is a most inspiring story that speaks to patience, persistence, partnership, love, and, most of all, a horse named Hope.

You just need to believe; you can never, never, never give up. Where there is life there is hope, and where there is hope anything—and I mean anything—is possible.

This leads us directly to the next and concluding chapter, which describes how I came to discover what I have come to call unrealistic optimism. You will also learn about the powerful influence Bernie Siegel, M.D., has had upon my thoughts and my life, for which I will always be grateful.

In Sum

Never in our wildest imaginations, while we were in the thick of Cancerville, did my family ever conceive of such a healing trip to Africa or our daughter's marriage to Zev in Tanzania among the Maasai tribe. Nor, did we ever conceive of their conceiving a child.

Life, as we have all learned, is unpredictable, not just in terribly scary and sad ways, but also in happy ways. For now, please try to see that there can be "happily ever after" times after the unhappy times in Cancerville.

My family went from the bleak darkness of Cancerville to the heart of darkness, as Africa has been called, where the sunny blue skies with swirling white clouds looked like a bright and beautiful work of art. Similarly, our beloved granddaughter is a beautiful work of nature's art too.

As Bernie Siegel, M.D., said in the Foreword, "You are always a work in progress, and as long as you are alive the canvas is never finished, as there is always more color on the palette." Our family enjoyed a most exciting, happy, and beautiful addition to our canvas, for which there was much to be thankful.

Life unfolds like a movie drama; fact is truly stranger than fiction. Try your best to assume and believe in some form or other that sunny skies lie on your family's horizon as well. Know that life is full of surprises and *bashert* moments of excitement and tears of joy. Try to look beyond this Cancerville moment and see a much more positive future. It is my sincere and heartfelt hope that you can also enjoy warm and positive experiences to salve your wounds from Cancerville. Toward that goal, I most sincerely wish you well!

I have come to learn that we need to open ourselves— our minds, hearts, and souls—to miraculous possibilities of all kinds. This subject is the topic of the next and last chapter—an ideal way to conclude our journey together.

CHAPTER 26

My mind remains open to all possibilities.

On Becoming
Even More Empowered

mpowerment involves just about everything we have
talked about previously. As we have seen, some people arrive in Cancerville already empowered; their
genes and their scenes have programmed them well. Some,
like Eileen and her family, with their strength intact, glide into
Cancerville like beautiful, rainbow-colored, graceful butterflies.

Then again, there are people like me whose genes and
scenes have programmed us to fall flat on our emotional

faces. They are the ones for whom this book was written—"I have written the book I needed to read that day at Sloan-Kettering." Those like me crash-land and initially burn up in a cess-based maelstrom of pain and perplexity.

But we can learn. We can slowly become "DAM STRONG!" We too can become strong, beautiful, rainbow-colored, graceful butterflies. It just takes us longer to adjust, adapt, cope, and learn to glide. We may be slow, but we eventually figure it out. In that context, my goal has been to help you become pumped, positive, and proactive.

Cancerville challenges each of us in our own unique ways. In reality, Cancerville is like a Rorschach inkblot—we see it from our individual perspectives. We engage with it on our own terms, in our own way, and with our own sensitivities and strengths. Your goal is to lead with your strengths, and find ways to soothe yourself when you struggle during challenging times.

We are all different and all become empowered by different approaches and in a variety of ways. I so want you to become empowered in your personalized way. Let your shirt or blouse of empowerment have your personal monogram clearly embroidered on it, right near your heart. Mine says, "DAM STRONG!" What do you want yours to say?

In this chapter, I also want to share with you how I have come to stretch and embrace that which lies beyond the realm of rational and realistic. Undeniably, there are forces in our universe that we don't understand and cannot see, forces that operate pretty much on the periphery. Whether we call them God's influence; miracles; angels; the power of our minds; meant-to-be experiences; or, as a person in my office said today, "a lucky punch," there is no denying they exist. If you don't believe me, just ask Bernie Siegel, M.D. His highly scientific mind has been able to embrace and teach us all about less than scientific, but no less possible, opportunities to see beyond our rigid and limited views of reality.

The Influence Bernie Siegel, M.D., Had on Me

Even before I met Bernie Siegel, M.D., on a beautiful sunny spring day at his home, he had a profound influence on me. I read his book *Love, Medicine & Miracles* in the 1980s and was excited by this surgeon's warm and loving heart. Throughout the years, I have given his wonderful book to many, many people with health challenges. They all reported it helped and inspired them.

I wrote the first sentence of this section about six weeks before Bernie and I actually met. Friends who read an early draft asked, "What will you do if it isn't a sunny day?" My response was, "Even if it is pouring down rain, it will be a sunny day for me, but I think it will be warm and sunny." And it was a spectacularly sunny spring day. In my mind's eye, I can still see Bernie's face glowing in the sunlight—and my inner sunshine was glowing too. Part of becoming empowered involves developing and strengthening your inner sunshine so that no matter what the outside weather or life circumstances, you can feel the warmth of that internally generated spirit.

It was neither an accident nor a coincidence that Bernie and I met. I needed him to walk me through the core of his beliefs in person and he graciously did—he accompanied me down the Miracle Mile! And we laughed like old high school buddies the whole journey through, even though we were total strangers.

Something very powerful happened as we got up from his lawn chairs in the backyard. The webbing on his chair had been ripping slowly the entire time we were sitting there. As he stood up, his less than supportive chair caused him to lose his balance; it appeared that he was about to fall backward, head over heals into his lovely garden. I quickly extended my left arm and steadied his balance for a few seconds. Clearly, we supported each other that bright and sunny spring day; that is the way all relationships are supposed to be—harmonious and balanced. That is the way both Bernie and I have dealt with our families, the people we have helped, and people in general. When we are kind-hearted, it usually pays multiple dividends, both in our dealings and in our inner feelings.

Truth be told, when I first read *Love, Medicine & Miracles,* I bypassed the "miracles" and focused on the "love and medicine." For me, as a young therapist and counselor, it was about "verbal medicine," which is a territory Bernie knows well. At that time in my life, my concrete, semi-scientific mind could not embrace the idea of miracles. Even today it is a bit of a stretch, but I have evolved like a fine bottle of aged wine and am now able to reach toward them. Reading Bernie's books, *A Book of Miracles* and *Faith, Hope & Healing,* has paved the way for me to be more accepting of these potentials. Miracles may not happen every day, but they do happen. I am very proud and grateful that Bernie welcomed me into his home and his mind, and guided me along this path, as well as writing the Foreword for this book.

Call it a Miracle/ God's Blessing/ Good Fortune/ Lucky Punch/ Whatever

The previous chapter, "A Modern Day Fairy Tale," was undeniably all of the above. Jodi, Zev, Ronnie, and I journeyed from the outhouse of Cancerville to the penthouse and pinnacle of life—Jodi and Zev getting married in a Maasai village was undeniably everything listed in this subhead title and more. Instead of being surrounded by patients and medical personnel in a hospital, we were surrounded by tribesmen and women in a celebration. If dancing a Hora with the entire hotel staff in Tanzania, in a spontaneous celebration of love, is not a magical moment, then what is? If you haven't watched the video at cancerville.com, go there immediately and click on "A Modern Day Fairy Tale." It is awesome, amazing, and miraculous, and I bet you will watch it twice.

Bernie teaches us that we can all make miracles happen through believing in them and maintaining an open mind and loving heart. I truly believe that my daughter's fairy tale wedding demonstrated that. We needed to open our minds and our hearts, take the chance and bid on the trip, and then we needed to believe we would be safe there. We drew from our newly created philosophy of realistic optimism, and you need to do the same by believing that you will safely navigate your way through Cancerville and beyond.

Jodi and Zev opened their minds and their hearts and took the chance of asking to be married in East Africa, while going with the flow of the unknown in their desire to share and commit to their love. Cancerville definitely teaches you how to tolerate and flow with the unknown. By "flowing" through Cancerville, and at times even treading water, or walking across a "bridge over troubled waters," you might just find a blessing coming your way. Bernie likes to say, "In every curse there are blessings to be found." He encourages us to look for them, find them, and embrace them fully.

From personal experience, I know that it is undeniably difficult to see beyond the "curse," but once we do, whole new fields of flowers appear, as if by magic. This is how the cognitive tools I spoke of in Chapter 17 expand our vision and provide a much brighter view. I could never have imagined the Maasai wedding in 2005, but I could have looked for a more positive future. You can do the same.

Try your hardest to see beyond "now" to "then"—and it is more likely that "then" will happen in one form or another. Ultimately, we need to give more weight to the hidden blessings than the curses that are part of life for all of us. Trumping the miracle of Jodi and Zev's African wedding, was opening their bodies, minds, and hearts to having a child. In so doing, they achieved their miracle.

On the Subject of Angels/Spiritual Guides/ Healers/Higher Powers/ Other Special Forces

Bernie also tells us to be on the alert for angels, who bring miracles and blessings with them. My first response to embracing angels was "Oy Vey!" I didn't know if my "fine wine" had evolved quite that far, so perhaps I needed more time in the barrel! Or perhaps I had unwittingly stumbled into a pickle barrel! But Bernie is one smooth, unassuming, and gentle salesman.

I soon came to realize that there have been many special forces in my life that have positively influenced my journey. Some have been real people and some that were invisible have worked in the periphery to help guide me along. In this regard, isn't there an angel or two perched on each of my shoulders as I pounded away at the keyboard to write this book? Aren't there special forces guiding my Cancerville journey to find all of the fine people I have had the privilege to meet and interview for the "Real People Facing Cancer" sections?

Wasn't an angel involved in having Bernie open his heart and the door to his home to me? His response was unexpected for someone of his stature—most people like him would not even have returned an email. Was that his angel or mine, I wonder? Mine I think! Bernie could have lived the rest of his life without meeting me, but could I have done as well or understood as much without meeting him?

Haven't I been a special force to so many who have sought my guidance and support? Often people have said of my encouraging and inspiring words, "From your mouth to God's ears!" My immediate response has always been, "It usually works that way!" I am not being cocky in these situations—I have just come to observe that many positive things I believe in and encourage ultimately come to be.

I have come to believe in angels—some are people you have known and some just wander on by; perhaps some are truly invisible, but guide your way nonetheless. Be on the look-out for them and be aware when you are in their presence. They can make amazing things happen for you although they cannot always save your life. Sometimes they do that, and sometimes they do other things that can help too.

So many intriguing things have become part of my life now that I have my mind wide open to amazing potentials. I have come to realize that the more I put myself "out there," the more "out there" responds in kind. I encourage you to allow yourself to consider communicating with "out there" in some way and see what happens. It is possible that you will receive a response—not always immediately, but eventually—not always clearly, but sometimes subtly or symbolically.

Dr. DuPree's warm, healing, and spiritually eye-opening book previously referenced, *The Healing Consciousness* opens many doors and windows to other dimensions. She says:

> Accepting that there are forces at work in the universe beyond those under my control required a certain amount of letting go. I was truly beginning to surrender to a higher power that exists in the universe. I had many experiences where I felt I had encountered angels on earth, but now I was open to a new world of communication with the angels above.

My sense is that Dr. DuPree is one of those angels here on earth.

Perhaps you are wondering how I can reconcile my philosophy of realistic optimism with these less than realistic ideas. Are there times in our lives when we might embrace beliefs that require leaps of faith—something we might call unrealistic optimism? That is a matter of your personal choosing.

Dr. Seligman, whom I discussed in Chapter 12, would likely feel that you have nothing to lose. There is no cost to being hopeful against all odds, as long as you simultaneously prepare yourself for the possibility of not having any special force assist you. It takes us right back to the Powerball lottery; everyone has a shot, but the odds are low, so don't spend the rent money. Then again, a couple of bucks might be worth the risk—so might a couple of prayers to a higher power in whatever way works for you.

Doctors as a Source of Empowerment

Doctors can be a source of added empowerment too. In Bernie's book *Faith, Hope & Healing,* another Cindy told of her mother being diagnosed with cancer when Cindy was eight years old. She overheard her mother's doctor say her mom had six months to live. Cindy says, "The memory of that day was vividly branded upon the core of my child-brain." It sounds like a major and traumatic cesspool deposit to me!

Her dad searched for another doctor and found one at Yale—New Haven Hospital. The doctor told her mom, "I can't tell you how long you are going to live any more than I can predict my own life span, but I can tell you this: In six months from now, you will not be dead. In six months you will be dancing again." In fact, that is exactly what happened. Six months after that doctor's prediction, Cindy's mom and dad danced like teens; her mom lived three years more. The doctor ordered new treatments and medicine but most importantly fed her large doses of confidence and hope. Cindy said, "I think of him as a very special angel in my life." A most interesting choice of words!

In Bernie's comments he commends this doctor, whom he calls "Doctor Hope," who obviously rides in on the horse I promote. Bernie says, "What has frustrated me for decades is that doctors do not receive training about how to care for people and not just treat their disease. Doctors keep their power by predicting when their patients will die?"

Isn't it time for doctors and patients alike to stop predicting death? Shouldn't we all strive to promote hope and optimism? Amazing unanticipated results have the potential to extend people's lives, but need the fertilizer of positive self-talk that is often stimulated or inhibited by others' talk. My point is simply that when doctors encourage optimism, it often translates into a more positive result. We saw this in Jack's comment ("You hang on every word.") in Chapter 18 and we will come upon this issue again soon.

If you should ever receive a less than favorable diagnosis, take it seriously and do whatever your doctors recommend. At the same time, your challenge is to allow those words to evaporate, while replacing them with hope. As importantly, try to live each day fully, just as Randy Pausch (*The Last Lecture*) did in the months before he passed on.

Marty, whom you met in Chapter 19, shared a relevant story upon reading a draft of this chapter. In the course of his work as a PA-C psychiatrist and psychologist, he had encountered a twenty-five year old woman with two different kinds of brain cancer. Her doctor had told her she would only live for five more years at best. She focused on the "death sentence" he had delivered and decided she would rather die than wait for the doctor's prediction to come true. Marty's intervention was direct and supportive:

> I told her that the doctor had no idea how long she would live. I helped her to see that by accepting his prognosis she gave up her own power. I told her she would live until she would die and encouraged her to live that time to the fullest— to find some things worthwhile to live for and get on with it. She bought into those ideas and has come to experience life as never before.

The simple truth is that no one can predict the future—no one! As part of becoming empowered, predict a long one for yourself. Do your best not to allow anyone to dampen your life spirit. Bernie has repeatedly encouraged people and patients to try to be happy and live each day to the fullest. My mother, who lived to 100 years against all odds, used to say the same thing. Her morning happiness and gratitude came from simply waking up. Clearly, it is not the amount of time that is of importance but that we use each day to the fullest. Life, no matter how long one lives, goes by quickly, and much rests in the qualitative choices that we make and the special opportunities that we take.

Let me be as clear here as I possibly can be. Do you remember my cousin Marilyn, who had Stage IV lung cancer and was given only weeks to live? I lit a candle in my mind, said a prayer, and hoped for a miracle, unlikely as that might have been. When it didn't happen, I was sad yet accepted it as not meant to be. The same is true of my cousin Debby. With Susan, who had Stage IV ovarian cancer, we were shooting for a miracle—realistic or unrealistic—from day one, until we had no choice but to accept a difficult reality. Death is always sad, but it is also inevitable. As I have previously said, "There are many paths to Heaven, only one of which is cancer."

When I met with Bernie, he encouraged me to read *Cancer Ward* by Alexander Solzhenitsyn.[39] Sitting there in the sunlight, he quoted from memory the following passage from that great work:

> There was a stir throughout the ward. It was as though 'self-induced healing' had fluttered out of the great open book like a rainbow-colored butterfly for everyone to see, and they all held up their foreheads and cheeks for its healing touch as it flew past.

As I previously said, you can learn to become that rainbow-colored butterfly and glide much more positively and comfortably through the challenges that Cancerville demands. This is precisely what your becoming empowered will enable.

Real People Facing Cancer

Jake and Chase

There are only two stories that belong in this concluding chapter about miracles and the like. The first story is the one that lit the fuse for me to write *How to Cope Better When Someone You Love Has Cancer*. It is the story of Jake and Chase, whom you already met—but haven't heard about all of the details and detours that tried their hardest to derail these strong young boys.

When Jake's grandfather Phil, our friend of fifty-plus years, emailed me about Jake's diagnosis, I cried bitterly as I knew they were heading into Cancerville. It is one wild bronco ride, especially for an eight-year-old child. It is every parent's worst nightmare. But by the next day, I was back in action mode and reached out to Rob, Jake's dad, via email. That led to an ongoing communication as one father who had been to Cancerville to another who had just entered. I encouraged his positive and optimistic beliefs whenever I could.

After Jake's four rounds of chemo failed to put him into remission, I have no doubt that Rob was less than pleased when I said we needed a Hail Mary pass. The doctors needed to get the leukemia blasts close to zero for Chase's magic bone marrow bullets to take out his cancer once and for all. That's just what we faced at that delicate and scary moment. That Jake and his family got that Hail Mary pass for which we all prayed is yet another example of a miracle and blessing.

In his inimitable fashion, Rob organized several prayer vigils all over the world on particular days at specific times as treatment progressed. No matter where we were or what time zone we were in, we were all praying at the same time—from all different religious perspectives. In one instance, when Ronnie and I were in Australia, we had the hotel call us in the middle of the night to make sure we joined the group prayer.

We believe that those prayers helped the doctors hike the ball to Jake's fraternal twin brother, Chase, who threw the ball high in the air. They were all attempting a play called "the miracle" based upon "Chase the Ace's" perfect bone marrow match. "Jake the Snake" bravely ran into the "non-end zone," caught the ball and beat cancer. Jake is alive and well today and can tell you about that amazing grace football catch himself, even though his sport of choice is Hockey. That play went against all odds and was undeniably a blessed miracle. Truth!

In this regard, I want to tell you a story that always makes me tear up and angry at the same time. It takes us back to Bernie's beef about doctors not encouraging their patients hopefully. I'm not sure why he was present, but at one very important doctor meeting, Jake asked a simple question of the doctor: "Am I going to die?" The doctor didn't respond. The doctor didn't what? Are you kidding me? The F-bomb needs to be dropped right before the words "respond," "what," and "kidding," so feel free. Phil said, "Of course not!" and went on to reassure his grandson when he realized that the doctor wasn't going to answer.

Why couldn't the doctor have answered him in a positive and encouraging way? Has a malpractice suit ever been filed because a doctor was unrealistically optimistic? I doubt it and I seriously doubt such a case would stand up in court. Here is what the doctor needed to say:

> You have the best doctors in the world for this problem. You are in the best hospital in the world for this problem. We are doing everything we can to help you get rid of the problem and get you back to your happy life. We are sorry that to help you, we have to make you miserable, but we are making your problem cells miserable too and that is the goal. I think you are strong and young and will make it through. I don't think you will die from this.

Why not promote Jake's hopes with optimism, and open the doors and windows of this young patient's mind and heart to possible positive potentials? Why just pretend to not hear this child's understandable plea and terror-stricken panic? Doc, you helped saved his life, so bless you for that, but you failed to give him hope at a critical time. In my respectful opinion, you need to rethink your strategy and find words of support that are comfortable for you. Don't even wait for the question to be asked—write the hopeful script from the very beginning. While I am encouraging a change in your script, please never say to parents, "Sometimes children just die." I think you can easily find more helpful and more healing words. For example, "We are doing everything we can to save your child's life. In addition to what we are doing medically, let's pray hard for a miracle."

Everything was wrong with the doctor's silence at Jake's question, and her words to Jake's parents. Unfortunately, similar silences happen many times a day. Doctors are afraid to help their patients and families up onto the horse named Hope. Some seem to prefer to offer grim statistics that portend a visit from the grim reaper. Why, in heaven's name, would they not try to project realistic or even unrealistic optimism? Though miracles are not guaranteed, they are more likely when hope is in the air and in the minds of their patients. Bernie has tried very hard to teach his colleagues this, but some just haven't listened. How about this simple statement that a doctor can say:

> I'm not going to pull any punches. You have a serious disease. The odds aren't exactly with us. But this is my expertise. I am devoting all of my energies and efforts to getting you well. My power is a force with which your cancer cells must reckon. SO IS YOURS! Mobilize your energies—cope, hope, and do everything in your power to fight this battle and heal your body by drawing from the sling shot of your mind.

If you don't hear words like that from your doctor(s), please find ones that will (like Cindy's father did when he searched for a different doctor), or give them to yourself. You will feel and do much better in Cancerville when you ride through it on a horse named Hope! I guarantee it.

There is yet another wild twist to Jake's tale. Even after going into remission, Jake has continued to visit Memorial Sloan-Kettering every week and more recently every two weeks. Therefore, the metiport that they implanted near his right collarbone when his ordeal began remained in place and is still used as an alternative to injections. He is no longer on chemo, but needs meds to counter the ill effects of the chemo. Jake has been though the proverbial mill, much more than I care to think about, but he is alive and doing well.

As reported to me by Rob, Jake was at the hospital for a routine visit. Cristina and Phil took Jake to the hospital, while Rob worked about 25 blocks away in Manhattan. As soon as he heard his Dad's voice on the phone around 11:30 a.m., Rob knew there was trouble. He had heard Phil's grave tone many times before since this all began. Rob literally ran through the streets of Manhattan to the hospital, as no cabs were available.

For reasons unknown, when the nurse practitioner placed the needle into the port, it broke loose from the catheter that ran into Jake's artery. A piece of the catheter had traveled down the artery toward Jake's heart, stopping only one inch away. Had it continued on its route, Jake would have died. Jake's family was not told of the severity of the situation until it was time for surgery; they did, however, sense the tension from the seriousness of the doctors who were involved.

Because Jake had eaten a tangerine on his ride to the hospital, they had to wait two hours before they could anesthetize him. Right before the surgery was to begin, Cristina and Rob had to sign a paper acknowledging that the piece of catheter was close to Jake's heart, and could move at any moment, especially when the interventional radiologist made a grab for it.

For understandable reasons, Rob froze in emotional paralysis—he hyperventilated and could not breathe easily because they were right back in crunch and crisis time. A routine visit had exploded unexpectedly into emergency surgery.

That scene took him back to the late night email he had sent me so long ago: "What if Jake is going to die in a few months? Should we tell him before and, if so, when?" he had asked. My immediate response was to "take that thought off the table and out of your mind, or it will drive you out of your mind." But in this elongated moment, Cristina and Rob were once again faced with the possibility of losing their son. No one should ever have to go through this once, let alone twice, but life is a strange and sometimes twisted journey. So there they were, needing a Hail Mary pass. How many miracles can one ask for in life? I guess as many as one needs.

Adding to the drama of this terrifying time was the operating room itself. As was their habit in other previous minor procedures, Cristina and Rob would go into the room just before anesthesia to give their son a hug and kiss and reassure him that all would be well. Before they stepped inside this OR, the surgeon cautioned them not to be intimidated by the room—but how could they not be? It was an amphitheater of an OR with large plasma TVs all over that showed just about every inch of Jake's X-rayed body from just about every angle. The ceiling was twenty feet high and the room seemed enormous compared to the small procedure rooms they had been in previously. In addition to the twenty doctors, nurses, and technicians near the operating table, there were twenty more behind a glass partition looking at even more plasma TVs. It was, to say the least, overwhelming and terrifying—this was undeniably a big deal, rather than a slam-dunk!

Clearly, they needed a miracle and there was no time to organize a prayer vigil. The good news is that Jake caught that pass in the "non-end zone" once again—this time thrown by the Lord above and the medical team. About twenty minutes after the procedure began, the surgeon texted Jake's family. Their cell phone screens and their minds simultaneously lit up at the picture showing the piece of catheter lying on a table with the words, "It's out. He's safe!" Miraculous!

Jake was released that night. His family was both relieved and grateful, and Jake was back for the last day of school. All's well that ends well, thank the Lord, the fine medical team and their techno-magic, and young Jake, who once again rose to the challenge and caught another play called "the miracle!" No one will ever know what prevented that piece of shrapnel from entering Jake's heart. Therein lies the miracle of all miracles!

In Sum

Be on the lookout for all kinds of amazing and miraculous blessings within whatever challenges you are facing and fighting. As Bernie would say, "It's not about the fight because sometimes that can be counterproductive and draining, but the slow and steady healthy healing of yourself—physically, emotionally, and spiritually. Your mind is a very powerful force and influence on how your healing proceeds. You need to find balance, harmony, and inner peace." Seek, he would encourage, and you shall find! Toward that empowering goal, I wish you well.

A Closing Letter of Caring

Dear Survivor,

We have been walking together for a while now. You have come to know a great deal about me, while I have not had the opportunity to get to know you. Such is the nature of book communication. Feel free to email me to let me know how things are going with you. Your feedback about this book is welcome as well.

I am hopeful your situation in Cancerville has gone well. I am sincerely sad and sorry if it has not. My goal was to write a clear, supportive, and elegant book about a confusing, overwhelming, and inelegant place. I have tried my best to guide you through this difficult land I call Cancerville. I hope you were able to feel my hand of support reaching out across the miles. I also hope, at least at times, that you were able to replace your frowns with smiles. I am very hopeful that you learned some things about yourself and others that apply to life in general, as well as to Cancerville.

I believe that how you let Cancerville shape you is ultimately within your control. You have the power to process your experience as you choose. You can't change what happened in Cancerville and all that you have gone through and may continue to go through. You can, however, deal with it in a way that frees you rather than causes you to be a perpetual prisoner.

If your power has been weakened by the journey, there are many resources available to help you regain your strength and be able to rebound soon. These include counselors, support groups, spiritual guides, family and friends, websites, books, and anything else that might be helpful to you. In addition to the above, sometimes just a getaway to a spa or other relaxing place helps to clear your mind and recharge worn and depleted batteries of body, mind, and spirit.

Cancerville has already taken so much from you, even if the outcome was successful. Try your hardest not to let it suck you dry and take away your energy and zest for living. Find ways to heal and to reclaim yourself—you are worth it! Even though Cancerville sucks, life, in my opinion, does not.

As I have said, one of the many lessons we learn in Cancerville is that we never know what's coming around the corner. Life is unpredictable and we are all vulnerable to unanticipated happenings that can be positive or negative. In that context, we need to live our lives fully. We need to treat ourselves kindly, and we need to eventually bounce back resiliently from the trauma of Cancerville.

It will take you some time to neutralize the newly acquired cess from Cancerville, but you can do it; I am optimistic that you will. I leave you with one of the very best prayers I have ever encountered. It works for all areas of life, including Cancerville, and for all religions as well:

THE SERENITY PRAYER

God, grant me the serenity to accept the things
I cannot change,
Courage to change the things I can,
And wisdom to know the difference.

I sincerely hope that this book and your own life experiences have helped you find that important wisdom. It is not always easy to know that, but Cancerville does make it a little clearer.

Here is a personal pledge that I wrote when dealing with my own mental misery in the 1970s, which you can draw from as well:

MY PERSONAL PLEDGE

I pledge allegiance to myself,
and the united state of my being,
and to the resilience with which I stand,
One person, under strain, with consideration and
compassion for ME.

Obviously, I cannot conclude by saying it has been a pleasure to go through Cancerville with you. There is no pleasure in being there. However, I am honored that you allowed me to walk by your side and take and talk you through its rough terrain.

I now slowly and gently withdraw my hand and leave you to go the rest of the way on your own, strengthened from our time together. Here is a fist bump coming at you to acknowledge the strength, courage, and dignity you displayed. Of course, you can always visit me online, read weekly posts on our cancerville.com Facebook page, or return to this book and grasp my hand whenever you might need to feel that symbolic but strong support. It will always be there for you.

I want to leave you with an image I observed a few years ago. It was Thanksgiving Day. Our entire family was at our house, which is always special. I wandered out to the backyard to water my new red impatiens plants. Jodi and Zev were near the canal, fun-fishing for bass. They were goofing around, teasing and laughing about who was the better fisherperson. Actually, Jodi often is, much to Zev's chagrin. I stopped and took in that tranquil and happy scene. I breathed in deeply and let it out very slowly. I let that joyful moment wash all over my Cancerville cess for a while. These are the simple times for which I will always feel so grateful!

I had the thought that, like plants and flowers, people need the emotional equivalent of sunshine, water, fertilizer, and weeding. We also need positive images to replace those that are not so pretty. We need to focus on the now so we can get rid of, or at least lessen, the harsh times of the then. My family and I have much for which to be thankful, all things considered. I sincerely hope you do, too, and wish you and your family the very best in all respects and good health from now on.

I dubbed this writing my *mitzvah* (good deed) project. I hope it has touched and helped you in the way I had envisioned. The lovely thing about good deeds is that they come back at us in all kinds of unanticipated ways. Please try to do a *mitzvah* every day and enjoy the multiple dividends that they offer. If nothing else, they will fill your pride bank and, frankly, that is payday enough for me, and I hope for you as well.

God bless all those who have ever been to Cancerville in the past, those who are there now, and those who will be entering it soon or in the future. God bless the researchers, doctors, nurses, and medical teams all over the world. God bless all of us who deserve to be among the blessed. With these blessings, I choose to hope, pray, and believe that you will be a survivor of this experience.

I sincerely thank you for reading my book. I hope it helped you—and that it was the "home run" I strived to hit!

Your Cancerville friend for life,

Bill

REFERENCES

1) Penzer, William. *How to Cope Better When Someone You Love Has Cancer.* Esperance Press Inc: Ft. Lauderdale, 2011.
2) Mukherjee, Siddhartha. *The Emperor of all Maladies: A Biography of Cancer.* Scribner Book Company: New York, 2010.
3) Siegel, Bernie, M.D. and Dander, Jennifer. *Faith, Hope & Healing.* Wiley: New York, 2009.
4) Seligman, Martin. *Learned Optimism.* Pocket Books: New York, 1990.
5) Siegel, Bernie. *Love, Medicine & Miracles.* Perennial Library: New York, 1988.
6) Penzer, William. *Getting Back Up from an Emotional Down.* Esperance Publishing: Ft. Lauderdale, 1989.
7) Pausch, Randy. *The Last Lecture.* Hyperion: New York, 2008.
8) Hope, Lori. *Help Me Live: 20 Things People with Cancer Want You to Know.* Celestial Arts: New York, 2011.
9) Lucas, Geralyn. *Why I Wore Lipstick to My Mastectomy.* St. Martin's Press: New York, 2004.

10) Armstrong, Lance. *It's Not About the Bike*. Berkley Publishing Group: New York, 2001.

11) Siegel, Bernie. *How to Live Between Office Visits*. Harper Collins: New York, 1994.

12) Cousins, Norman. *Anatomy of an Illness as Perceived By the Patient*. Bantam: Toronto, 1981.

13) Brinker, Nancy. *How a Sister's Love Launched the Global Movement to End Breast Cancer*. Random House: New York, 2010.

14) Kansas, George. *iCanSir!* Journey Press: New York, 2011.

15) Siegel, Bernie and August, Yosaif. *Help Me to Heal*. Hay House: Carlsbad, 2003.

16) Rubin, Theodore. Compassion and Self-Hate: An Alternative to Despair, Simon and Shuster: New York, 1998.

17) Byrne, Rhonda. *The Secret*. Simon and Shuster: New York, 2006.

18) Siegel, Bernie. *A Book of Miracles*. New World Library: Novato, 2011.

19) Holland, Jimmie and Lewis, Sheldon. *The Human Side of Cancer*. Harper Collins: New York, 2000.

20) Simonton, O. Carl, Matthews-Simonton, Stephanie and Creighton, James. *Getting Well Again*. Bantam: New York, 1978.

21) Peale, Norman Vincent. *The Power of Positive Thinking*. Simon and Shuster: New York, 2003.

22) Ellis, Albert and Harper, Robert. *A Guide to Rational Living*. Wilshire Book Company: Chatsworth, 1997.

23) Seligman, Martin. *Flourish*. Simon and Shuster: New York, 2011.

24) Radner, Gilda. *It's Always Something*. Avon: New York, 1989.

25) Pecorino, Lauren. *Why Millions Survive Cancer*. Oxford: New York, 2011.

26) DuPree, Beth. *The Healing Consciousness*: A Doctor's Journey to Healing. Woven Word Press: Boulder, 2006.

27) Achatz, Grant and Kokonas, Nick. *Life, on the Line*. Gotham: New York, 2011.

28) Ebert, Roger. *Life Itself: A Memoir*. Grand Central Publishing: New York, 2011.

29) Carr, Kris. *Crazy, Sexy Cancer Tips*. Skirt: Guilford, 2007.

30) Kreamer, Ann. *It's Always Personal: Emotions in the New Work Place*. Random House: New York, 2011.

31) Kushner, Harold. *When Bad Things Happen to Good People*. Avon: New York, 1981.

32) Rollins, Betty. *First, You Cry*. Harper Collins: New York, 1976.

33) Goodheart, Annette. *Laughter Therapy*. Less Stress Press: Santa Barbara, 1994.

34) Provine, Robert. *Laughter: A Scientific Investigation*. Viking Penguin: New York, 2000.

35) Klein, Allen. *The Healing Power of Humor*. Tarcher: Los Angeles, 1989.

36) Gray, John. *Men are From Mars Women are from Venus*. Harper Collins: New York, 2004.

37) Becker, Earnest. *The Denial of Death*. Simon and Shuster: New York, 1973.

38) Nouwen, Henri. *Turn My Morning into Dancing*. Thomas Nelson: Nashville, 2001.

39) Solzhenitsyn, Alexander. *Cancer Ward*. Bantam: New York, 1981.